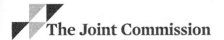
The Joint Commission

MW00606995

2022

Standards for
Ambulatory Care

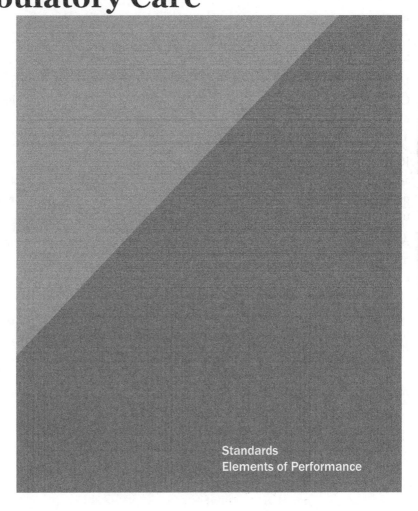

Standards
Elements of Performance

The Joint Commission Mission

The mission of The Joint Commission is to continuously improve health care for the public, in collaboration with other stakeholders, by evaluating health care organizations and inspiring them to excel in providing safe and effective care of the highest quality and value.

© 2022 The Joint Commission

Published by Joint Commission Resources
Oak Brook, Illinois 60523 USA
https://www.jcrinc.com

Joint Commission Resources, Inc. (JCR), a not-for-profit affiliate of The Joint Commission, has been designated by The Joint Commission to publish publications and multimedia products. JCR reproduces and distributes these materials under license from The Joint Commission.

JCR educational programs and publications support, but are separate from, the accreditation activities of The Joint Commission. Attendees at JCR educational programs and purchasers of JCR publications receive no special consideration or treatment in, or confidential information about, the accreditation process.

ISBN: 978-1-63585-242-4
ISSN: 1096-455X

Printed in the U.S.A.

For more information about The Joint Commission, please visit https://www.jointcommission.org.

Contents

2022

SAC

Introduction
(INTRO)

Introduction (INTRO)

The *2022 Standards for Ambulatory Care* (*SAC*) aims to keep accreditation leaders, managers, and frontline staff up to date with the requirements necessary to achieve and maintain Joint Commission ambulatory care accreditation. This abridged version of the *Comprehensive Accreditation Manual for Ambulatory Care* (*CAMAC*) provides all ambulatory care standards, elements of performance (EPs), National Patient Safety Goals® (NPSGs), and Accreditation Participation Requirements (APRs) effective **January 1, 2022**.

The *CAMAC* and the E-dition® available on your organization's *Joint Commission Connect®* extranet site include policies, procedures, and other information about the ambulatory care accreditation process. These are not provided in this book.

Chapter Structure

The *SAC* includes the information your organization needs for continuous performance improvement. Each chapter in this book is set up as follows:

- An *overview* explains the chapter's purpose and the principles on which the standards were built.
- The *chapter outline* shows you exactly how the chapter is laid out and provides a frame of reference for the numbering of standards.
- *Introductions* at the beginning of some standards (or cluster of standards) provide information about the standard's origin and any issues that surround it.
- The *standards* (also known as requirements) are statements that define the performance expectations and/or structures or processes that must be in place for your organization to provide safe, quality care, treatment, or services.
- A *rationale* is additional background, justification, or information about a standard to explain its purpose. In some cases, the rationale for a requirement is self-evident. Therefore, not every requirement has a written rationale. Rationales are not scored.
- *References* (placed in parentheses following the requirement) identify related requirements, whether they are in the same chapter or a different chapter. These references should help you more quickly find related standards on a particular topic.

- *EPs*, or elements of performance, are statements that detail the specific performance expectations and/or structures or processes that must be in place in order for an organization to provide quality care, treatment, or services. EPs are scored and determine an organization's overall compliance with a standard.
- *Notes* provide organizations and surveyors with additional or clarifying information about a specific EP.

The *SAC* also includes the "Standards Applicability Process" (SAP) chapter, a Glossary, and an Index.

Description of Icons

The following icons can be found in this book:

- The documentation icon Ⓓ indicates when written documentation is required to demonstrate compliance with an EP. A documentation icon is used to identify data collection and documentation requirements that are beyond information required to be included in the clinical record. For example, an EP that requires a written procedure will include a Ⓓ, but the icon is not applied to an EP that contains the required list of components of the clinical record. Other examples in which the documentation icon is used are for EPs that require a policy, a written plan, bylaws, a license, evidence of testing, data, performance improvement reports, medication labels, safety data sheets, or meeting minutes.
- The risk icon Ⓡ identifies specific risks assessed by a system's proximity to the patient, probability of harm, severity of harm, and number of patients at risk. Risk categories identified by The Joint Commission are related to NPSGs, accreditation program–specific risk areas, and RFIs identified during current accreditation cycle survey events. This book will show a single icon at the EP level for the NPSGs and accreditation program–specific risk areas that are required to be addressed during the Intracycle Monitoring (ICM) process through the Focused Standards Assessment (FSA). The third risk category—related to an organization's own RFIs—will appear only in the ICM Profile on the organization's *Joint Commission Connect* extranet site.

Standard
A statement that, when achieved, facilitates safe, quality care, treatment, or services

Rationale
Additional text that describes the purpose of the requirement/standard

Standard MM.01.01.03

The organization safely manages high-alert and hazardous medications.

Rationale for MM.01.01.03

High-alert medications are those medications that bear a heightened risk of causing significant patient harm and/or sentinel events when they are used in error and, as a result, require special safeguards to reduce the risk of errors. Examples of high-alert medications include opioids, insulin, anticoagulants, and neuromuscular blocking agents. Lists of high-alert medications are available from organizations such as the Institute for Safe Medication Practices (ISMP).

Hazardous drugs and medications are those in which studies in animals or humans indicate that exposure to them has a potential for causing cancer, developmental or reproductive toxicity, genotoxicity, or harm to organs. An example of a hazardous drug is one that contains antineoplastic agents or other ingredients that cause the aforementioned risks. Lists of hazardous drugs are available from the National Institute for Occupational Safety and Health (NIOSH).

Element of Performance
Identifies performance expectations—only the elements of performance are scored

For safe management, the organization needs to develop its own lists of both high-alert medications and hazardous drugs. These should be based on the organization's unique utilization patterns, its own internal data about medication errors and sentinel events, and known safety issues published in professional literature. It is up to the organization to determine whether medications that are new to the market are high alert or hazardous. In addition, the organization may separately choose to include other drugs that require special precautions such as investigational medications, controlled substances, and psychotherapeutic medications.

Note: *For a list of high-alert medications, see https://www.ismp.org/recommendations. For a list of hazardous drugs, see https://www.cdc.gov/niosh/docs/2016-161/pdfs/2016-161.pdf.*

Elements of Performance for MM.01.01.03

1. Ⓓ The organization identifies, in writing, its high-alert and hazardous medications. ℝ

Documentation Icon Ⓓ
Indicates when written documentation is required beyond that in the medical record

Risk Icon ℝ
Indicates an identified risk for the purposes of the Focused Standards Assessment

Figure 1. *Components of a standards chapter. The components are further described in the "Chapter Structure" and "Description of Icons" sections.*

Accreditation Participation Requirements (APR)

Overview

This chapter consists of specific requirements for participation in the accreditation process and for maintaining an accreditation award.

For an organization seeking accreditation for the first time, compliance with most of the Accreditation Participation Requirements (APRs) is assessed during the initial survey, including the Early Survey Policy Option. Please note that APR.09.01.01 and APR.09.02.01 are not assessed during the initial survey. For the accredited organization, compliance with the APRs is assessed throughout the accreditation cycle through on-site surveys, the Focused Standards Assessment (FSA), Evidence of Standards Compliance (ESC), and periodic updates of organization-specific data and information. Organizations are either compliant or not compliant with the APRs. When an organization does not comply with an APR, the organization will be assigned a Requirement for Improvement (RFI) in the same context that noncompliance with a standard or element of performance generates an RFI. However, refusal to permit performance of a survey (APR.02.01.01) will lead to a denial of accreditation. Falsification of information (APR.01.02.01) will lead to preliminary denial of accreditation. All RFIs can impact the accreditation decision and follow-up requirements, as determined by established accreditation decision rules. Failure to resolve an RFI can ultimately lead to loss of accreditation.

Chapter Outline

I. Submission of Information to The Joint Commission
   A. Timely Submission of Information (APR.01.01.01)
   B. Accuracy of Information (APR.01.02.01)
   C. Changes in Information (APR.01.03.01)

II. Performance of Survey
   A. Performance of Survey at The Joint Commission's Discretion (APR.02.01.01)

III. Not applicable to ambulatory care

IV. Performance Measurement — Not applicable to ambulatory care

V. External Evaluations
   A. Sharing Results of External Evaluations with The Joint Commission (APR.05.01.01)

VI. Accreditation-Related Consulting Services
   A. Prohibiting Use of Joint Commission Employees (APR.06.01.01)

VII. Survey Observations
   A. Joint Commission Management and Leadership Observing Surveys (APR.07.01.01)

VIII. Representation of Accreditation Status
   A. Accurately Representing Accreditation Status (APR.08.01.01)

IX. Reporting of Safety and Quality Concerns
   A. Notifying the Public about Reporting Safety and Quality Concerns (APR.09.01.01)
   B. Notifying Individuals Who Provide Care, Treatment, or Services about Reporting Safety and Quality Concerns (APR.09.02.01)
   C. Adhering to Joint Commission Guidelines for Describing Information in the Quality Report (APR.09.03.01)
   D. Providing Care, Treatment, Services, and an Environment That Pose No Risk of an Immediate Threat to Health or Safety (APR.09.04.01)

Requirements, Rationales, and Elements of Performance

APR.01.01.01

The organization submits information to The Joint Commission as required.

Elements of Performance for APR.01.01.01

1. The organization meets all requirements for timely submissions of data and information to The Joint Commission.

   Note 1: *The Joint Commission will impose the following consequence for failure to comply with this APR:*

   If the organization consistently fails to meet the requirements for the timely submission of data and information to The Joint Commission, the organization will be required to undergo an Accreditation with Follow-up Survey. Failure to resolve this issue at the time of the Accreditation with Follow-up Survey may result in an accreditation decision change.

   Note 2: *The proposed consequences address only compliance with the requirement itself. They do not address the content of the organization's submissions to The Joint Commission. For example, if information in an organization's electronic application for accreditation (E-App) leads to inaccuracies in the appropriate length of the survey and a longer survey is required, the organization will incur the additional costs of the longer survey. In addition, if there is evidence that the organization has intentionally falsified the information submitted to The Joint Commission, the requirement at APR.01.02.01, EP 1 and its consequences will apply.*

   (*See also* APR.01.02.01, EP 1)

APR.01.02.01

The organization provides accurate information throughout the accreditation process.

Rationale for APR.01.02.01

The Joint Commission requires each organization seeking accreditation to engage in the accreditation process in good faith. Sound business practices require transparency in all reporting procedures to ensure the safety of the public and the people who work in the organization. Any organization that fails to participate in good faith by falsifying information or neglecting to exercise due care and diligence in ensuring the accuracy of such information may have its accreditation denied or removed by The Joint Commission.

Elements of Performance for APR.01.02.01

1. The organization provides accurate information throughout the accreditation process.

   Note 1: *Information may be received in any of the following ways:*
   - *Provided verbally*
   - *Obtained through direct observation by, or in an interview or any other type of communication with, a Joint Commission employee*
   - *Derived from documents supplied by the organization to The Joint Commission*
   - *Submitted electronically by the organization to The Joint Commission*

   Note 2: *For the purpose of this requirement, falsification is defined as the fabrication, in whole or in part, and through commission or omission, of any information provided by an applicant or accredited organization to The Joint Commission. This includes redrafting, reformatting, or deleting document content. However, the organization may submit supporting material that explains the original information submitted to The Joint Commission. These additional materials must be properly identified, dated, and accompanied by the original documents.*

   (*See also* APR.01.01.01, EP 1)

APR.01.03.01

The organization reports any changes in the information provided in the application for accreditation and any changes made between surveys.

Elements of Performance for APR.01.03.01

1. Ⓓ The organization notifies The Joint Commission in writing within 30 days of a change in ownership, control, location, capacity, or services offered.

   Note: *When the organization changes ownership, control, location, capacity or services offered, it may be necessary for The Joint Commission to survey the organization again. If the organization does not provide written notification to The Joint Commission within 30 days of these changes, the organization may be denied accreditation.*

2. Ⓓ **For ambulatory surgical centers that elect to use The Joint Commission deemed status option:** The organization notifies The Joint Commission immediately upon receiving notice from the Centers for Medicare & Medicaid

Services (CMS) that its deemed status has been removed due to Medicare condition-level noncompliance identified during a recent CMS complaint or validation survey.

APR.02.01.01 ▬▬▬▬▬▬▬▬▬▬▬▬▬▬▬

The organization permits the performance of a survey at The Joint Commission's discretion.

Elements of Performance for APR.02.01.01

1. The organization permits the performance of a survey at The Joint Commission's discretion.

APR.05.01.01 ▬▬▬▬▬▬▬▬▬▬▬▬▬▬▬

The organization allows The Joint Commission to review the results of external evaluations from publicly recognized bodies.

Rationale for APR.05.01.01

In order to conduct a meaningful accreditation survey, The Joint Commission collects information on many aspects of the organization's performance. External bodies other than The Joint Commission also evaluate areas related to safety and quality. These evaluations complement accreditation reviews but may have a different focus or emphasis. These evaluations may contain information The Joint Commission needs to make accreditation decisions.

Elements of Performance for APR.05.01.01

1. Ⓓ When requested, the organization provides The Joint Commission with all official records and reports of licensing, examining, reviewing, or planning bodies.

APR.06.01.01 ▬▬▬▬▬▬▬▬▬▬▬▬▬▬▬

Applicants and accredited organizations do not use Joint Commission employees to provide accreditation-related consulting services.

Elements of Performance for APR.06.01.01

1. The organization does not use Joint Commission employees to provide any accreditation-related consulting services.

APR.07.01.01 ▬▬▬▬▬▬▬▬▬▬▬▬▬▬▬

The organization accepts the presence of Joint Commission surveyor management staff or a Board of Commissioners member in the role of observer of an on-site survey.

Elements of Performance for APR.07.01.01

1. The organization allows Joint Commission surveyor management staff or a member of the Board of Commissioners to observe the on-site survey.

    Note 1: *The observer will not participate in the on-site survey process, including the scoring of standards compliance. Surveyor management staff will only participate in the survey process if they feel it is necessary to bring any potential findings or observations to the attention of the surveyor and the organization.*

    Note 2: *The organization will not incur any additional survey fees because an observer(s) is present.*

APR.08.01.01

The organization accurately represents its accreditation status and the programs and services to which Joint Commission accreditation applies.

Elements of Performance for APR.08.01.01

1. The organization's advertising accurately reflects the scope of programs and services that are accredited by The Joint Commission.

2. The organization does not engage in any false or misleading advertising about its accreditation award.

APR.09.01.01

The organization notifies the public it serves about how to contact its organization management and The Joint Commission to report concerns about patient safety and quality of care.

Note: *Methods of notice may include, but are not limited to, distribution of information about The Joint Commission, including contact information in published materials such as brochures and/or posting this information on the organization's website.*

Elements of Performance for APR.09.01.01

1. The organization informs the public it serves about how to contact its management to report concerns about patient safety and quality of care.

2. The organization informs the public it serves about how to contact The Joint Commission to report concerns about patient safety and quality of care.

APR.09.02.01

Any individual who provides care, treatment, or services can report concerns about safety or the quality of care to The Joint Commission without retaliatory action from the organization.

Rationale for APR.09.02.01

Any individual who provides care, treatment, or services should be free to raise concerns to The Joint Commission when the organization has not adequately prevented or corrected problems that can have or have had a serious adverse impact on patients. To support this culture of safety, the organization must communicate to staff that such reporting is permitted. Furthermore, the organization must make it clear to staff that no formal disciplinary actions (for example, demotions, reassignments, or change in working conditions or hours) or informal punitive actions (for example, harassment, isolation, or abuse) will be threatened or carried out in retaliation for reporting concerns to The Joint Commission.

Elements of Performance for APR.09.02.01

1. The organization educates its staff and other persons who provide care, treatment, or services that concerns about the safety or quality of care provided in the organization may be reported to The Joint Commission.

2. The organization informs its staff that it will take no disciplinary or punitive action because an employee or other individual who provides care, treatment, or services reports safety or quality-of-care concerns to The Joint Commission.

3. The organization takes no disciplinary or punitive action against employees or other individuals who provide care, treatment, or services when they report safety or quality-of-care concerns to The Joint Commission.

APR.09.03.01

The organization is truthful and accurate when describing information in its Quality Report to the public.

Elements of Performance for APR.09.03.01

1. The organization adheres to The Joint Commission's published guidelines for how it describes information in its Quality Report.

APR.09.04.01

The organization provides care, treatment, services, and an environment that pose no risk of an "Immediate Threat to Health or Safety."

Elements of Performance for APR.09.04.01

1. The organization provides care, treatment, services, and an environment that pose no risk of an "Immediate Threat to Health or Safety."

Environment of Care (EC)

Overview

The goal of this chapter is to promote a safe, functional, and supportive environment within the organization so that quality and safety are preserved. The environment of care is made up of the following three basic elements:

- The building or space, including how it is arranged and special features that protect patients, visitors, and staff
- Equipment used to support patient care or to safely operate the building or space
- People who work within the organization, patients, and anyone else who enters the environment, all of whom have a role in minimizing risks

This chapter stresses the importance of managing risks in the environment of care, which are different from the risks associated with the provision of care, treatment, or services. Any organization, regardless of its size or location, faces risks in the environment, including those associated with safety and security, fire, hazardous materials and waste, medical equipment, and utility systems. When staff are educated about the elements of a safe environment, they are more likely to follow processes for identifying, reporting, and taking action on environmental risks.

About This Chapter

The standards are organized around the concepts of planning, implementing, and evaluating of results. The chapter calls for written plans for managing risks in each of these areas. Organizations may choose to address all required components of the environment in a single management plan or in several different plans. If an organization has multiple sites, it may have separate management plans for each of its locations, or it may choose to have one comprehensive set of plans. In any case, the organization must address specific risks and the unique conditions at each of its sites.

The standards address the need to identify someone to manage environmental risks as well as to intervene when situations threaten people or property; both responsibilities may be assigned to one person. It is important to remember that the standards in this chapter do not prescribe a particular structure (such as a safety committee) or individual (such as one employee hired to be a safety officer) for managing the environment, nor do they prescribe how required planning activities are conducted.

Important aspects of the environment addressed in the standards include the following:

- Safety and security. This section addresses risks in the physical environment, access to security-sensitive areas, product recalls, and smoking.
- Hazardous materials and waste. This section addresses risks associated with hazardous chemicals, radioactive materials, hazardous energy sources, hazardous medications, and hazardous gases and vapors.
- Fire safety. This section addresses risks from fire, smoke, and other products of combustion; fire response plans; fire drills; management of fire detection, alarm, and suppression equipment and systems; and measures to implement during construction or when the *Life Safety Code®** cannot be met.
- Medical equipment. This section addresses selection, testing, and maintenance of medical equipment and contingencies when equipment fails.
- Utilities. This section addresses inspection and testing of operating components, control of airborne contaminants, and management of disruptions (refer to Standard IM.01.01.03).

Note: *Emergency management standards are located in a separate chapter.*

Other Issues for Consideration

1. The organization that provides care, treatment, or services in space it does not own (for example, in leased or complimentary space) may want to communicate with the property owner about maintenance expectations for building equipment and features not under its control. For example, an organization may need access to the maintenance documents. This organization and the property owner may want to discuss any building or equipment problems that could adversely affect the safety or health of patients, staff, and other people coming to the organization, as well as the property owner's plan to resolve such issues.

2. A number of elements of performance describe time frames for completing certain tasks or functions. The Joint Commission recognizes that it will not always be possible to meet the exact time frames cited in the requirements. For evaluation purposes, therefore, the following intervals are acceptable:
   - Every 36 months/every 3 years = 36 months from the last event, plus or minus 45 days
   - Annually/every 12 months/once a year/every year = 1 year from the last event, plus or minus 30 days

---

* *Life Safety Code*® is a registered trademark of the National Fire Protection Association, Quincy, MA.

- Every 6 months = 6 months from the last event, plus or minus 20 days
- Quarterly/every quarter = every 3 months, plus or minus 10 days
- Monthly/30-day intervals/every month = 12 times a year, once per calendar month
- Every week = once per calendar week

Chapter Outline

I.   Plan (EC.01.01.01)

II. Implement
     A. Safety and Security (EC.02.01.01, EC.02.01.03)
     B. Hazardous Materials and Waste (EC.02.02.01)
     C. Fire Safety (EC.02.03.01, EC.02.03.03, EC.02.03.05)
     D. Medical Equipment (EC.02.04.01, EC.02.04.03)
     E. Utilities (EC.02.05.01, EC.02.05.03, EC.02.05.05, EC.02.05.07, EC.02.05.09)
     F. Other Physical Environment Requirements (EC.02.06.01, EC.02.06.05)

III. Staff Demonstrate Competence (EC.03.01.01)

IV. Monitor and Improve (EC.04.01.01, EC.04.01.03, EC.04.01.05)

Standards, Rationales, and Elements of Performance

Standard EC.01.01.01

The organization plans activities to minimize risks in the environment of care.

Note 1: *One or more persons can be assigned to manage risks associated with the management plans described in this standard.*

Note 2: *For ambulatory surgical centers that elect to use The Joint Commission deemed status option: The organization complies with the 2012 edition of NFPA 99: Health Care Facilities Code. Chapters 7, 8, 12, and 13 of the Health Care Facilities Code do not apply.*

Note 3: *For further information on waiver and equivalency requests, see https://www.jointcommission.org/resources/patient-safety-topics/the-physical-environment/life-safety-code-information-and-resources/ and NFPA 99-2012: 1.4.*

Rationale for EC.01.01.01

Risks are inherent in the environment because of the types of care provided and the equipment and materials that are necessary to provide that care. The best way to manage these risks is through a systematic approach that involves the proactive evaluation of the harm that could occur. By identifying one or more individuals to coordinate and manage risk assessment and reduction activities—and to intervene when conditions immediately threaten life and health—organizations can be more confident that they have minimized the potential for harm.

Risks in the environment include safety and security for people, equipment, and other material; the handling of hazardous materials and waste; the potential for fire; the use of medical equipment; and utility systems. Written management plans help the organization manage risks. These plans are not the same as operational plans, but they do provide a framework for managing the environment of care. These plans should also address the scope and objectives of risk assessment and management, describe the responsibilities of individuals or groups, and give time frames for specific activities identified in the plan.

Note: *It is not necessary to have a separate plan for each of the areas identified in the standard; the plans may all be contained in a single document.*

Elements of Performance for EC.01.01.01

1. Leaders identify an individual(s) to manage risk, coordinate risk reduction activities in the physical environment, collect deficiency information, and disseminate summaries of actions and results.

   Note: *Deficiencies include injuries, problems, or use errors.*

3. The organization has a library of information regarding inspection, testing, and maintenance of its equipment and systems.

   Note: *This library includes manuals, procedures provided by manufacturers, technical bulletins, and other information.*

The organization has a written plan for managing the following:

4. Ⓓ The environmental safety of everyone who enters the organization's facilities.

5. Ⓓ The security of everyone who enters the organization's facilities.

6. Ⓓ Hazardous materials and waste.

7. Ⓓ Fire safety.

8. Ⓓ Medical equipment.

9. Ⓓ Utility systems.

Standard EC.02.01.01 ▬▬▬▬▬▬▬▬▬▬▬▬▬▬▬▬

The organization manages safety and security risks.

Rationale for EC.02.01.01

Safety and security risks are present in most health care environments. These risks affect all individuals in the organization—patients, visitors, and those who work in the organization. It is important to identify these risks in advance so the organization can prevent or effectively respond to incidents. In some organizations, safety and security are treated as a single function, although in others they are treated as separate functions.

Safety risks may arise from the structure of the physical environment, from the performance of everyday tasks, or from situations beyond the organization's control, such as the weather. Safety incidents are most often accidental. On the other hand, security incidents are often intentional. Security protects individuals and property against harm or loss. Examples of security risks include workplace violence, theft, and unrestricted access to medications. Security incidents are caused by individuals from either outside or inside the organization.

Elements of Performance for EC.02.01.01

1. ⑩ The organization implements its process to identify safety and security risks associated with the environment of care that could affect patients, staff, and other people coming to the organization's facilities.

    Note: *Risks are identified from internal sources such as ongoing monitoring of the environment, results of root cause analyses, results of proactive risk assessments of high-risk processes, and from credible external sources such as Sentinel Event Alerts.*

3. The organization takes action to minimize identified safety and security risks in the physical environment.

5. **For ambulatory surgical centers that elect to use The Joint Commission deemed status option:** The organization maintains all grounds and equipment.

6. The organization manages safety risks related to entering and exiting the organization.

8. The organization controls access to and from areas it identifies as security sensitive.

11. The organization responds to product notices and recalls.

    (*See also* MM.05.01.17, EPs 1, 3, 4)

14. The organization manages magnetic resonance imaging (MRI) safety risks associated with the following:
    - Patients who may experience claustrophobia, anxiety, or emotional distress
    - Patients who may require urgent or emergent medical care
    - Patients with medical implants, devices, or imbedded metallic foreign objects (such as shrapnel)
    - Ferromagnetic objects entering the MRI environment
    - Acoustic noise

16. The organization manages magnetic resonance imaging (MRI) safety risks by doing the following:

- Restricting access of everyone not trained in MRI safety or screened by staff trained in MRI safety from the scanner room and the area that immediately precedes the entrance to the MRI scanner room.
- Making sure that these restricted areas are controlled by and under the direct supervision of staff trained in MRI safety.
- Posting signage at the entrance to the MRI scanner room that conveys that potentially dangerous magnetic fields are present in the room. Signage should also indicate that the magnet is always on except in cases where the MRI system, by its design, can have its magnetic field routinely turned on and off by the operator.

Standard EC.02.01.03

The organization prohibits smoking.

Elements of Performance for EC.02.01.03

1. Smoking is not permitted in the organization.

   Note: *The scope of this EP is concerned with all smoking types—tobacco, electronic, or other.*

Standard EC.02.02.01

The organization manages risks related to hazardous materials and waste.

Rationale for EC.02.02.01

Hazardous materials and waste cause harm if they are not managed properly. Examples of such materials include chemicals (for example cleaning products, solvents, pesticides), compressed gases, and hazardous energy sources. Federal, state, or local regulations often guide the handling, use, and storage of hazardous materials and waste. The organization identifies materials it uses that need special handling to minimize the risks of unsafe use and improper disposal.

Note: *This standard does not address oxygen because it is not a "hazardous material." Oxygen is addressed under the safety standard (see EC.02.01.01). However, other substances such as blood are covered by this standard.*

Elements of Performance for EC.02.02.01

1. Ⓓ The organization maintains a written, current inventory of hazardous materials and waste that it uses, stores, or generates. The only materials that need to be included on the inventory are those whose handling, use, and storage are addressed by law and regulation.

    (*See also* MM.01.01.03, EP 1)

3. Ⓓ The organization has written procedures, including the use of precautions and personal protective equipment, to follow in response to hazardous material and waste spills or exposures.

    (*See also* IC.02.01.01, EP 2)

4. The organization implements its procedures in response to hazardous material and waste spills or exposures.

5. The organization minimizes risks associated with selecting, handling, storing, transporting, using, and disposing of hazardous chemicals.

6. The organization minimizes risks associated with selecting, handling, storing, transporting, using, and disposing of radioactive materials.

7. The organization minimizes risks associated with the selection and use of hazardous energy sources.

    Note 1: *Hazardous energy is produced by both ionizing equipment (for example, radiation and x-ray equipment) and nonionizing equipment (for example, lasers and MRIs).*

    Note 2: *This includes the use of proper shielding during fluoroscopic procedures.*

8. The organization minimizes risks associated with disposing of hazardous medications.

    (*See also* MM.01.01.03, EP 2)

9. The organization minimizes risks associated with selecting, handling, storing, transporting, using, and disposing of hazardous gases and vapors.

    Note: *Hazardous gases and vapors include, but are not limited to, ethylene oxide and nitrous oxide gases; vapors generated by glutaraldehyde; cauterizing equipment, such as lasers; waste anesthetic gas disposal (WAGD); and laboratory rooftop exhaust. (For full text, refer to NFPA 99-2012: 9.3.8; 9.3.9)*

10. The organization monitors levels of hazardous gases and vapors to determine that they are in safe range. **R**

    Note: *Law and regulation determine the frequency of monitoring hazardous gases and vapors as well as acceptable ranges.*

11. Ⓓ For managing hazardous materials and waste, the organization has the permits, licenses, manifests, and safety data sheets required by law and regulation.

12. The organization labels hazardous materials and waste. Labels identify the contents and hazard warnings.[†]

    (*See also* IC.02.01.01, EP 6)

14. Ⓓ **For ambulatory surgical centers that elect to use The Joint Commission deemed status option:** The ambulatory surgical center checks radiology staff, according to time frames it defines, for radiation exposure, using exposure meters or badge tests. The dates of the checks and amount of exposure are documented.

15. **For ambulatory surgical centers that elect to use The Joint Commission deemed status option:** The radiologic services, including ionizing radiology procedures, are free from hazards for patients and staff.

17. **For organizations that provide computed tomography (CT), positron emission tomography (PET), nuclear medicine (NM), or fluoroscopy services:** The results of dosimetry monitoring are reviewed at least quarterly by the radiation safety officer, diagnostic medical physicist, or health physicist to assess whether staff radiation exposure levels are "as low as reasonably achievable" (ALARA) and below regulatory limits.

    Note 1: *For the definition of ALARA, please refer to US Nuclear Regulatory Commission federal regulation 10 CFR 20.1003.*

    Note 2: *This element of performance does not apply to dental cone beam CT radiographic imaging studies performed for diagnosis of conditions affecting the maxillofacial region or to obtain guidance for the treatment of such conditions.*

[†] The Occupational Safety and Health Administration's (OSHA) Bloodborne Pathogens and Hazard Communications Standards and the National Fire Protection Association (NFPA) provide details on labeling requirements.

Standard EC.02.03.01 ▬▬▬▬▬▬▬▬▬▬▬▬▬▬▬▬▬

The organization manages fire risks.

Elements of Performance for EC.02.03.01

1. The organization minimizes the potential for harm from fire, smoke, and other products of combustion. 🄡

4. The organization maintains free and unobstructed access to all exits. 🄡

    Note: *This requirement applies to all buildings classified as business occupancy. The "Life Safety" (LS) chapter addresses the requirements for all other occupancy types.*

9. Ⓓ The organization has a written fire response plan that describes the specific roles of staff and licensed independent practitioners during a fire, including when and how to sound fire alarms, how to contain smoke and fire, how to use a fire extinguisher, how to assist and relocate patients, and how to evacuate to areas of refuge. Staff and licensed independent practitioners are periodically instructed on and kept informed of their duties under the plan. A copy of the plan is readily available with the telephone operator or security.

    Note: *For full text, refer to NFPA 101-2012: 20/21.7.1; 7.2.*

11. Periodic evaluations, as determined by the organization, are made of potential fire hazards that could be encountered during surgical procedures. Written fire prevention and response procedures, including safety precautions related to the use of flammable germicides or antiseptics, are established.

12. When flammable germicides or antiseptics are used during surgeries utilizing electrosurgery, cautery, or lasers, the following are required:
    ■ Nonflammable packaging
    ■ Unit-dose applicators
    ■ Preoperative "time-out" prior to the initiation of any surgical procedure to verify the following:
       ❏ Application site is dry prior to draping and use of surgical equipment
       ❏ Pooling of solution has not occurred or has been corrected
       ❏ Solution-soaked materials have been removed from the operating room prior to draping and use of surgical devices

    (For full text, refer to NFPA 99-2012: 15.13)

13. The organization meets all other Health Care Facilities Code fire protection requirements, as related to NFPA 99-2012: Chapter 15.

Standard EC.02.03.03

The organization conducts fire drills.

Rationale for EC.02.03.03

The organization's plan for fire response is an important part of achieving a fire-safe environment. It is important that this response be evaluated in drill scenarios or actual fire situations in order to assess performance of staff and fire safety equipment. Testing the fire response plan should involve realistic situations, although actual evacuation of patients during the drills is not required.

Elements of Performance for EC.02.03.03

1. Ⓓ The organization conducts quarterly fire drills in each building defined as an ambulatory health care occupancy by the *Life Safety Code.*

    Note 1: *Evacuation of patients during drills is not required.*

    Note 2: *When drills are conducted between 9:00* P.M. *and 6:00* A.M., *the organization may use alternative methods to notify staff instead of activating audible alarms.*

    Note 3: *In leased or rented facilities, drills need be conducted only in areas of the building that the organization occupies.*

    (*See also* LS.01.02.01, EP 11)

2. Ⓓ The organization conducts fire drills every 12 months from the date of the last drill in each area that is defined as a business occupancy by the *Life Safety Code* and in which care, treatment, or services are provided, or quarterly for ambulatory surgical centers seeking accreditation for Medicare certification.

    Note 1: *In leased or rented facilities, drills need be conducted only in areas of the building that the organization occupies.*

    Note 2: *In sites that are used on average 70 hours or less per month, the organization may choose either to review the fire response plan or to conduct a fire drill every 12 months. This note does not apply to ambulatory surgical centers that elect to use The Joint Commission deemed status option.*

3. When quarterly fire drills are required, they are unannounced and held at unexpected times and under varying conditions. Fire drills include transmission of fire alarm signal and simulation of emergency fire conditions.

Note 1: *When drills are conducted between 9:00* P.M. *and 6:00* A.M., *the organization may use alternative methods to notify staff instead of activating audible alarms.*

Note 2: *For full text, refer to NFPA 101-2012: 20/21: 7.1; 7.2; 7.3.*

5. Ⓓ The organization critiques fire drills.

Standard EC.02.03.05

The organization maintains fire safety equipment and fire safety building features.

Note: *This standard does not require organizations to have the types of fire safety equipment and building features described below. However, if these types of equipment or features exist within the building, then the following maintenance, testing, and inspection requirements apply.*

Elements of Performance for EC.02.03.05

1. Ⓓ At least quarterly, the organization tests supervisory signal devices on the inventory (except valve tamper switches). The results and completion dates are documented.

    Note 1: *For additional guidance on performing tests, see NFPA 72-2010: Table 14.4.5.*

    Note 2: *Supervisory signals include the following: control valves; pressure supervisory; pressure tank, pressure supervisory for a dry pipe (both high and low conditions), steam pressure; water level supervisory signal initiating device; water temperature supervisory; and room temperature supervisory.*

2. Ⓓ Every 6 months, the organization tests vane-type and pressure-type water flow devices and valve tamper switches on the inventory. The results and completion dates are documented.

    Note 1: *For additional guidance on performing tests, see NFPA 72-2010: Table 14.4.5.*

    Note 2: *Mechanical water-flow devices (including, but not limited to, water motor gongs) should be tested quarterly. The results and completion dates are documented. (For full text, refer to NFPA 25-2011: Table 5.1.1.2)*

3. Ⓓ Every 12 months, the organization tests duct detectors, heat detectors, manual fire alarm boxes, and smoke detectors on the inventory. The results and completion dates are documented.

    Note: *For additional guidance on performing tests, see NFPA 72-2010: Table 14.4.5; 17.14.*

4. Ⓓ Every 12 months, the organization tests visual and audible fire alarms, including speakers and door-releasing devices on the inventory. The results and completion dates are documented. Ⓡ

    Note: *For additional guidance on performing tests, see NFPA 72-2010: Table 14.4.5.*

5. Ⓓ Every 12 months the organization tests fire alarm equipment on the inventory for notifying off-site fire responders. The results and completion dates are documented.

    Note: *For additional guidance on performing tests, see NFPA 72-2010: Table 14.4.5.*

6. Ⓓ **For automatic sprinkler systems:** The organization tests electric motor–driven fire pumps monthly and diesel engine–driven fire pumps every week under no-flow conditions. The results and completion dates are documented.

    Note: *For additional guidance on performing tests, see NFPA 25-2011: 8.3.1; 8.3.2.*

7. Ⓓ **For automatic sprinkler systems:** Every six months, the organization tests water-storage tank high- and low-water level alarms. The results and completion dates are documented.

    Note: *For additional guidance on performing tests, see NFPA 25-2011: 9.3; Table 9.1.1.2.*

8. Ⓓ **For automatic sprinkler systems:** Every month during cold weather, the organization tests water-storage tank temperature alarms. The results and completion dates are documented.

    Note: *For additional guidance on performing tests, see NFPA 25-2011: 9.2.4; Table 9.1.1.2.*

9.   ⓓ **For automatic sprinkler systems:** Every 12 months, the organization tests main drains at system low point or at all system risers. The results and completion dates are documented.

   Note: *For additional guidance on performing tests, see NFPA 25-2011: 13.2.5; 13.3.3.4; Table 13.1.1.2; Table 13.8.1.*

10.   ⓓ **For automatic sprinkler systems:** Every quarter, the organization inspects all fire department water supply connections. The results and completion dates are documented.

   Note: *For additional guidance on performing tests, see NFPA 25-2011: 13.7; Table 13.1.1.2.*

11.   ⓓ **For automatic sprinkler systems:** Every 12 months, the organization tests fire pumps under flow. The results and completion dates are documented. **Ⓡ**

   Note: *For additional guidance on performing tests, see NFPA 25-2011: 8.3.3.*

12.   ⓓ Every 5 years, the organization conducts hydrostatic and water-flow tests for standpipe systems. The results and completion dates are documented.

   Note: *For additional guidance on performing tests, see NFPA 25-2011: 6.3.1; 6.3.2; Table 6.1.1.2.*

14.   ⓓ Every 12 months, the organization tests carbon dioxide and other gaseous automatic fire-extinguishing systems. The results and completion dates are documented.

   Note 1: *Discharge of the fire-extinguishing systems is not required.*

   Note 2: *For full text, refer to NFPA 12-2011: 4.8.3 and NFPA 12A-2009: Chapter 6.*

15.   ⓓ At least monthly, the organization inspects portable fire extinguishers. The results and completion dates are documented.

   Note 1: *There are many ways to document the inspections, such as using bar-coding equipment, using check marks on a tag, or using an inventory.*

   Note 2: *Inspections involve a visual check to determine correct type of and clear and unobstructed access to a fire extinguisher, in addition to a check for broken parts and full charge.*

Note 3: *For additional guidance on inspection of fire extinguishers,* see *NFPA 10-2010: 7.2.2; 7.2.4.*

16.   ⓓ Every 12 months, the organization performs maintenance on portable fire extinguishers, including recharging. Individuals performing annual maintenance on extinguishers are certified. The results and completion dates are documented.

Note 1: *There are many ways to document the maintenance, such as using barcoding equipment, using check marks on a tag, or using an inventory.*

Note 2: *For additional guidance on maintaining fire extinguishers,* see *NFPA 10-2010: 7.1.2; 7.2.2; 7.2.4; 7.3.1.*

17.   ⓓ The organization conducts hydrostatic tests on standpipe occupant hoses 5 years after installation and every 3 years thereafter. The results and completion dates are documented.

Note: *For additional guidance on hydrostatic testing,* see *NFPA 1962-2008: Chapter 7 and NFPA 25-2011: Chapter 6.*

18.   ⓓ The organization operates fire and smoke dampers one year after installation and then at least every four years to verify that they fully close. The results and completion dates are documented.

Note: *For additional guidance on performing tests,* see *NFPA 90A-2012: 5.4.8; NFPA 80-2010: 19.4; NFPA 105-2010: 6.5.*

19.   ⓓ Every 12 months, the organization tests automatic smoke-detection shutdown devices for air-handling equipment. The results and completion dates are documented. **R**

Note: *For additional guidance on performing tests,* see *NFPA 90A-2012: 6.4.1.*

20.   ⓓ Every 12 months, the organization tests sliding and rolling fire doors, smoke barrier sliding or rolling doors, and sliding and rolling fire doors in corridor walls and partitions for proper operation and full closure. The results and completion dates are documented.

Note: *For full text, refer to NFPA 80-2010: 5.2.14.3; NFPA 105-2010: 5.2.1; 5.2.2.*

25.   ⒹThe organization has annual inspection and testing of fire door assemblies by individuals who can demonstrate knowledge and understanding of the operating components of the door being tested. Testing begins with a pre-test visual inspection; testing includes both sides of the opening.

Note 1: *Nonrated doors, including corridor doors to patient care rooms and smoke barrier doors, are not subject to the annual inspection and testing requirements of either NFPA 80 or NFPA 105.*

Note 2: *For ambulatory surgical centers that elect to use The Joint Commission deemed status option: Nonrated doors should be routinely inspected and maintained in accordance with the facility maintenance program.*

Note 3: *For additional guidance on testing of door assemblies, see NFPA 101-2012: 7.2.1.5.10.1; 7.2.1.5.11; 7.2.1.15; NFPA 80-2010: 4.8.4; 5.2.1; 5.2.3; 5.2.4; 5.2.6; 5.2.7; 6.3.1.7; NFPA 105-2010: 5.2.1.*

27.   ⒹElevators with firefighters' emergency operations are tested monthly. The test completion dates and results are documented. (For full text, refer to NFPA 101-2012: 9.4.3; 9.4.6)

28.   ⒹDocumentation of maintenance, testing, and inspection activities for EC.02.03.05, EPs 1–20, 25 (including fire alarm and fire protection features) includes the following:
- Name of the activity
- Date of the activity
- Inventory of devices, equipment, or other items
- Required frequency of the activity
- Name and contact information, including affiliation, of the person who performed the activity
- NFPA standard(s) referenced for the activity
- Results of the activity

Note: *For additional guidance on documenting activities, see NFPA 25-2011: 4.3; 4.4; NFPA 72-2010: 14.2.1; 14.2.2; 14.2.3; 14.2.4.*

Standard EC.02.04.01 ━━━━━━━━━━━━━━━━━━━━━━

The organization manages medical equipment risks.

Elements of Performance for EC.02.04.01

2. Ⓓ The organization maintains either a written inventory of all medical equipment or a written inventory of selected equipment categorized by physical risk associated with use (including all life-support equipment) and equipment incident history. The organization evaluates new types of equipment before initial use to determine whether they should be included in the inventory. **Ⓡ**

   For ambulatory surgical centers and outpatient surgical departments that elect to use The Joint Commission deemed status option: The organization maintains a written inventory of all medical equipment.

3. Ⓓ The organization identifies the activities and frequencies for maintaining, inspecting, and testing for all medical equipment on the inventory. Various maintenance strategies may be used to ensure reliable performance (for example, predictive maintenance, reliability-centered maintenance, interval-based inspections, corrective maintenance, or metered maintenance). Defined intervals may be based on criteria such as manufacturers' recommendations, risk levels, and current organization experience.

   For ambulatory surgical centers and outpatient surgical departments that elect to use The Joint Commission deemed status option: The organization identifies the activities and frequencies for maintaining, inspecting, and testing for all medical equipment on the inventory. These activities and frequencies must follow manufacturers' recommendations or other federal or state requirements.

5. Ⓓ The organization monitors and reports all incidents in which medical equipment is suspected in or attributed to the death, serious injury, or serious illness of any individual, as required by the Safe Medical Devices Act of 1990.

6. Ⓓ The organization has written procedures to follow when medical equipment fails, including using emergency clinical interventions and backup equipment.

10. The organization identifies quality control and maintenance activities to maintain the quality of the diagnostic computed tomography (CT), positron emission tomography (PET), magnetic resonance imaging (MRI), and nuclear medicine (NM) images produced. The organization identifies how often these activities should be conducted.

Standard EC.02.04.03 ━━━━━━━━━━━━━━━━━━━━━━━━

The organization inspects, tests, and maintains medical equipment.

Elements of Performance for EC.02.04.03

1. Before initial use of medical equipment on the medical equipment inventory, the organization performs safety, operational, and functional checks.

2. Ⓓ The organization inspects, tests, and maintains all high-risk equipment. These activities are documented. **R**

    Note: *High-risk equipment includes life-support equipment.*

3. Ⓓ The organization inspects, tests, and maintains non-high-risk equipment identified on the medical equipment inventory. These activities are documented.

4. Ⓓ The organization conducts performance testing of and maintains all sterilizers. These activities are documented. **R**

    (*See also* IC.02.02.01, EP 2)

5. Ⓓ The organization performs equipment maintenance and chemical and biological testing of water used in hemodialysis. These activities are documented. **R**

8. Equipment listed for use in oxygen-enriched atmospheres is clearly and permanently labeled (withstands cleaning/disinfecting) as follows:
    - Oxygen-metering equipment, pressure-reducing regulators, humidifiers, and nebulizers are labeled with name of manufacturer or supplier.
    - Oxygen-metering equipment and pressure reducing regulators are labeled "OXYGEN–USE NO OIL."
    - Labels on flowmeters, pressure-reducing regulators, and oxygen-dispensing apparatuses designate the gases for which they are intended.
    - Cylinders and containers are labeled in accordance with Compressed Gas Association (CGA) C-7.

    (For full text, refer to NFPA 99-2012: 11.5.3.1)

    Note: *Color coding is not utilized as the primary method of determining cylinder or container contents.*

10. All occupancies containing hyperbaric facilities comply with construction, equipment, administration, and maintenance requirements of NFPA 99-2012: Chapter 14.

18. The organization maintains the quality of the diagnostic computed tomography (CT), positron emission tomography (PET), magnetic resonance imaging (MRI), and nuclear medicine (NM) images produced.

19. **For ambulatory surgical centers that elect to use The Joint Commission deemed status option:** Emergency equipment is maintained by qualified staff.

20. Ⓓ **For diagnostic computed tomography (CT) services:** At least annually, a diagnostic medical physicist does the following:
    - Measures the radiation dose (in the form of volume computed tomography dose index [CTDIvol]) produced by each diagnostic CT imaging system for the following four CT protocols: adult brain, adult abdomen, pediatric brain, and pediatric abdomen. If one or more of these protocols is not used by the organization, other commonly used CT protocols may be substituted.
    - Verifies that the radiation dose (in the form of CTDIvol) produced and measured for each protocol tested is within 20 percent of the CTDIvol displayed on the CT console. The dates, results, and verifications of these measurements are documented.

    Note 1: *This element of performance is only applicable for systems capable of calculating and displaying radiation doses.*

    Note 2: *This element of performance does not apply to dental cone beam CT radiographic imaging studies performed for diagnosis of conditions affecting the maxillofacial region or to obtain guidance for the treatment of such conditions.*

    Note 3: *Medical physicists are accountable for these activities. They may be assisted with the testing and evaluation of equipment performance by individuals who have the required training and skills, as determined by the physicist. (For more information, refer to HR.01.02.01, EP 1; HR.01.02.07, EPs 1 and 2; HR.01.06.01, EP 1; LD.03.06.01, EP 4.)*

21. Ⓓ **For diagnostic computed tomography (CT) services:** At least annually, a diagnostic medical physicist conducts a performance evaluation of all CT imaging equipment. The evaluation results, along with recommendations for correcting any problems identified, are documented. The evaluation includes the use of phantoms to assess the following imaging metrics:
    - Image uniformity
    - Scout prescription accuracy
    - Alignment light accuracy

- Table travel accuracy
- Radiation beam width
- High-contrast resolution
- Low-contrast detectability
- Geometric or distance accuracy
- CT number accuracy and uniformity
- Artifact evaluation

Note 1: *This element of performance does not apply to dental cone beam CT radiographic imaging studies performed for diagnosis of conditions affecting the maxillofacial region or to obtain guidance for the treatment of such conditions.*

Note 2: *Medical physicists are accountable for these activities. They may be assisted with the testing and evaluation of equipment performance by individuals who have the required training and skills, as determined by the physicist. (For more information, refer to HR.01.02.01, EP 1; HR.01.02.07, EPs 1 and 2; HR.01.06.01, EP 1; LD.03.06.01, EP 4.)*

22. ⓓ At least annually, a diagnostic medical physicist or magnetic resonance imaging (MRI) scientist conducts a performance evaluation of all MRI imaging equipment. The evaluation results, along with recommendations for correcting any problems identified, are documented. The evaluation includes the use of phantoms to assess the following imaging metrics:
    - Image uniformity for all radiofrequency (RF) coils used clinically
    - Signal-to-noise ratio (SNR) for all coils used clinically
    - Slice thickness accuracy
    - Slice position accuracy
    - Alignment light accuracy
    - High-contrast resolution
    - Low-contrast resolution (or contrast-to-noise ratio)
    - Geometric or distance accuracy
    - Magnetic field homogeneity
    - Artifact evaluation

Note: *Medical physicists or MRI scientists are accountable for these activities. They may be assisted with the testing and evaluation of equipment performance by individuals who have the required training and skills, as determined by the medical physicist or MRI scientist. (For more information, refer to HR.01.02.01, EP 1; HR.01.02.07, EPs 1 and 2; HR.01.06.01, EP 1; LD.03.06.01, EP 4.)*

23. Ⓓ At least annually, a diagnostic medical physicist or nuclear medicine physicist conducts a performance evaluation of all nuclear medicine imaging equipment. The evaluation results, along with recommendations for correcting any problems identified, are documented. The evaluations are conducted for all of the image types produced clinically by each NM scanner (for example, planar and/or tomographic) and include the use of phantoms to assess the following imaging metrics:
    - Image uniformity/system uniformity
    - High-contrast resolution/system spatial resolution
    - Sensitivity
    - Energy resolution
    - Count-rate performance
    - Artifact evaluation

    Note 1: *The following test is recommended, but not required: Low-contrast resolution or detectability for non-planar acquisitions.*

    Note 2: *The medical physicist or nuclear medicine physicist is accountable for these activities. They may be assisted with the testing and evaluation of equipment performance by individuals who have the required training and skills, as determined by the medical physicist or nuclear medicine physicist. (For more information, refer to HR.01.02.01, EP 1; HR.01.02.07, EPs 1 and 2; HR.01.06.01, EP 1; LD.03.06.01, EP 4.)*

24. Ⓓ At least annually, a diagnostic medical physicist conducts a performance evaluation of all positron emission tomography (PET) imaging equipment. The evaluation results, along with recommendations for correcting any problems identified, are documented. The evaluations are conducted for all of the image types produced clinically by each PET scanner (for example, planar and/or tomographic) and include the use of phantoms to assess the following imaging metrics:
    - Image uniformity/system uniformity
    - High-contrast resolution/system spatial resolution
    - Low-contrast resolution or detectability (not applicable for planar acquisitions)
    - Artifact evaluation

    Note 1: *The following tests are recommended, but not required, for PET scanner testing: sensitivity, energy resolution, and count-rate performance.*

Note 2: *Medical physicists are accountable for these activities. They may be assisted with the testing and evaluation of equipment performance by individuals who have the required training and skills, as determined by the medical physicist. (For more information, refer to HR.01.02.01, EP 1; HR.01.02.07, EPs 1 and 2; HR.01.06.01, EP 1; LD.03.06.01, EP 4.)*

25. **For computed tomography (CT), positron emission tomography (PET), nuclear medicine (NM), or magnetic resonance imaging (MRI) services:** The annual performance evaluation conducted by the diagnostic medical physicist or MRI scientist (for MRI only) includes testing of image acquisition display monitors for maximum and minimum luminance, luminance uniformity, resolution, and spatial accuracy.

     Note 1: *This element of performance does not apply to dental cone beam CT radiographic imaging studies performed for diagnosis of conditions affecting the maxillofacial region or to obtain guidance for the treatment of such conditions.*

     Note 2: *Medical physicists or MRI scientists are accountable for these activities. They may be assisted with the testing and evaluation of equipment performance by individuals who have the required training and skills, as determined by the physicist or MRI scientist. (For more information, refer to HR.01.02.01, EP 1; HR.01.02.07, EPs 1 and 2; HR.01.06.01, EP 1; LD.03.06.01, EP 4.)*

26. The organization performs equipment maintenance on the anesthesia apparatus(es). An apparatus is tested at the final path to patient after any adjustment, modification, or repair. Before the apparatus is returned to service, each connection is checked to verify proper gas flow and an oxygen analyzer is used to verify oxygen concentration. Areas designated for servicing of oxygen equipment are clean and free of oil, grease, or other flammables. (For full text, refer to NFPA 99-2012: 11.4.1.3; 11.5.1.3; 11.6.2.5; 11.6.2.6)

27. The organization meets NFPA 99-2012: Health Care Facilities Code requirements related to electrical equipment in the patient care vicinity. (For full text, refer to NFPA 99-2012: Chapter 10)

     Note: *For ambulatory surgical centers that elect to use The Joint Commission deemed status option: The organization meets the applicable provisions of the Health Care Facilities Code Tentative Interim Amendment (TIA) 12-5.*

34. Ⓓ **For organizations that provide fluoroscopic services:** At least annually, a diagnostic medical physicist conducts a performance evaluation of fluoroscopic imaging equipment. The evaluation results, along with recommendations for correcting any problems identified, are documented. The evaluation includes an assessment of the following:
- Beam alignment and collimation
- Tube potential/kilovolt peak (kV/kVp) accuracy
- Beam filtration (half-value layer)
- High-contrast resolution
- Low-contrast detectability
- Maximum exposure rate in fluoroscopic mode
- Displayed air-kerma rate and cumulative-air kerma accuracy (when applicable)

Note 1: *Medical physicists conducting performance evaluations may be assisted with the testing and evaluation of equipment performance by individuals who have the required training and skills, as determined by the physicist.*

Note 2: *This element of performance does not apply to fluoroscopy equipment used for therapeutic radiation treatment planning or delivery.*

Standard EC.02.05.01

The organization manages risks associated with its utility systems.

Elements of Performance for EC.02.05.01

2. New building systems and modifications to existing building systems are designed to meet the National Fire Protection Association's Categories 1–4 requirements. (For full text, refer to NFPA 99-2012: Chapter 4 for descriptions of the four categories related to gas, vacuum, electrical, and electrical equipment.)

4. Ⓓ The organization identifies the activities and frequencies for maintaining, inspecting, and testing for all operating components of utility systems. Various maintenance strategies may be used to ensure reliable performance (for example, predictive maintenance, reliability-centered maintenance, interval-based inspections, corrective maintenance, or metered maintenance). Defined intervals may be based on criteria such as manufacturers' recommendations, risk levels, and current organization experience.

For ambulatory surgical centers and outpatient surgical departments that elect to use The Joint Commission deemed status option: The organization identifies the activities and frequencies for maintaining, inspecting, and testing for all operating components of utility systems. These activities and frequencies must follow manufacturers' recommendations or other federal or state requirements.

5. **For ambulatory surgical centers and outpatient surgical departments that elect to use The Joint Commission deemed status option:** The organization provides ventilation, temperature, and humidity levels in accordance with the levels established in the American Society of Heating, Refrigerating and Air Conditioning Engineers (ASHRAE) standards followed during initial construction or subsequent major renovations, alterations, or modernizations of the facility.

7. ⒹIn areas designed to control airborne contaminants (such as biological agents, gases, fumes, dust), the ventilation system provides appropriate pressure relationships, air-exchange rates, filtration efficiencies, relative humidity, and temperature. **R**

   Note: *Areas designed for control of airborne contaminants include spaces such as all classes of operating rooms, special procedure rooms that require a sterile field, caesarean delivery rooms, rooms for patients diagnosed with or suspected of having airborne communicable diseases (for example, airborne infection isolation rooms, rooms for patients with pulmonary or laryngeal tuberculosis, bronchoscopy treatment rooms), patients in "protective environment" rooms (for example, rooms for patients receiving bone marrow transplants), laboratories, pharmacies, sterile supply/processing rooms, and other sterile spaces. For further information, refer to Guidelines for Design and Construction of Health Care Facilities, 2014 edition, administered by the Facility Guidelines Institute and published by the American Society for Healthcare Engineering (ASHE).*

8. ⒹThe organization maps the distribution of its utility systems.

9. The organization labels utility system controls to facilitate partial or complete emergency shutdowns.

   Note 1: *Examples of utility system controls that should be labeled are utility source valves, utility system main switches and valves, and individual circuits in an electrical distribution panel.*

Note 2: *For example, the fire alarm system's circuit is clearly labeled as Fire Alarm Circuit; the disconnect method (that is, the circuit breaker) is marked in red; and access is restricted to authorized personnel. Information regarding the dedicated branch circuit for the fire alarm panel is located in the control unit. For additional guidance, see NFPA 101-2012: 20/21.3.4.1; 9.6.1.3; NFPA 72-2010: 10.5.5.2.*

10. Ⓓ The organization has written procedures for responding to utility system disruptions.

11. The organization's procedures address shutting off the malfunctioning system and notifying staff in affected areas.

12. The organization's procedures address performing emergency clinical interventions during utility system disruptions.

13. The organization responds to utility system disruptions as described in its procedures. 🆁

16. In non–critical care areas, the ventilation system provides required pressure relationships, temperature, and humidity.

    Note: *Examples of non–critical care areas are general care nursing units; clean and soiled utility rooms in acute care areas; laboratories, pharmacies, diagnostic and treatment areas, food preparation areas, and other support departments.*

18. Medical gas storage rooms and transfer and manifold rooms comply with NFPA 99-2012: 9.3.7.

19. The emergency power supply system's equipment and environment are maintained per manufacturers' recommendations, including ambient temperature not less than 40°F; ventilation supply and exhaust; and water jacket temperature (when required). (For full text, refer to NFPA 99-2012: 9.3.10)

20. Ⓓ Operating rooms are considered wet procedure locations, unless otherwise determined by a risk assessment authorized by the facility governing body. Operating rooms defined as wet locations are protected by either isolated power or ground-fault circuit interrupters. A written record of the risk assessment is maintained and available for inspection. (For full text, refer to NFPA 99-2012: 6.3.2.2.8.4; 6.3.2.2.8.7; 6.4.4.2)

21. Electrical distribution in the organization is based on the following categories:

- Category 1: Critical care rooms served by a Type 1 essential electrical system (EES) in which electrical system failure is likely to cause major injury or death to patients, including all rooms where electric life support equipment is required.

- Category 2: General care rooms served by a Type 1 or Type 2 EES in which electrical system failure is likely to cause minor injury to patients.

- Category 3: Basic care rooms in which electrical system failure is not likely to cause injury to patients. Patient care rooms are required to have a Type 3 EES where the life safety branch has an alternate source of power that will be effective for 1½ hours.

(For full text, refer to NFPA 99-2012: 3.3.138; 6.3.2.2.10; 6.6.2.2.2; 6.6.3.1.1)

22. Hospital-grade receptacles at patient bed locations and where deep sedation or general anesthesia is administered are tested after initial installation, replacement, or servicing. In pediatric locations, receptacles in patient rooms (other than nurseries), bathrooms, play rooms, and activity rooms are listed tamper-resistant or have a listed tamper-resistant cover. Electrical receptacles or cover plates supplied from the life safety and critical branches have a distinctive color or marking. (For full text, refer to NFPA 99-2012: 6.3.2; 6.3.3; 6.3.4; 6.4.2.2.6; 6.5.2.2.4.2; 6.6.2.2.3.2)

23. Power strips in a patient care vicinity are only used for components of movable electrical equipment used for patient care that have been assembled by qualified personnel. These power strips meet UL 1363A or UL 60601-1. Power strips used outside of a patient care vicinity, but within the patient care room, meet UL 1363. In non–patient care rooms, power strips meet other UL standards. (For full text, refer to NFPA 99-2012: 10.2.3.6; 10.2.4; NFPA 70-2011: 400-8; 590.3(D); Tentative Interim Amendment [TIA] 12-5)

24. Extension cords are not used as a substitute for fixed wiring in a building. Extension cords used temporarily are removed immediately upon completion of the intended purpose. (For full text, refer to NFPA 99-2012: 10.2.3.6; 10.2.4; NFPA 70-2011: 400-8; 590.3(D); Tentative Interim Amendment [TIA] 12-5)

25. Areas designated for administration of general anesthesia (specifically, inhaled anesthetics) using medical gases or vacuum are in accordance with NFPA 101-2012: 8.7 and NFPA 99-2012 as follows:

- Zone valves are located immediately outside each anesthetizing location for medical gas or vacuum, readily accessible in an emergency, and arranged so shutting off any one anesthetizing location will not affect others.
- Area alarm panels are installed to monitor all medical gas, medical-surgical vacuum, and piped waste anesthetic gas disposal (WAGD) systems. Alarm panels include visual and audible sensors and are in locations that provide for surveillance, including medical gas pressure decreases of 20% and vacuum decreases of 12-inch gauge HgV (mercury vacuum).
- Alarm sensors are installed either on the source side of individual room zone valve box assemblies or on the patient/use side of each of the individual zone valve box assemblies.

(For full text, refer to NFPA 101-2012: 20/21.3.2.3; NFPA 99-2012: 5.1.4.8.7; 5.1.9.3)

26. Areas designated for administration of general anesthesia (specifically, inhaled anesthetics) using medical gases or vacuum are in accordance with NFPA 101-2012: 8.7 and NFPA 99-2012 as follows: The essential electrical system's (EES) critical branch supplies power for task illumination, fixed equipment, select receptacles, and select power circuits. The EES equipment system supplies power to the ventilation system. (For full text, refer to NFPA 101-2012: 20.21.3.2.3; NFPA 99-2012: 6.4.2.2.4.2)

27. Areas designated for administration of general anesthesia (specifically, inhaled anesthetics) using medical gases or vacuum have the following characteristics:
- Heating, cooling, and ventilation are in accordance with ASHRAE 170. Medical supply and equipment manufacturers' instructions are considered before reducing humidity levels to those allowed by ASHRAE.
- Existing smoke control systems automatically vent smoke, prevent the recirculation of smoke originating within the surgical suite, and prevent the circulation of smoke entering the system intake without interfering with exhaust function. New occupancies have no smoke control requirement.
- **For ambulatory surgical centers that elect to use The Joint Commission deemed status option:** Existing smoke control systems are maintained according to the edition of NFPA 101 adopted by the Centers for Medicare & Medicaid Services at the time of installation.

(For full text, refer to NFPA 101-2012: 20/21.3.2.3; NFPA 99-2012: 9.3.1)

Note: *Smoke evacuation by smoke control systems refers to by-products of combustion from a fire; it does not refer to medical plume caused by thermal destruction of tissue, which is addressed in EC.02.02.01, EP 9.*

Standard EC.02.05.03 ▬▬▬▬▬▬▬▬▬▬▬▬▬▬▬

The organization has a reliable emergency electrical power source.

Elements of Performance for EC.02.05.03

1. **For ambulatory surgical centers and outpatient surgical departments that elect to use The Joint Commission deemed status option:** For facilities that were constructed, or had a change in occupancy type, or have undergone an electrical system upgrade since 1983, the organization has a Type 1 or Type 3 essential electrical system in accordance with NFPA 99, 2012 edition. This essential electrical system must be divided into three branches, including the life safety branch, critical branch, and equipment branch. Both the life safety branch and the critical branch are kept independent of all other wiring and equipment, and they transfer within 10 seconds of electrical interruption. Each branch has at least one automatic transfer switch. For additional guidance, *see* NFPA 99-2012: 6.4.2.2.

The organization provides emergency power within 10 seconds for the following:

2. Alarm systems, as required by the *Life Safety Code*. **R**

   Note: *For guidance in establishing a reliable emergency power system (that is, an essential electrical distribution system), see NFPA 99-2012: 6.4.1.1; 6.4.2.2; 6.4.4.1.1; NFPA 110-2010: 4.1; Table 4.1(b).*

3. Exit route and exit sign illumination, as required by the *Life Safety Code*. **R**

   Note: *For guidance in establishing a reliable emergency power system (that is, an essential electrical distribution system), see NFPA 99-2012: 6.4.1.1.6; 6.4.2.2; NFPA 110-2010: 4.1; Table 4.1(b).*

4. New buildings equipped with or requiring the use of life support systems (electro-mechanical or inhalation anesthetics) have illumination of means of egress, emergency lighting equipment, exit, and directional signs supplied by the life safety branch of the electrical system described in NFPA 99. (For full text, refer to NFPA 101-2012: 18.2.9.2; 18.2.10.5; NFPA 99-2012: 6.4.2.2)

The organization provides emergency power within 10 seconds for the following:

5.   Emergency communication systems, as required by the *Life Safety Code.* **R**

   Note: *For guidance in establishing a reliable emergency power system (that is, an essential electrical distribution system), see NFPA 99-2012: 6.4.2.2; NFPA 110-2010: 4.1; Table 4.1(b).*

6.   Equipment that could cause patient harm when it fails, including life-support systems; blood, bone, and tissue storage systems; medical air compressors; and medical and surgical vacuum systems. **R**

   Note: *For ambulatory surgical centers and outpatient surgical departments that elect to use The Joint Commission deemed status option:* *See NFPA 99-2012: 6.4.1.1; 6.4.2.2; NFPA 110-2010: 4.1; Table 4.1(b) for guidance in establishing a reliable emergency power system (that is, an essential electrical distribution system).*

7.   Areas in which loss of power could result in patient harm, including operating rooms and recovery rooms. **R**

   Note: *For guidance in establishing a reliable emergency power system (that is, an essential electrical distribution system), see NFPA 99-2012: 6.4.1.1; 6.4.2.2; NFPA 110-2010: 4.1; Table 4.1(b).*

11.   Emergency lighting at emergency generator locations. The organization's emergency power system (EPS) has a remote manual stop station (with identifying label) to prevent inadvert or unintentional operation. A remote annunciator (powered by storage battery) is located outside the EPS location.

    Note: *For guidance in establishing a reliable emergency power system (that is, an essential electrical distribution system), refer to NFPA 99-2012: 6.4.1.1.6; 6.4.1.1.17; 6.4.2.2; NFPA 110-2010: 5.6.5.6; 7.3.1.*

12.   Equipment designated to be powered by emergency power supply is energized by the organization's design. Staging of equipment startup is permissible. (For full text, refer to NFPA 99-2012: 6.4.2.2)

14. ⒟ The organization implements a policy to provide emergency backup for essential medication dispensing equipment identified by the organization, such as automatic dispensing cabinets, medication carousels, and central medication robots.

Note: *Examples of emergency backup can include emergency power, battery-based indoor generators, or other actions describing how dispensing and administration of medications will continue when emergency backup is needed.*

15. ⒟ The organization implements a policy to provide emergency backup for essential refrigeration for medications identified by the organization, such as designated refrigerators and freezers.

Note: *Examples of emergency backup can include emergency power, battery-based indoor generators, or other actions describing how refrigeration of medications will continue when emergency backup is needed.*

Standard EC.02.05.05

The organization inspects, tests, and maintains utility systems.

Note: *At times, maintenance is performed by an external service. In these cases, organizations are not required to possess maintenance documentation but must have access to such documentation during survey and as needed.*

Elements of Performance for EC.02.05.05

1. When performing repairs or maintenance activities, the organization has a process to manage risks associated with air-quality requirements; infection control; utility requirements; noise, odor, dust, vibration; and other hazards that affect care, treatment, or services for patients, staff, and visitors.

2. ⒟ The organization tests utility system components before initial use. The completion dates and test results are documented.

The organization inspects, tests, and maintains the following:

3. ⒟ Utility systems. The completion dates and test results are documented.

7. Ⓓ Line isolation monitors (LIM), if installed, are tested at least monthly by actuating the LIM test switch per NFPA 99-2012: 6.3.2.6.3.6, which activates both visual and audible alarms. For LIM circuits with automated self-testing, a manual test is performed at least annually. LIM circuits are tested per NFPA 99-2012: 6.3.3.3.2 after any repair or renovation to the electric distribution system. Records are maintained of required tests and associated repairs or modifications, containing date, room or area tested, and results. (For full text, refer to NFPA 99-2012: 6.3.2; 6.3.3; 6.3.4)

8. The organization meets NFPA 99-2012: Health Care Facilities Code requirements related to electrical systems and heating, ventilation, and air conditioning (HVAC). (For full text, refer to NFPA 99-2012: Chapters 6 and 9)

   Note: *For ambulatory surgical centers that elect to use The Joint Commission deemed status option: The organization meets the applicable provisions of the Health Care Facilities Code Tentative Interim Amendments (TIAs) 12-2 and 12-3.*

Standard EC.02.05.07

The organization inspects, tests, and maintains emergency power systems.

Note: *This standard does not require organizations to have the types of emergency power equipment discussed below. However, if these types of equipment exist within the building, then the following maintenance, testing, and inspection requirements apply.*

Rationale for EC.02.05.07

Emergency electrical power supply systems may fail during a power disruption, leaving the organization unable to deliver safe care, treatment, or services to patients. Testing these systems for sufficient lengths of time at regular frequencies increases the likelihood of detecting reliability problems and reduces the risk of losing this critical resource when it is most needed.

Elements of Performance for EC.02.05.07

1. Ⓓ At least monthly, the organization performs a functional test of emergency lighting systems and exit signs required for egress and task lighting for a minimum duration of 30 seconds, along with a visual inspection of other exit signs. The test results and completion dates are documented. (For full text, refer to NFPA 101-2012: 7.9.3; 7.10.9; NFPA 99-2012: 6.3.2.2.11.5)

2.   ⓓ Every 12 months, the organization performs a functional test of battery-powered lights on the inventory required for egress and exit signs for a duration of 1½ hours. For new construction, renovation, or modernization, battery-powered lighting in locations where deep sedation and general anesthesia are administered is tested annually for 30 minutes. The test results and completion dates are documented. (For full text, refer to NFPA 101-2012: 7.9.3; 7.10.9; NFPA 99-2012: 6.3.2.2.11.5)

3.   ⓓ The organization performs a functional test of Level 1 stored emergency power supply systems (SEPSS) on a monthly basis and performs a test of Level 2 SEPSS on a quarterly basis. Test duration is for five minutes or as specified for its class (whichever is less). The organization performs an annual test at full load for 60% of the full duration of its class. The test results and completion dates are documented.

Note 1: *Non–SEPSS battery backup emergency power systems that the organization has determined to be critical for operations during a power failure (for example, laboratory equipment or electronic clinical records) should be properly tested and maintained in accordance with manufacturers' recommendations.*

Note 2: *Level 1 SEPSS are intended to automatically supply illumination or power to critical areas and equipment essential for safety to human life. Included are systems that supply emergency power for such functions as illumination for safe exiting, ventilation where it is essential to maintain life, fire detection and alarm systems, public safety communications systems, and processes where the current interruption would produce serious life safety or health hazards to patients, the public, or staff.*

Note 3: *Class defines the minimum time for which the SEPSS is designed to operate at its rated load without being recharged.*

Note 4: *For additional guidance on operational inspection and testing, see NFPA 111-2010: 8.4.*

4.   ⓓ Every week, the organization inspects the emergency power supply system (EPSS), including all associated components and batteries. The results and completion dates of the inspections are documented. (For full text, refer to NFPA 110-2010: 8.3.1; 8.3.3; 8.3.4; 8.4.1)

5.   ⓓ At least monthly, the organization tests each emergency generator beginning with a cold start under load for at least 30 continuous minutes. The cooldown period is not part of the 30 continuous minutes. The test results and completion dates are documented. (For full text, refer to NFPA 99-2012: 6.4.4.1) **R**

6.   ⓓ The monthly tests for diesel-powered emergency generators are conducted with a dynamic load that is at least 30% of the nameplate rating of the generator or meets the manufacturer's recommended prime movers' exhaust gas temperature. If the organization does not meet either the 30% of nameplate rating or the recommended exhaust gas temperature during any test in EC.02.05.07, EP 5, then it must test the emergency generator once every 12 months using supplemental (dynamic or static) loads of 50% of nameplate rating for 30 minutes, followed by 75% of nameplate rating for 60 minutes, for a total of 1½ continuous hours. (For full text, refer to NFPA 99-2012: 6.4.4.1) **R**

Note: *Tests for non-diesel-powered generators need only be conducted with available load.*

7.   ⓓ At least monthly, the organization tests all automatic and manual transfer switches on the inventory. The test results and completion dates are documented. (For full text, refer to NFPA 99-2012: 6.4.4.1) **R**

8.   ⓓ At least annually, the organization tests the fuel quality to ASTM standards. The test results and completion dates are documented.

Note: *For additional guidance, see NFPA 110-2010: 8.3.8.*

9.   ⓓ At least once every 36 months, organizations with a generator providing emergency power test each emergency generator for a minimum of 4 continuous hours. The test results and completion dates are documented. **R**

Note: *For additional guidance, see NFPA 110-2010, Chapter 8.*

10.   ⓓ The 36-month diesel-powered emergency generator test uses a dynamic or static load that is at least 30% of the nameplate rating of the generator or meets the manufacturer's recommended prime movers' exhaust gas temperature. **R**

Note 1: *Tests for non-diesel-powered generators need only be conducted with available load.*

Note 2: *For additional guidance, see NFPA 110-2010, Chapter 8.*

Standard EC.02.05.09 ━━━━━━━━━━━━

The organization inspects, tests, and maintains medical gas and vacuum systems.

Note 1: *This standard does not require organizations to have the medical gas and vacuum systems discussed below. However, if an organization has these types of systems, then the following inspection, testing, and maintenance requirements apply.*

Note 2: *Piped medical gas systems include oxygen, nitrous oxide, medical air, carbon dioxide, helium, nitrogen, instrument air and mixtures thereof. Piped vacuum systems include both medical-surgical vacuum and waste anesthetic gas disposal (WAGD) systems.*

Rationale for EC.02.05.09

Medical gas and vacuum systems must be reliable. Testing these systems increases the likelihood of detecting reliability problems and reduces the risk of losing this critical resource.

Elements of Performance for EC.02.05.09

1. Medical gas, medical air, surgical vacuum, waste anesthetic gas disposal (WAGD), and air supply systems are designated as follows:
    - Category 1: Systems in which failure is likely to cause major injury or death.
    - Category 2: Systems in which failure is likely to cause minor injury to patients.
    - Category 3: Systems in which failure is not likely to cause injury but can cause discomfort to patients. Deep sedation and general anesthesia are not administered when using Category 3 medical gas systems.
    - Category 4: Systems in which failure would have no impact on patient care.

    (For full text, refer to NFPA 99-2012: 5.1.1.1; 5.2.1; 5.3.1.1; 5.3.1.5; 5.1.14.2)

2. All master, area, and local alarm systems used for medical gas and vacuum systems comply with the category 1–3 warning system requirements. (For full text, refer to NFPA 99-2012: 5.1.9; 5.2.9; 5.3.6.2.2)

3. Containers, cylinders, and tanks are designed, fabricated, tested, and marked in accordance with NFPA 99-2012: 5.1.3.1.1–5.1.3.1.7.

4. Locations containing positive pressure gases, other than oxygen or medical air, have doors labeled "Positive Pressure Gases: NO Smoking or Open Flame. Room May Have Insufficient Oxygen. Open Door and Allow Room to Ventilate Before Entering." Locations containing central supply systems or cylinders only containing oxygen or medical air have doors labeled "Medical Gases: NO Smoking or Open Flame." (For full text, refer to NFPA 99-2012: 5.1.3.1.8 and 5.1.3.1.9)

5. A precautionary sign readable from 5 feet away is on each door or gate of a cylinder storage room, where the sign, at a minimum, includes the wording "CAUTION: OXIDIZING GAS(ES) STORED WITHIN. NO SMOKING." Storage is planned so cylinders are used in the order they are received from the supplier. Only gas cylinders and reusable shipping containers and their accessories are permitted to be stored in rooms containing central supply systems or gas cylinders.

6. When the organization uses cylinders with an integral pressure gauge, a threshold pressure considered empty is established when the volume of stored gases is as follows:

    ■ When more than 300 but less than 3,000 cubic feet, the storage locations are outdoors in an enclosure or within an enclosed interior space of non- or limited-combustible construction, with door (or gates outdoors) that can be secured. Oxidizing gases are not stored with flammables and are separated from combustibles by 20 feet (5 feet if sprinklered) or enclosed in a cabinet of noncombustible construction having a minimum ½-hour fire protection rating.

    ■ When less than 301 cubic feet in a single smoke compartment, individual cylinders available for immediate use in patient care areas with an aggregate volume of less than or equal to 300 cubic feet are not required to be stored in an enclosure. Cylinders must be handled with precautions as specified in NFPA 99-2012: 11.6.2.

    (For full text, refer to NFPA 99-2012: 5.1.3.1; 5.1.3.2.3; 5.2.3.1; 5.3.10; 11.3; 11.6.5.2.1)

7. ⓓ In time frames defined by the organization, the organization inspects, tests, and maintains critical components of piped medical gas and vacuum systems, waste anesthetic gas disposal (WAGD), and support gas systems on the inventory. This inventory of critical components includes at least all source subsystems, control valves, alarms, manufactured assemblies containing patient gases, and inlets and outlets. Activities, dates, and results are documented. Persons maintaining the systems are qualified by training and certification to the requirements of the American Society of Sanitary Engineers (ASSE) 6030 or 6040. (For full text, refer to NFPA 99-2012: 5.1.14.2; 5.1.15; 5.2.14; 5.3.13) Ⓡ

8. When the organization has bulk oxygen systems above ground, they are in a locked enclosure (such as a fence) at least 10 feet from vehicles and sidewalks. There is permanent signage stating "OXYGEN – NO SMOKING – NO OPEN FLAMES."

    Note: *For additional guidance, refer to NFPA 99-2012: 5.1.3.5.12.*

9. The organization's emergency oxygen supply connection is installed in a manner that allows a temporary auxiliary source to connect to it.

    Note: *For additional guidance, refer to NFPA 99-2012: 5.1.3.5.13.*

10. ⓓ The organization tests piped medical gas and vacuum systems for purity, correct gas, and proper pressure when these systems are installed, modified, or repaired. The test results and completion dates are documented. (For full text, refer to NFPA 99-2012: 5.1.2; 5.1.4; 5.1.14.4.1; 5.1.14.4.6; 5.2.13) Ⓡ

11. The organization makes main supply valves and area shutoff valves for piped medical gas and vacuum systems accessible and clearly identifies what the valves control. Piping is labeled by stencil or adhesive markers identifying the gas or vacuum system, including the name of system or chemical symbol, color code (*see* NFPA 99-2012: Table 5.1.11), and operating pressure if other than standard. Labels are at intervals of 20 feet or less and are in every room, at both sides of wall penetrations, and on every story traversed by riser. Piping is not painted. Shutoff valves are identified with the name or chemical symbol of the gas or vacuum system, room or area served, and caution to not use the valve except in emergency. (For full text, refer to NFPA 99-2012: 5.1.4; 5.1.11.1; 5.1.11.2; 5.1.14.3; 5.2.11; 5.3.13.3; 5.3.11)

12. The organization implements a policy on all cylinders within the organization that includes the following:

- Labeling, handling, and transporting (for example, in carts, attached to equipment, on racks) in accordance with NFPA 99-2012: 11.5.3.1 and 11.6.2
- Physically segregating full and empty cylinders from each other in order to assist staff in selecting the proper cylinder
- Adaptors or conversion fittings are prohibited
- Oxygen cylinders, containers, and associated equipment are protected from contamination, damage, and contact with oil and grease
- Cylinders are kept away from heat and flammable materials and do not exceed a temperature of 130°F
- Nitrous oxide and carbon dioxide cylinders do not reach temperatures lower than manufacturer recommendations or -20°F
- Valve protection caps (if supplied) are secured in place when cylinder is not in use
- Labeling empty cylinders
- Prohibiting transfilling in any compartment with patient care

(For full text, refer to NFPA 99-2012: 11.6.1; 11.6.2; 11.6.5; 11.7.3)

13. At no time is transfilling done in any patient care room. A designated area is used away from any section of the organization where patients are housed, treated, or examined. The designated area is separated by a barrier of at least 1-hour fire-resistant construction from any patient care areas. Transfilling cylinders is only of the same gas (no mixing of different compressed gases). Transfilling of liquid oxygen is only done in an area that is mechanically ventilated, sprinklered, and has ceramic or concrete flooring. Storage and use of liquid oxygen in base reservoir containers and portable containers comply with sections NFPA 99-2012: 11.7.2–11.7.4. (For full text, refer to NFPA 99-2012: 11.5.2.2; 11.5.2.3.1; 11.5.2.3.2; 11.7.2–11.7.4)

14. The organization meets all other NFPA 99-2012: Health Care Facilities Code requirements related to gas and vacuum systems and gas equipment. (For full text, refer to NFPA 99-2012: Chapters 5 and 11)

Note: *For ambulatory surgical centers that elect to use The Joint Commission deemed status option:* *The organization meets the applicable provisions of the Health Care Facilities Code Tentative Interim Amendments (TIAs) 12-4 and 12-6.*

Introduction to Standard EC.02.06.01

Features of the organization's space influence patient outcomes and satisfaction and promote patient safety. The physical space also affects families, staff, and others in the organization. These features of the environment of care include the following:

- Quality of natural and artificial light
- Privacy
- Size and configuration of space
- Security for patients and their belongings
- Clear access to internal and external doors
- Level of noise
- Space that allows staff to work efficiently

When designed into and managed as part of the environment, these elements create safe and suitable surroundings that support patient dignity and allow ease of interaction.

The standards do not specifically address all these features. However, organizations may wish to consider these aspects of the environment when they design and manage spaces. Decisions on what features to pursue should be based on data, such as patient satisfaction information, data collected from staff, and evidence-based design guidelines.

Standard EC.02.06.01

The organization establishes and maintains a safe, sanitary, and functional environment.

Elements of Performance for EC.02.06.01

1. Interior spaces meet the needs of the patient population and are safe and suitable to the care, treatment, or services provided.

7. **For ambulatory surgical centers and outpatient surgical departments that elect to use The Joint Commission deemed status option:** The organization provides separate waiting and postanesthesia recovery areas.

11. Lighting is suitable for care, treatment, or services.

20. Areas used by patients are clean and sanitary. **R**

Standard EC.02.06.05

The organization manages its space during demolition, renovation, or new construction.

Note: *These elements of performance are applicable to all occupancy types.*

Rationale for EC.02.06.05

In addition to fire safety, there are other hazards and risks resulting from demolition, renovation, or new construction that must be addressed. It is important to plan and conduct risk assessments before construction begins. Authoritative guidelines and state regulations can provide valuable information to guide demolition, renovation, or new construction.

Elements of Performance for EC.02.06.05

1. When planning for new, altered, or renovated space, the organization uses one of the following design criteria:
    - State rules and regulations
    - Guidelines for Design and Construction of Outpatient Facilities, 2018 edition, published by the Facility Guidelines Institute

    When the above rules, regulations, and guidelines do not meet specific design needs, use other reputable standards and guidelines that provide equivalent design criteria.

2. When planning for demolition, construction, renovation, or general maintenance, the organization conducts a preconstruction risk assessment for air quality requirements, infection control, utility requirements, noise, vibration, and other hazards that affect care, treatment, and services.

    Note: See *LS.01.02.01 for information on fire safety procedures to implement during construction or renovation.*

3. The organization takes action based on its assessment to minimize risks during demolition, construction, renovation, or general maintenance. 🆁

4. **For computed tomography (CT), positron emission tomography (PET), or nuclear medicine (NM) services:** Prior to installation of new imaging equipment, replacement of existing imaging equipment, or modification to rooms where ionizing radiation will be emitted or radioactive materials will be stored (such as scan rooms or hot labs), a medical physicist or health physicist conducts a structural shielding design‡ assessment to specify required radiation shielding.

---

‡ For additional guidance on shielding designs and radiation protection surveys, *see* National Council on Radiation Protection and Measurements Report No. 147 (NCRP-147).

Note: *This element of performance does not apply to dental cone beam CT radiographic imaging studies performed for diagnosis of conditions affecting the maxillofacial region or to obtain guidance for the treatment of such conditions.*

6. **For computed tomography (CT), positron emission tomography (PET), or nuclear medicine (NM) services:** After installation of imaging equipment or construction in rooms where ionizing radiation will be emitted or radioactive materials will be stored, a medical physicist or health physicist conducts a radiation protection survey to verify the adequacy of installed shielding.[‡] This survey is conducted prior to clinical use of the room.

    Note: *This element of performance does not apply to dental cone beam CT radiographic imaging studies performed for diagnosis of conditions affecting the maxillofacial region or to obtain guidance for the treatment of such conditions.*

Standard EC.03.01.01

Staff and licensed independent practitioners are familiar with their roles and responsibilities relative to the environment of care.

Rationale for EC.03.01.01

People are the key to successfully managing risks in the physical environment. Plans and procedures are of no value if those who work in the organization do not know how to follow them. Everyone who works in the organization is responsible for safety, and it is important for them to know how to identify and minimize risks, what actions to take when an incident occurs, and how to report it.

Elements of Performance for EC.03.01.01

1. Staff responsible for the maintenance, inspection, testing, and use of medical equipment, utility systems and equipment, fire safety systems and equipment, and safe handling of hazardous materials and waste are competent and receive continuing education and training.

2. Staff and licensed independent practitioners can describe or demonstrate actions to take in the event of an environment of care incident.

Introduction to Standard EC.04.01.01

Most organizations are able to manage their physical spaces because they typically use all areas on a daily basis, making it easier for staff to monitor environment of care issues. Monitoring includes keeping track of injuries to patients or others accessing the organization; occupational illness and injuries to staff; property damage or loss; security incidents involving patients, staff, or others accessing the organization; hazardous materials and waste spills and exposures; and fire safety equipment and utility management problems, failures, or use errors.

Quickly identifying and resolving actual and potential environment of care problems is crucial. Organizations are often able to resolve environmental issues without formal reporting processes. However, when reporting processes are more informal, the organization faces a greater risk of overlooking important patterns or trends. Staff reports and their resolution can be a sign of how comprehensively and effectively the risk assessments, as described in the management plans, have been conducted. Consistently investigating and resolving staff reports about environmental issues can lead to safer delivery of care, treatment, or services.

Standard EC.04.01.01 ━━━━━━━━━━━━━━━━━━━━━━━━━━

The organization collects information to monitor conditions in the environment.

Elements of Performance for EC.04.01.01

1. The organization establishes a process(es) for continually monitoring, internally reporting, and investigating the following:
   - Problems and incidents related to risks addressed in the environment of care management plans
   - Injuries to patients or others within the organization's facilities
   - Occupational illnesses and staff injuries
   - Incidents of damage to its property or the property of others

   Note 1: *All the incidents and issues listed above may be reported to staff in quality assessment, improvement, or other functions. A summary of such incidents may also be shared with the person designated to coordinate safety management activities.*

   Note 2: *Review of incident reports often requires that legal processes be followed to preserve confidentiality. Opportunities to improve care, treatment, or services, or to prevent similar incidents, are not lost as a result of following the legal process.*

   Based on its process(es), the organization reports and investigates the following:

2. Problems and incidents related to each of the environment of care management plans.

3. Injuries to patients or others within the organization's facilities.

4. Occupational illnesses and staff injuries.

5. Incidents of damage to its property or the property of others.

15. Ⓓ Every 12 months, the organization evaluates each environment of care management plan, including a review of the plan's objectives, scope, performance, and effectiveness. 🅁

Standard EC.04.01.03 ▬▬▬▬▬▬▬▬▬▬

The organization analyzes identified environment of care issues.

Elements of Performance for EC.04.01.03

2. The organization uses the results of data analysis to identify opportunities to resolve environmental safety issues.

Standard EC.04.01.05 ▬▬▬▬▬▬▬▬▬▬

The organization improves its environment of care.

Elements of Performance for EC.04.01.05

1. The organization takes action on the identified opportunities to resolve environmental safety issues.

Emergency Management (EM)

Overview

Emergencies can be threats to any health care organization. A single emergency can temporarily disrupt services; however, multiple emergencies that occur concurrently or sequentially can adversely impact patient safety and the organization's ability to provide care, treatment, or services for an extended length of time. This is particularly true in situations where the community cannot adequately support the organization. Power failures, water and fuel shortages, flooding, and communication breakdowns are just a few of the hazards that can disrupt patient care and pose risks to staff and the organization.

About This Chapter

The "Emergency Management" (EM) chapter is organized to allow organizations to plan to respond to the effects of potential emergencies that fall on a continuum from disruptive to disastrous. Planning involves those activities that must be done in order to put together a comprehensive Emergency Management Plan (EMP). This planning results in the EMP document, which may reflect response strategies that range from continuing a full scope of services, to rescheduling non-urgent appointments, to closing temporarily. After the EMP is in place, it must be tested through staged emergency response exercises in order to evaluate its effectiveness. Adjustments to the EMP can then be made.

The four phases of emergency management are mitigation, preparedness, response, and recovery. They occur over time; mitigation and preparedness generally occur before an emergency, and response and recovery occur during and after an emergency. The planning activities described in Standard EM.01.01.01 help the organization to focus its strategy for mitigating the potential effects of emergencies, as well as the approach to preparedness that will help it to organize and mobilize its essential resources. The organization will use its EMP (described in Standard EM.02.01.01 and subsequent standards) to define its response to emergencies and to help position it for recovery after the emergency has passed.

Organizations should identify the types of emergencies that could impact the organization's capacity to provide care, treatment, or services for its patients. This assessment is designed to assist organizations in gaining a realistic understanding of their vulnerabilities in order to help them mitigate and respond to emergencies and their subsequent impact. No organization can predict the nature of a future emergency, nor can it predict the date of its arrival. However, organizations can plan for managing the following critical areas of their organizations so that they can respond effectively regardless of the cause(s) of an emergency:

- Communications
- Resources and assets
- Safety and security
- Staff responsibilities
- Utilities
- Patient clinical and support activities

When organizations consider their capabilities in these areas, they are taking an approach to emergency management that supports a level of preparedness sufficient to address a range of emergencies. This approach lays the foundation for developing an Emergency Management Plan that is scalable to emergencies that may escalate in complexity, scope, or duration. For the most extreme type of emergencies—disasters—additional human resources may be necessary. Organizations can choose to assign responsibilities to volunteer practitioners or to privilege volunteer licensed independent practitioners when such volunteers are essential for meeting patient care needs. Organizations should test their EMPs through exercise scenarios so that they can use the lessons learned to improve the effectiveness of their response strategies.

Additional standards in other chapters are integral to organizationwide emergency preparedness, including processes for the following:

- Maintaining continuity of information (refer to Standard IM.01.01.03)
- Responding to outbreaks of infectious disease (refer to Standard IC.01.06.01)

Chapter Outline

Standards, Rationales, and Elements of Performance

Standard EM.01.01.01

The organization engages in planning activities prior to developing its Emergency Management Plan.

Note: *An emergency is an unexpected or sudden event that significantly disrupts the organization's ability to provide care, or the environment of care itself, or that results in a sudden, significantly changed or increased demand for the organization's services. Emergencies can be either human-made (for example, an electrical system failure or cyberattack) or natural (for example, a tornado or an infectious disease outbreak such as Ebola, Zika, influenza), or a combination of both, and they exist on a continuum of severity. A disaster is a type of emergency that, due to its complexity, scope, or duration, threatens the organization's capabilities and requires outside assistance to sustain patient care, safety, or security functions.*

Rationale for EM.01.01.01

An emergency in a health care organization can suddenly and significantly affect demand for its services or its ability to provide those services. Therefore, the organization needs to engage in planning activities that prepare it to form its Emergency Management Plan. These activities include identifying risks, and considering its potential emergencies in developing strategies for preparedness. Because some emergencies that impact an organization originate in the community, the organization needs to take advantage of opportunities, where possible, to collaborate with relevant parties in the community.

Elements of Performance for EM.01.01.01

1. The organization's leaders participate in planning activities prior to developing an Emergency Management Plan.

2. The organization identifies potential emergencies and the direct and indirect effects that these emergencies may have on the need for its services or its ability to provide those services.

    Note 1: *Some organizations refer to this process as a hazard vulnerability analysis.*

    Note 2: *If the organization identifies a surge in infectious patients as a potential emergency, this issue is addressed in the "Infection Prevention and Control" (IC) chapter.*

(*See also* IC.01.06.01, EP 4)

3. The organization prioritizes the potential emergencies it has identified.

4. The organization determines what its role will be, if any, in the community response plan.

    Note: *A community response plan is the response plan of the organization's city, county, region, or state, whichever plan is activated by community leadership.*

5. The organization uses its prioritized emergencies as a basis for defining mitigation activities (that is, activities designed to reduce the risk of and potential damage from an emergency).

    Note: *Mitigation, preparedness, response, and recovery are the four phases of emergency management. They occur over time: Mitigation and preparedness generally occur before an emergency, and response and recovery occur during and after an emergency.*

6. The organization uses its prioritized emergencies as a basis for defining the preparedness activities that will organize and mobilize essential resources.

    (*See also* IM.01.01.03, EPs 1, 2)

9. ⒟ **For ambulatory surgical centers that elect to use The Joint Commission deemed status option:** The Emergency Management Plan includes documentation of potential risks in the community that could impact the organization's ability to provide care for its patients.

10. ⒟ **For rural health clinics and federally qualified health centers:** The Emergency Management Plan includes documentation of potential risks in the community that could impact the organization's ability to provide care for its patients.

Standard EM.02.01.01 ▬▬▬▬▬▬▬▬▬▬▬▬▬▬

The organization has an Emergency Management Plan.

Note: *The organization's Emergency Management Plan (EMP) is designed to coordinate its communications, resources and assets, safety and security, staff responsibilities, utilities, and patient clinical and support activities during an emergency. Although emergencies have many causes, the effects on these areas of the organization and the required response effort may be similar. This all-hazards approach supports a general response capability that is sufficiently nimble to address a range of emergencies of different duration, scale, and cause. For this reason, the plan's response procedures address the prioritized emergencies but are also adaptable to other emergencies that the organization may experience.*

Rationale for EM.02.01.01

A successful response effort relies on a comprehensive and flexible Emergency Management Plan that guides decision making regarding how the organization will respond to emergencies, including plans to continue to serve patients or to close in specified circumstances. The plan also supports decision making at the onset of an emergency and as an emergency evolves. While the Emergency Management Plan can be formatted in a variety of ways, it must address response procedures that are adaptable in supporting key areas (such as communications and patient care) that might be affected by emergencies of different causes.

Elements of Performance for EM.02.01.01

1. The organization's leaders participate in the development of the Emergency Management Plan.

2. Ⓓ The organization has a written Emergency Management Plan that describes the response procedures to follow when emergencies occur.

    Note: *The response procedures address the prioritized emergencies but can also be adapted to other emergencies that the organization may experience. Response procedures could include the following:*
    - *Maintaining or expanding services*
    - *Conserving resources*
    - *Curtailing services*
    - *Supplementing resources from outside the local community*
    - *Closing the organization to new patients*
    - *Staged evacuation*
    - *Total evacuation*

4. ⓓ The organization has a written Emergency Management Plan that describes the recovery strategies, actions, and individual responsibilities necessary to restore the organization's care, treatment, or services after an emergency.

5. The Emergency Management Plan describes the processes for initiating and terminating the organization's response and recovery phases of an emergency, including under what circumstances these phases are activated.

   Note: *Mitigation, preparedness, response, and recovery are the four phases of emergency management. They occur over time: Mitigation and preparedness generally occur before an emergency, and response and recovery occur during and after an emergency.*

6. The Emergency Management Plan identifies the individual(s) responsible for activating the response and recovery phases of the emergency response.

7. ⓓ **For ambulatory surgical centers that elect to use The Joint Commission deemed status option:** The Emergency Management Plan identifies alternative sites for care, treatment, and services that meet the needs of the organization's patients during emergencies.

8. If the organization experiences an actual emergency, the organization implements its response procedures related to care, treatment, or services for its patients. ⓡ

10. ⓓ **For ambulatory surgical centers that elect to use The Joint Commission deemed status option:** The Emergency Management Plan, including the communication plan, must be reviewed and updated at least every two years.

11. ⓓ **For ambulatory surgical centers that elect to use The Joint Commission deemed status option:** The Emergency Management Plan describes the patient population served by the organization and the extent to which additional populations may be cared for during an emergency based on the organization's capabilities (staff, space, supplies, equipment).

12. ⓓ **For ambulatory surgical centers that elect to use The Joint Commission deemed status option:** The Emergency Management Plan includes a continuity of operations strategy that covers the following:
    - Continuity of facilities and communications to support organizational functions at the original site or alternate site(s), in case the original site is incapacitated

- A succession plan that lists who replaces the key leader(s) during an emergency if the leader is not available to carry out their duties
- A delegation of authority plan that describes the decisions and policies that can be implemented by authorized successors during an emergency and criteria or triggers that initiate this delegation

Note: *A continuity of operations strategy is an essential component of emergency management planning. The goal of emergency management planning is to provide care to individuals who are incapacitated by emergencies in the community or in the organization. A continuity of operations strategy focuses on the organization, with the goal of protecting the organization's physical plant, information technology systems, business and financial operations, and other infrastructure from direct disruption or damage so that it can continue to function throughout or shortly after an emergency. When the organization itself becomes, or is at risk of becoming, a victim of an emergency (power failure, fire, flood, bomb threat, and so forth), it is the continuity of operations strategy that provides the resilience to respond and recover.*

14. Ⓓ **For ambulatory surgical centers that elect to use The Joint Commission deemed status option:** The ambulatory surgical center has a procedure for requesting an 1135 waiver for care and treatment at an alternative care site.

Note: *During disasters, organizations may need to request 1135 waivers to address care and treatment at an alternate care site identified by emergency management officials. The 1135 waivers are granted by the federal government during declared public health emergencies; these waivers authorize modification of certain federal regulatory requirements (for example, Medicare, Medicaid, Children's Health Insurance Program, Health Insurance Portability and Accountability Act) for a defined time period during response and recovery.*

15. Ⓓ **For ambulatory surgical centers that elect to use The Joint Commission deemed status option: For organizations that plan to provide services during an emergency:** The Emergency Management Plan addresses a means to shelter staff and volunteers on site who remain in the organization, including essential space, utilities, and supplies, and criteria for who can be sheltered on site.

20. Ⓓ **For rural health clinics and federally qualified health centers:** The Emergency Management Plan, including the communication plan, must be reviewed and updated at least every two years.

21. ⓓ **For rural health clinics and federally qualified health centers:** The Emergency Management Plan describes the patient population served by the organization and the extent to which additional populations may be cared for during an emergency based on the organization's capabilities (staff, space, supplies, equipment).

22. ⓓ **For rural health clinics and federally qualified health centers:** The Emergency Management Plan includes a continuity of operations strategy that covers the following:
    - Continuity of facilities and communications to support organizational functions at the original site or alternate site(s), in case the original site is incapacitated
    - A succession plan that lists who replaces the key leader(s) during an emergency if the leader is not available to carry out their duties
    - A delegation of authority plan that describes the decisions and policies that can be implemented by authorized successors during an emergency and criteria or triggers that initiate this delegation

Note: *A continuity of operations strategy is an essential component of emergency management planning. The goal of emergency management planning is to provide care to individuals who are incapacitated by emergencies in the community or in the organization. A continuity of operations strategy focuses on the organization, with the goal of protecting the organization's physical plant, information technology systems, business and financial operations, and other infrastructure from direct disruption or damage so that it can continue to function throughout or shortly after an emergency. When the organization itself becomes, or is at risk of becoming, a victim of an emergency (power failure, fire, flood, bomb threat, and so forth), it is the continuity of operations strategy that provides the resilience to respond and recover.*

Standard EM.02.02.01

As part of its Emergency Management Plan, the organization prepares for how it will communicate during emergencies.

Rationale for EM.02.02.01

The organization maintains reliable communication capabilities for the purpose of communicating response efforts to staff, patients, and external organizations. The organization establishes backup communication processes and technologies (for example, cell phones, landlines, bulletin boards, fax machines, satellite phones, amateur radio, text messages) to communicate essential information if primary communication systems fail.

Elements of Performance for EM.02.02.01

1. The Emergency Management Plan describes how staff will be notified that emergency response procedures have been initiated.

3. The Emergency Management Plan describes how the organization will notify external authorities that emergency response measures have been initiated.

For ambulatory surgical centers that elect to use The Joint Commission deemed status option: The Emergency Management Plan describes the following:

4. Ⓓ How the organization will communicate with external authorities during an ongoing emergency.

7. Ⓓ How the organization will communicate with suppliers of essential services, equipment, and supplies during an emergency.

12. Ⓓ How, and under what circumstances, the organization will communicate information about patients to third parties (such as other health care organizations, the state health department, police, and the Federal Bureau of Investigation [FBI]).

14. The organization establishes backup communication systems or technologies for use in the event that internal or external systems fail during an emergency.

17. The organization implements the components of its Emergency Management Plan that require advance preparation to support communications during an emergency.

20. Ⓓ **For ambulatory surgical centers that elect to use The Joint Commission deemed status option:** As part of its communication plan, the organization maintains the names and contact information of the following:
    - Staff
    - Physicians
    - Volunteers

■ Other potential response partners (depending upon services provided, these may be rural health clinics, federally qualified health centers, or other sources of collaboration or assistance)

■ Entities providing services under arrangement

■ Relevant federal, state, tribal, regional, and local emergency preparedness staff

21. ⓓ **For ambulatory surgical centers that elect to use The Joint Commission deemed status option:** The Emergency Management Plan describes the following:

■ The organization's primary and alternate means of communicating with staff and federal, state, tribal, and local emergency management agencies

■ Process for communicating information about the general condition and location of patients under the organization's care to public and private entities assisting with disaster relief

■ How the organization will communicate information about its needs and ability to provide assistance to the authority having jurisdiction, the incident command center, or designee

Note: *Depending upon the type of emergency, the authority having jurisdiction might be the municipal, county, or state health department, or another governmental entity.*

22. ⓓ **For ambulatory surgical centers that elect to use The Joint Commission deemed status option:** The organization has a process for cooperation and collaboration with the local, state, tribal, regional, and federal emergency preparedness officials' efforts to maintain an integrated response during a disaster or emergency situation.

23. ⓓ **For ambulatory surgical centers that elect to use The Joint Commission deemed status option:** The Emergency Management Plan describes the following:

■ The organization's arrangements for communicating necessary clinical information on patients under the organization's care with other health care providers in order to maintain continuity of care

■ A method, in the event of an evacuation, to release patient information to family or others designated by the patient, as permitted under law and regulation at 45 CFR 164.510(b)(1)(ii)

For rural health clinics and federally qualified health centers: The Emergency Management Plan describes the following:

30.   ⓓ How the organization will communicate with suppliers of essential services, equipment, and supplies during an emergency.

31.   ⓓ How, and under what circumstances, the organization will communicate information about patients to third parties (such as other health care organizations, the state health department, police, and the Federal Bureau of Investigation [FBI]).

32.   ⓓ **For rural health clinics and federally qualified health centers:** As part of its communication plan, the organization maintains the names and contact information of the following:

- Staff
- Physicians
- Volunteers
- Other potential response partners (depending upon services provided, these may be rural health clinics, federally qualified health centers, or other sources of collaboration or assistance)
- Entities providing services under arrangement
- Relevant federal, state, tribal, regional, and local emergency preparedness staff

33.   ⓓ **For rural health clinics and federally qualified health centers:** The Emergency Management Plan describes the following:

- The organization's primary and alternate means of communicating with staff and federal, state, tribal, and local emergency management agencies
- Process for communicating information about the general condition and location of patients under the organization's care to public and private entities assisting with disaster relief
- How the organization will communicate information about its needs and ability to provide assistance to the authority having jurisdiction, the incident command center, or designee

Note: *Depending upon the type of emergency, the authority having jurisdiction might be the municipal, county, or state health department, or another governmental entity.*

34.   ⓓ **For rural health clinics and federally qualified health centers:** The organization has a process for cooperation and collaboration with the local, state, tribal, regional, and federal emergency preparedness officials' efforts to maintain an integrated response during a disaster or emergency situation.

Standard EM.02.02.03 ▬▬▬▬▬▬▬▬▬▬▬▬▬▬▬▬▬▬

As part of its Emergency Management Plan, the organization prepares for how it will manage resources and assets during emergencies.

Note: *All organizations are required to respond to a patient's immediate care and safety needs if an emergency occurs with patients on site.*

Rationale for EM.02.02.03

The organization that continues to provide care, treatment, or services to its patients during emergencies needs to determine how resources and assets (that is, supplies, equipment, and facilities) will be managed internally and, when necessary, solicited and acquired from external sources. The organization should also recognize the risk that some resources may not be available from planned sources, particularly in emergencies of long duration or broad geographic scope, and that contingency plans will be necessary for critical supplies. This situation may occur when multiple organizations are vying for a limited supply from the same vendor.

Elements of Performance for EM.02.02.03

1. **For organizations that plan to provide service during an emergency:** The Emergency Management Plan describes how the organization will obtain and replenish medications and related supplies that will be required in response to an emergency.

2. **For organizations that plan to provide service during an emergency:** The Emergency Management Plan describes how the organization will obtain and replenish medical supplies that will be required in response to an emergency.

3. **For organizations that plan to provide service during an emergency:** The Emergency Management Plan describes how the organization will obtain and replenish nonmedical supplies (including food, bedding, and other provisions consistent with the organization's plan for sheltering on site) that will be required in response to an emergency.

For ambulatory surgical centers that elect to use The Joint Commission deemed status option: The Emergency Management Plan describes the following:

9. Ⓓ The organization's arrangements for transporting some or all patients; their requisite medications, supplies, and equipment; and staff to an alternative care site(s) when the organization's environment cannot support care, treatment, and services.

(*See also* EM.02.02.11, EP 3)

12. **For organizations that plan to provide service during an emergency:** The organization implements the components of its Emergency Management Plan that require advance preparation to provide for resources and assets during an emergency.

Standard EM.02.02.05

As part of its Emergency Management Plan, the organization prepares for how it will manage security and safety during an emergency.

Rationale for EM.02.02.05

Although patients are ambulatory and in most cases are able to provide for their own safety during an emergency, organization staff have a responsibility to take action to protect patients if an emergency occurs while patients are on site. This includes protecting patients from exposure to hazardous conditions or materials and making provisions for isolation and decontamination, when appropriate.

Elements of Performance for EM.02.02.05

1. The Emergency Management Plan describes how internal security and safety will be provided during an emergency.

5. **For organizations that plan to provide services during an emergency:** The Emergency Management Plan describes how the organization will provide for radioactive, biological, and chemical isolation and decontamination.

10. The organization implements the components of its Emergency Management Plan that require advance preparation to support internal security and safety during an emergency.

Standard EM.02.02.07

As part of its Emergency Management Plan, the organization prepares for how it will manage staff during an emergency.

Rationale for EM.02.02.07

To provide safe and effective patient care during an emergency, staff roles are well defined in advance, and staff are oriented in their assigned responsibilities. Staff roles and responsibilities may be documented in the Plan using a variety of formats (for example, job action sheets, checklists, flowcharts).

Elements of Performance for EM.02.02.07

The Emergency Management Plan describes the following:

 1. How the organization will manage staff during emergencies.

 2. Ⓓ The roles and responsibilities of staff during an emergency.

 3. The process for assigning staff to all essential staff functions.

4. The Emergency Management Plan identifies the individual(s) to whom staff report in emergencies.

7. Ⓓ **For ambulatory surgical centers that elect to use The Joint Commission deemed status option:** The organization trains staff for their assigned emergency response roles.

9. **For organizations that plan to provide services during an emergency:** The Emergency Management Plan describes how the organization will identify licensed independent practitioners, staff, and authorized volunteers during emergencies.

   Note: *This identification could include identification cards, wristbands, vests, hats, or badges.*

   (*See also* EM.02.02.13, EP 3; EM.02.02.15, EP 3)

10. The organization implements the components of its Emergency Management Plan that require advance preparation to manage staff during an emergency.

11. Ⓓ **For ambulatory surgical centers that elect to use The Joint Commission deemed status option:** The organization has a system to track the location of on-duty staff during an emergency.

12. Ⓓ **For rural health clinics and federally qualified health centers:** The Emergency Management Plan describes how volunteers and state and federally designated health care professionals will be incorporated into the staffing strategy for addressing a surge in needs during an emergency. The staffing strategy will vary depending on the type of emergency, whether the organization chooses to use volunteers, and the organization's role, if any, in community response plans.

13.   Ⓓ **For ambulatory surgical centers that elect to use The Joint Commission deemed status option:** The organization provides emergency preparedness training to staff, volunteers, and individuals providing on-site services under arrangement at the following intervals:
- Initial training
- At least every two years
- When roles or responsibilities change
- When policies and procedures are significantly updated

This training is documented.

Note: *Staff demonstrate knowledge of emergency procedures through participation in drills and exercises, as well as post-training tests, participation in instructor-led feedback (for example, questions and answers), or other methods determined and documented by the organization.*

14.   Ⓓ **For ambulatory surgical centers that elect to use The Joint Commission deemed status option:** The Emergency Operations Plan describes the use of volunteers in an emergency, including emergency staffing strategies, such as the role and process for integration of state or federally designated health care professionals to address surge needs during an emergency.

18.   Ⓓ **For rural health clinics and federally qualified health centers:** The organization trains staff for their assigned emergency response roles.

19.   Ⓓ **For rural health clinics and federally qualified health centers:** The organization has a system to track the location of on-duty staff during an emergency.

20.   Ⓓ **For rural health clinics and federally qualified health centers:** The organization provides emergency preparedness training to staff, volunteers, and individuals providing on-site services under arrangement at the following intervals:
- Initial training
- At least every two years
- When roles or responsibilities change
- When policies and procedures are significantly updated

This training is documented.

Note: *Staff demonstrate knowledge of emergency procedures through participation in drills and exercises, as well as post-training tests, participation in instructor-led feedback (for example, questions and answers), or other methods determined and documented by the organization.*

21. Ⓓ **For ambulatory surgical centers that elect to use The Joint Commission deemed status option:** The organization has an emergency preparedness training program based on its Emergency Management Plan. This training program is reviewed and updated at least every two years.

Standard EM.02.02.09 ▬▬▬▬▬▬▬▬▬▬▬▬▬▬▬▬▬▬▬▬

As part of its Emergency Management Plan, the organization prepares for how it will manage utilities during an emergency.

Rationale for EM.02.02.09

Different types of emergencies can have the same detrimental impact on an organization's utility systems. For example, brush fires, ice storms, and industrial accidents can all result in a loss of utilities required for care, treatment, services, and building operations. Organizations, therefore, must have alternative means of providing for essential utilities (for example, alternative equipment at the organization; negotiated relationships with the primary suppliers; provision through a parent entity; Memoranda of Understanding (MOU) with other organizations in the community). Organizations should determine how long they expect to remain open to care for patients and plan for their utilities accordingly.

Elements of Performance for EM.02.02.09

1. **For organizations that plan to provide services during an emergency:** The Emergency Management Plan describes how the organization will provide for alternative means of meeting essential building utility needs.

    Note: *Examples of potential utility problems might include disruptions to piped medical gas systems, failure of backup generators, and water pipe rupture.*

8. The organization implements the components of its Emergency Management Plan that require advance preparation to provide for utilities during an emergency.

Standard EM.02.02.11 ▬▬▬▬▬▬▬▬▬▬▬▬▬▬▬▬▬▬▬▬

As part of its Emergency Management Plan, the organization prepares for how it will manage patients during emergencies.

Rationale for EM.02.02.11

The fundamental goal of emergency management planning is to protect life and prevent disability. The manner in which care, treatment, or services are provided may vary by type of emergency. However, certain activities are so fundamental to patient safety (this can include decisions to modify or discontinue services, make referrals, or transport patients) that the organization should take a proactive approach in considering how they might be accomplished.

Elements of Performance for EM.02.02.11

1. ⒟ The Emergency Management Plan describes how the organization will manage activities related to patient care, treatment, or services.

   Note: *Activities related to care, treatment, or services might include scheduling, modifying, or discontinuing services; controlling information about patients; making referrals; transporting patients; and providing security.*

3. ⒟ The Emergency Management Plan describes how the organization will evacuate its occupied space.

   (*See also* EM.02.02.03, EP 9)

11. The organization implements the components of its Emergency Management Plan that require advance preparation to manage patients during an emergency.

12. ⒟ **For ambulatory surgical centers that elect to use The Joint Commission deemed status option:** The organization has a system to track the location of patients sheltered on site during an emergency. This system includes documentation of the name and location of the receiving facility or alternate site in the event a patient is relocated during the emergency.

    Note: *The name and location of receiving facilities or alternate sites may be defined in the emergency management plan, formal transfer agreements, or other accessible documents.*

13. ⒟ **For ambulatory surgical centers that elect to use The Joint Commission deemed status option:** Procedures for evacuating patients from the organization during an emergency address, at a minimum, the following:
    - Care and treatment needs of patients when deciding where they will be evacuated (for example, transfer to a higher level of care, transport to an alternative site in the community, discharge to home)

- Primary and alternate means of communication with external sources of assistance regarding patient care
- Transportation for the evacuated patient to an alternative site

15. Ⓓ **For rural health clinics and federally qualified health centers:** The organization has a system to track the location of patients sheltered on site during an emergency. This system includes documentation of the name and location of the receiving facility or alternate site in the event a patient is relocated during the emergency.

    Note: *The name and location of receiving facilities or alternate sites may be defined in the emergency management plan, formal transfer agreements, or other accessible documents.*

16. Ⓓ **For rural health clinics and federally qualified health centers:** Procedures for evacuating patients from the organization during an emergency address, at a minimum, the following:
    - Care and treatment needs of patients when deciding where they will be evacuated (for example, transfer to a higher level of care, transport to an alternative site in the community, discharge to home)
    - Primary and alternate means of communication with external sources of assistance regarding patient care
    - Transportation for the evacuated patient to an alternative site

Introduction to Standards EM.02.02.13 and EM.02.02.15

When the organization activates its Emergency Management Plan in response to a disaster and the immediate needs of its patients cannot be met, the organization can choose to rely on volunteer practitioners to meet these needs. These practitioners may be volunteer licensed independent practitioners or volunteer practitioners who are not licensed independent practitioners but who are required by law and regulation to have a license, certification, or registration to meet these needs. Under these circumstances, if the usual credentialing and privileging processes cannot be performed because of the disaster, the organization may use a modified credentialing and privileging process on a case-by-case basis for eligible volunteer practitioners. While this standard allows for a method to streamline the process for determining qualifications and competence, safeguards must be in place to assure that the volunteer practitioners are competent to provide safe and adequate care, treatment, or services. Even in a disaster, the integrity of two specific parts of the usual process for determining qualifications and competence must be maintained:

1. Verification of licensure, certification, or registration required to practice a profession
2. Oversight of the care, treatment, or services provided

A number of state and federal systems engaged in pre-event verification of qualifications can help facilitate the assigning of disaster privileges to volunteer licensed independent practitioners at the time of a disaster. Examples of such systems include the Emergency System for Advance Registration of Volunteer Health Professionals (ESAR-VHP) and the Medical Reserve Corps (MRC). The ESAR-VHP, created by the Health Resources and Services Administration (HRSA), allows for the advance registration and credentialing of health care professionals needed to augment a hospital or other medical facility to meet increased patient/victim care and increased surge capacity needs. MRC units are comprised of locally based medical and public health volunteers who can assist their communities during emergencies, such as an influenza epidemic, a chemical spill, or an act of terrorism.

Standard EM.02.02.13 ━━━━━━━━━━━━━━━━━━━━━━

During disasters, the organization may grant disaster privileges to volunteer licensed independent practitioners.

Note: *A disaster is an emergency that, due to its complexity, scope, or duration, threatens the organization's capabilities and requires outside assistance to sustain patient care, safety, or security functions.*

Elements of Performance for EM.02.02.13

1. The organization grants disaster privileges to volunteer licensed independent practitioners only when the Emergency Management Plan has been activated in response to a disaster and the organization is unable to meet immediate patient needs.

2. ⓓ The organization identifies, in writing, those individuals responsible for granting disaster privileges to volunteer licensed independent practitioners.

3. The organization determines how it will distinguish volunteer licensed independent practitioners from other licensed independent practitioners.

    (*See also* EM.02.02.07, EP 9)

4. ⓓ The organization describes, in writing, how it will oversee the performance of volunteer licensed independent practitioners who are granted disaster privileges (for example, by direct observation, mentoring, clinical record review).

5. Before a volunteer practitioner is considered eligible to function as a volunteer licensed independent practitioner, the organization obtains the volunteer practitioner's valid government-issued photo identification (for example, a driver's license or passport) and at least one of the following: **R**
    - A current picture identification card from a health care organization that clearly identifies professional designation
    - A current license to practice
    - Primary source verification of licensure
    - Identification indicating that the individual is a member of a Disaster Medical Assistance Team (DMAT), the Medical Reserve Corps (MRC), the Emergency System for Advance Registration of Volunteer Health Professionals (ESAR-VHP), or other recognized state or federal response organization or group
    - Identification indicating that the individual has been granted authority by a government entity to provide patient care, treatment, or services in disaster circumstances

- Confirmation by a licensed independent practitioner currently privileged by the organization or by a staff member with personal knowledge of the volunteer practitioner's ability to act as a licensed independent practitioner during a disaster

6. During a disaster, the organization oversees the performance of each volunteer licensed independent practitioner.

7. Based on its oversight of each volunteer licensed independent practitioner, the organization determines within 72 hours of the practitioner's arrival if granted disaster privileges should continue.

8. Ⓓ Primary source verification of licensure occurs as soon as the disaster is under control or within 72 hours from the time the volunteer licensed independent practitioner arrives at the organization, whichever comes first. If primary source verification of a volunteer licensed independent practitioner's licensure cannot be completed within 72 hours of the practitioner's arrival due to extraordinary circumstances, the organization documents all of the following:
   - Reason(s) it could not be performed within 72 hours of the practitioner's arrival
   - Evidence of the licensed independent practitioner's demonstrated ability to continue to provide adequate care, treatment, or services
   - Evidence of the organization's attempt to perform primary source verification as soon as possible

9. If, due to extraordinary circumstances, primary source verification of licensure of the volunteer licensed independent practitioner cannot be completed within 72 hours of the practitioner's arrival, it is performed as soon as possible.

   Note: *Primary source verification of licensure is not required if the volunteer licensed independent practitioner has not provided care, treatment, or services under the disaster privileges.*

Standard EM.02.02.15

During disasters, the organization may assign disaster responsibilities to volunteer practitioners who are not licensed independent practitioners, but who are required by law and regulation to have a license, certification, or registration.

Note: *While this standard allows for a method to streamline the process for verifying identification and licensure, certification, or registration, the elements of performance are intended to safeguard against inadequate care during a disaster.*

Elements of Performance for EM.02.02.15

1. The organization assigns disaster responsibilities to volunteer practitioners who are not licensed independent practitioners only when the Emergency Management Plan has been activated in response to a disaster and the organization is unable to meet immediate patient needs.

2. Ⓓ The organization identifies, in writing, those individuals responsible for assigning disaster responsibilities to volunteer practitioners who are not licensed independent practitioners.

3. The organization determines how it will distinguish volunteer practitioners who are not licensed independent practitioners from its staff.

   (*See also* EM.02.02.07, EP 9)

4. Ⓓ The organization describes, in writing, how it will oversee the performance of volunteer practitioners who are not licensed independent practitioners who have been assigned disaster responsibilities. Examples of methods for overseeing their performance include direct observation, mentoring, and clinical record review.

5. Before a volunteer practitioner who is not a licensed independent practitioner is considered eligible to function as a practitioner, the organization obtains the volunteer practitioner's valid government-issued photo identification (for example, a driver's license or passport) and one of the following: Ⓡ
   - A current picture identification card from a health care organization that clearly identifies professional designation
   - A current license, certification, or registration
   - Primary source verification of licensure, certification, or registration (if required by law and regulation in order to practice)
   - Identification indicating that the individual is a member of a Disaster Medical Assistance Team (DMAT), the Medical Reserve Corps (MRC), the Emergency System for Advance Registration of Volunteer Health Professionals (ESAR-VHP), or other recognized state or federal response organization or group

- Identification indicating that the individual has been granted authority by a government entity to provide patient care, treatment, or services in disaster circumstances
- Confirmation by organization staff with personal knowledge of the volunteer practitioner's ability to act as a qualified practitioner during a disaster

6. During a disaster, the organization oversees the performance of each volunteer practitioner who is not a licensed independent practitioner.

7. Based on its oversight of each volunteer practitioner who is not a licensed independent practitioner, the organization determines within 72 hours after the practitioner's arrival whether assigned disaster responsibilities should continue.

8. Ⓓ Primary source verification of licensure, certification, or registration (if required by law and regulation in order to practice) of volunteer practitioners who are not licensed independent practitioners occurs as soon as the disaster is under control or within 72 hours from the time the volunteer practitioner arrives at the organization, whichever comes first. If primary source verification of licensure, certification, or registration (if required by law and regulation in order to practice) for a volunteer practitioner who is not a licensed independent practitioner cannot be completed within 72 hours due to extraordinary circumstances, the organization documents all of the following:
   - Reason(s) it could not be performed within 72 hours of the practitioner's arrival
   - Evidence of the volunteer practitioner's demonstrated ability to continue to provide adequate care, treatment, or services
   - Evidence of the organization's attempt to perform primary source verification as soon as possible

9. If, due to extraordinary circumstances, primary source verification of licensure of the volunteer practitioner cannot be completed within 72 hours of the practitioner's arrival, it is performed as soon as possible.

   Note: *Primary source verification of licensure, certification, or registration is not required if the volunteer practitioner has not provided care, treatment, or services under their assigned disaster responsibilities.*

Standard EM.03.01.03

The organization evaluates the effectiveness of its Emergency Management Plan.

Rationale for EM.03.01.03

The organization conducts exercises to assess the Emergency Management Plan's appropriateness, adequacy, and effectiveness in regard to logistics, human resources, training, policies, procedures, and protocols. Exercises should stress the limits of the plan to support assessment of the organization's preparedness and performance. The design of the exercises should reflect likely disasters but should test the organization's ability to respond to the effects of emergencies on its capabilities to provide care, treatment, and services.

Elements of Performance for EM.03.01.03

3. Ⓓ The organization conducts an exercise to test the emergency plan at least annually. The organization is required to conduct either one community-based, full-scale exercise if available, or a facility-based, functional exercise, every other year. In the opposite year, the organization's annual exercise includes, but is not limited to, one of the following:
   - A second full-scale, community-based exercise
   - A second facility-based, functional exercise
   - Mock disaster drill
   - Tabletop exercise or workshop that is led by a facilitator and includes a group discussion using a narrated, clinically relevant emergency scenario and a set of problem statements, directed messages, or prepared questions designed to challenge an emergency plan.

   Note 1: *If the organization experiences an actual emergency (natural or man-made) that requires activation of the emergency plan, the organization is exempt from engaging in its next required full-scale, community-based exercise or facility-based, functional exercise following the onset of the emergency event.*

   Note 2: See *the Glossary for the definitions of community-based exercise, full-scale exercise, and functional exercise.*

5. Emergency response exercises incorporate likely disaster scenarios that allow the organization to evaluate its handling of communications, resources and assets, security, staff, utilities, and patients.

For ambulatory surgical centers that elect to use The Joint Commission deemed status option: During emergency response exercises, the organization monitors its management of the following:

   10. Staff roles and responsibilities.

13. Representatives from administrative, support, and clinical services participate in the evaluation of all emergency response exercises and all responses to actual emergencies.

14. Ⓓ The evaluation of all emergency response exercises and all responses to actual emergencies includes the identification of deficiencies and opportunities for improvement. This evaluation is documented.

16. The organization modifies its Emergency Management Plan based on its evaluation of emergency response exercises and responses to actual emergencies.

    Note: *When modifications requiring substantive resources cannot be accomplished by the next emergency response exercise, interim measures are put in place until final modifications can be made.*

17. Subsequent emergency response exercises reflect modifications and interim measures as described in the modified Emergency Management Plan.

For rural health clinics and federally qualified health centers: During emergency response exercises, the organization monitors its management of the following:

22. Staff roles and responsibilities.

Introduction to Standard EM.04.01.01

Each individual health care organization must have an emergency plan that reflects the risks facing the organization and the strategies, resources, and capabilities it can deploy to serve its patients safely during a time of disaster. Health care organizations in systems with integrated emergency preparedness programs can increase resilience through integrating their plans with the system and leveraging system expertise, resources, and other capabilities. System participation extends the ability of the organization to serve its patients, protect its facilities, mobilize its staff, and aid its system and/or community by serving more patients.

Depending on the organization's risks, services, and capabilities, some aspects of integration with the system may be at an early stage rather than an advanced stage. However, because disasters can occur at any time, the organization must implement communication procedures immediately in order to stand ready to actively use and align with the system's emergency response procedures.

In terms of format, the system's plan can be an annex to the organization's plan, the organization's individual emergency plan can be integrated into the system's plan, or there can be a single universal system plan that has sections for each organization—no specific format is prescribed. However, the organization must be able to readily access and use its individual plan for its preparedness, response, and recovery efforts. The organization must be able to readily access the system's plan and use it to carry out its role effectively within the system's integrated emergency preparedness program.

Standard EM.04.01.01

If the organization is part of a health care system that has an integrated emergency preparedness program, and it chooses to participate in the integrated emergency preparedness program, the organization participates in planning, preparedness, and response activities with the system.

Elements of Performance for EM.04.01.01

1.   ⒟ **For ambulatory surgical centers that elect to use The Joint Commission deemed status option:** The organization demonstrates its participation in the development of its system's integrated emergency preparedness program through the following:

  ■ Designation of a staff member(s) who will collaborate with the system in developing the program

  ■ Documentation that the organization has reviewed the community-based risk assessment developed by the system's integrated all-hazards emergency management program

  ■ Documentation that the organization's individual risk assessment is incorporated into the system's integrated program

  ■ Documentation that the organization's patient population, services offered, and any unique circumstances of the organization are reflected in the system's integrated program

  ■ Documentation of an integrated communication plan, including information on key contacts in the system's integrated program

  ■ Documentation that the organization participates in the review at least every two years of the system's integrated program

2.   ⒟ **For ambulatory surgical centers that elect to use The Joint Commission deemed status option:** The organization has implemented communication procedures for emergency planning and response activities in coordination with the system's integrated emergency preparedness program.

3. Ⓓ **For ambulatory surgical centers that elect to use The Joint Commission deemed status option:** The organization's integrated emergency management policies, procedures, or plans address the following:
   - Identification of the organization's emergency preparedness, response, and recovery activities that can be coordinated with the system's integrated program (for example, acquiring or storing clinical supplies, assigning staff to the local health care coalition to create joint training protocols, and so forth)
   - The organization's communication and/or collaboration with local, tribal, regional, state, or federal emergency preparedness officials through the system's integrated program
   - Coordination of continuity of operations planning with the system's integrated program
   - Plans and procedures for integrated training and exercise activities with the system's integrated program

5. Ⓓ **For rural health clinics and federally qualified health centers:** The organization demonstrates its participation in the development of its system's integrated emergency preparedness program through the following:
   - Designation of a staff member(s) who will collaborate with the system in developing the program
   - Documentation that the organization has reviewed the community-based risk assessment developed by the system's integrated all-hazards emergency management program
   - Documentation that the organization's individual risk assessment is incorporated into the system's integrated program
   - Documentation that the organization's patient population, services offered, and any unique circumstances of the organization are reflected in the system's integrated program
   - Documentation of an integrated communication plan, including information on key contacts in the system's integrated program
   - Documentation that the organization participates in a review at least every two years of the system's integrated program

6. Ⓓ **For rural health clinics and federally qualified health centers:** The organization has implemented communication procedures for emergency planning and response activities in coordination with the system's integrated emergency preparedness program.

7.   Ⓓ **For rural health clinics and federally qualified health centers:** The organization's integrated emergency management policies, procedures, or plans address the following:

- Identification of the organization's emergency preparedness, response, and recovery activities that can be coordinated with the system's integrated program (for example, acquiring or storing clinical supplies, assigning staff to the local health care coalition to create joint training protocols, and so forth)
- The organization's communication and/or collaboration with local, tribal, regional, state, or federal emergency preparedness officials through the system's integrated program
- Coordination of continuity of operations planning with the system's integrated program
- Plans and procedures for integrated training and exercise activities with the system's integrated program

Human Resources (HR)

Overview

The contribution that human resources management makes to an organization's ability to provide safe, quality care cannot be overestimated. The quality of the organization's staff and licensed independent practitioners will, in large part, determine the quality of the care, treatment, and services it provides.

The World Health Organization's Global Strategy on Human Resources for Health: Workforce 2030* asserts that the mere availability of staff is not sufficient to provide effective service coverage and emergency management; staff competence, motivation, and support are also important factors. The ability of health care organizations to respond effectively to modern priorities like community-based health services and evolving epidemiologic profiles is reliant on establishing a strong, effective workforce. After staff are hired and licensed independent practitioners are granted clinical privileges, even the smallest organization has a responsibility to see that staff and practitioners receive the education and training they need to provide quality care and to keep patients safe.

About This Chapter

The standards and elements of performance in this chapter address the organization's responsibility to establish and verify staff qualifications, orient staff, and provide staff with the training they need to support the care, treatment, or services the organization provides. After staff is on the job, the organization must provide for the assessment of staff competence and performance.

This chapter also addresses the organization's responsibility to credential and privilege licensed independent practitioners and provide them with orientation and a fair hearing and appeal process.

---

* World Health Organization (WHO). Global Strategy on Human Resources for Health: Workforce 2030. 2016

Chapter Outline

I. Staff
    A. Qualifications (HR.01.01.01, HR.01.02.07)
    B. Staffing (HR.01.02.05)
    C. Orientation (HR.01.04.01)
    D. Training and Education (HR.01.05.03)
    E. Competence (HR.01.06.01)
    F. Evaluation of Performance (HR.01.07.01)

II. Licensed Independent Practitioners
    A. Credentialing and Privileging (HR.02.01.03, HR.02.01.05)
    B. Orientation (HR.02.02.01)
    C. Fair Hearing and Appeal (HR.02.03.01)
    D. Additional Standards for Services Offered Through a Telemedical Link
        (HR.02.04.01, HR.02.04.03)

III. Primary Care Medical Home — Qualifications (HR.03.01.01)

Standards, Rationales, and Elements of Performance

Standard HR.01.01.01 ━━━━━━━━━━━━━━━━━━━━━━

The organization defines and verifies staff qualifications.

Elements of Performance for HR.01.01.01

1. The organization defines staff qualifications specific to their job responsibilities.

    Note: *Qualifications for infection control may be met through ongoing education, training, experience, and/or certification (such as that offered by the Certification Board for Infection Control).*

    (*See also* IC.01.01.01, EP 3)

2. Ⓓ The organization verifies and documents the following:
    - Credentials of care providers using the primary source when licensure, certification, or registration is required by law and regulation to practice their profession. This is done at the time of hire and at the time credentials are renewed.
    - Credentials of care providers (primary source not required) when licensure, certification, or registration is not required by law and regulation. This is done at the time of hire and at the time credentials are renewed.

    Note 1: *It is acceptable to verify current licensure, certification, or registration with the primary source via a secure electronic communication or by telephone, if this verification is documented.*

    Note 2: *A primary verification source may designate another agency to communicate credentials information. The designated agency can then be used as a primary source.*

    Note 3: *An external organization (for example, a credentials verification organization [CVO]) may be used to verify credentials information. A CVO must meet the CVO guidelines identified in the Glossary.*

3. Ⓓ The organization verifies and documents that the applicant has the education and experience required by the job responsibilities.

4. Ⓓ The organization obtains a criminal background check on the applicant as required by law and regulation or organization policy. Criminal background checks are documented.

5.   Ⓓ Staff comply with applicable health screening as required by law and regulation or organization policy. Health screening compliance is documented.

7.   Before providing care, treatment, or services, the organization confirms that nonemployees who are brought into the organization by a licensed independent practitioner to provide care, treatment, or services have the same qualifications and competencies required of employed individuals performing the same or similar services at the organization.

   Note 1: *This confirmation can be accomplished either through the organization's regular process or with the licensed independent practitioner who brought in the individual.*

   Note 2: *When the care, treatment, or services provided by the nonemployee are not currently performed by anyone employed by the organization, leadership consults the appropriate professional organization guidelines for the required credentials and competencies.*

32.   Ⓓ Technologists who perform diagnostic computed tomography (CT) exams have advanced-level certification by the American Registry of Radiologic Technologists (ARRT) or the Nuclear Medicine Technology Certification Board (NMTCB) in computed tomography or have one of the following qualifications:
   - State licensure that permits them to perform diagnostic CT exams and documented training on the provision of diagnostic CT exams or
   - Registration and certification in radiography by ARRT and documented training on the provision of diagnostic CT exams or
   - Certification in nuclear medicine technology by ARRT or NMTCB and documented training on the provision of diagnostic CT exams

   Note 1: *This element of performance does not apply to CT exams performed for therapeutic radiation treatment planning or delivery, or for calculating attenuation coefficients for nuclear medicine studies.*

   Note 2: *This element of performance does not apply to dental cone beam CT radiographic imaging studies performed for diagnosis of conditions affecting the maxillofacial region or to obtain guidance for the treatment of such conditions.*

   (*See also* HR.01.02.07, EPs 1, 2)

33.   Ⓓ The organization verifies and documents that diagnostic medical physicists who support computed tomography (CT) services have board certification in

diagnostic radiologic physics or radiologic physics by the American Board of Radiology, or in Diagnostic Imaging Physics by the American Board of Medical Physics, or in Diagnostic Radiological Physics by the Canadian College of Physicists in Medicine, or meet all of the following requirements:

- A graduate degree in physics, medical physics, biophysics, radiologic physics, medical health physics, or a closely related science or engineering discipline from an accredited college or university
- College coursework in the biological sciences with at least one course in biology or radiation biology and one course in anatomy, physiology, or a similar topic related to the practice of medical physics
- Documented experience in a clinical CT environment conducting at least 10 CT performance evaluations under the direct supervision of a board-certified medical physicist

Note: *This element of performance does not apply to dental cone beam CT radiographic imaging studies performed for diagnosis of conditions affecting the maxillofacial region or to obtain guidance for the treatment of such conditions.*

Standard HR.01.02.05

The organization has the necessary staff to support the care, treatment, or services it provides.

Elements of Performance for HR.01.02.05

10. **For ambulatory surgical centers that elect to use The Joint Commission deemed status option:** The organization directs and staffs nursing services to meet patient needs.

11. **For ambulatory surgical centers that elect to use The Joint Commission deemed status option:** The organization delineates patient care, treatment, or service responsibilities for all nursing personnel.

12. **For ambulatory surgical centers that elect to use The Joint Commission deemed status option:** Nursing services follow recognized standards of practice.

13. **For ambulatory surgical centers that elect to use The Joint Commission deemed status option:** A registered nurse is available to provide emergency treatment whenever a patient is present in the organization. **R**

   Note: *Available refers to on the premises and sufficiently free from other duties, allowing the registered nurse to respond rapidly to emergency situations.*

(*See also* PC.02.01.09, EP 4)

Standard HR.01.02.07 ━━━━━━━━━━━━━━━━━━

The organization determines how staff function within the organization.

Elements of Performance for HR.01.02.07

1. All staff who provide patient care, treatment, or services possess a current license, certification, or registration, in accordance with law and regulation.

    (*See also* HR.01.01.01, EP 32)

2. Staff who provide patient care, treatment, or services practice within the scope of their license, certification, or registration and as required by law and regulation.

    (*See also* HR.01.01.01, EP 32)

3. **For organizations that elect The Joint Commission Primary Care Medical Home option:** The primary care clinician and the interdisciplinary team members function within their scope of practice and in accordance with privileges granted. (For more information, refer to Standards HR.01.06.01 and HR.02.01.03)

5. Staff supervise students when they provide patient care, treatment, or services as part of their training.

Introduction to Standard HR.01.04.01

Orientation is a process that gives the organization the opportunity to inform staff and licensed independent practitioners about its values, culture, and procedures. It is very important that staff begin working with an understanding of how their jobs contribute to patient safety and the quality of care, treatment, or services the organization provides. Some important questions that can be answered for staff through orientation include how to prevent and control infections, exhibit sensitivity to cultural diversity, and respect patient rights.

Standard HR.01.04.01 ━━━━━━━━━━━━━━━━━━

The organization provides orientation to staff.

Elements of Performance for HR.01.04.01

1. Ⓓ The organization orients its staff to the key safety content it identifies before staff provides care, treatment, or services. Completion of this orientation is documented.

    Note: *Key safety content may include specific processes and procedures related to the provision of care, treatment, or services; the environment of care; and infection control.*

3. Ⓓ The organization orients staff on the following:
    - Relevant policies and procedures
    - Their specific job duties, including those related to infection prevention and control and assessing and managing pain
    - Sensitivity to cultural diversity based on their job duties and responsibilities
    - Patient rights, including ethical aspects of care, treatment, or services and the process used to address ethical issues based on their job duties and responsibilities

    Completion of this orientation is documented.

Introduction to Standard HR.01.05.03

Education and training are important because they help maintain a competent workforce. The standard uses the terms education and training because these words are often used interchangeably. Generally, education can be thought of as the development of knowledge and training as the development of skills. However, the standard does not contain requirements specific to education and requirements specific to training. Instead, it speaks to areas in which staff should receive education or training depending on staff and organization needs. These areas include education and training specific to changes in staff responsibilities, the needs of the patient population, and the need and way(s) to report unanticipated adverse events.

Education and training can be provided through in-person instruction, demonstration, or independent study and can, of course, make use of computer technology.

While not required by the standard, some things an organization may want to look at in order to identify areas for development of education and training include the following:
- Results of performance improvement initiatives that point to the need for staff

education and training
- Staff needs identified through competence assessments or performance evaluations
- Topics that are particularly critical to patient safety
- Changes in technology or practices

Standard HR.01.05.03 ━━━━━━━━━━━━━━━━━

Staff participate in ongoing education and training.

Elements of Performance for HR.01.05.03

1. Ⓓ Staff participate in ongoing education and training to maintain or increase their competency and, as needed, when staff responsibilities change. Staff participation is documented.
   For ambulatory surgical centers that elect to use The Joint Commission deemed status option: Staff participate in ongoing education and training with respect to their roles in the fire response plan. (For information on staff's roles in the fire response plan, *see* EC.02.03.01, EP 10.)

14. Ⓓ The organization verifies and documents that individuals who perform diagnostic computed tomography (CT) examinations participate in ongoing education that includes annual training on the following:
    - Radiation dose optimization techniques and tools for pediatric and adult patients addressed in the Image Gently® and Image Wisely® campaigns
    - Safe procedures for operation of the types of CT equipment they will use

    Note 1: *Information on the Image Gently and Image Wisely initiatives can be found online at http://www.imagegently.org and http://www.imagewisely.org, respectively.*

    Note 2: *This element of performance does not apply to CT systems used for therapeutic radiation treatment planning or delivery, or for calculating attenuation coefficients for nuclear medicine studies.*

    Note 3: *This element of performance does not apply to dental cone beam CT radiographic imaging studies performed for diagnosis of conditions affecting the maxillofacial region or to obtain guidance for the treatment of such conditions.*

25. Ⓓ The organization verifies and documents that technologists who perform magnetic resonance imaging (MRI) examinations participate in ongoing education that includes annual training on safe MRI practices in the MRI environment, including the following:
    - Patient screening criteria that address ferromagnetic items, electrically

conductive items, medical implants and devices, and risk for nephrogenic
systemic fibrosis (NSF)

- Proper patient and equipment positioning activities to avoid thermal injuries
- Equipment and supplies that have been determined to be acceptable for use in
  the MRI environment (MR safe or MR conditional)[†]
- MRI safety response procedures for patients who require urgent or emergent
  medical care
- MRI system emergency shutdown procedures, such as MRI system quench
  and cryogen safety procedures
- Patient hearing protection
- Management of patients with claustrophobia, anxiety, or emotional distress

Introduction to Standards HR.01.06.01 and HR.01.07.01

A close relationship exists between competence assessment and performance evaluation.
Sometimes this relationship can be confusing. Competence assessment lets the
organization know whether its staff have the ability to use specific skills and to employ
the knowledge necessary to perform their jobs.

When the organization defines specific competencies, it should consider the needs of its
patient population, the types of procedures conducted, conditions or diseases treated,
and the kinds of equipment it uses.

Where competency assessment focuses on specific knowledge, skill, and ability,
performance evaluations are broader in scope. Performance evaluations are not only
focused on a staff member's competence, they also include other expectations that have
been established for each staff member. For example, a performance evaluation might
include expectations relative to whether a staff member participates in education and
training offered by the organization or how well a staff member carries out job
responsibilities and manages time.

What competency assessments and performance evaluations share is the requirement

---

[†] Terminology for defining the safety of items in the magnetic resonance environment is provided in
ASTM F2503 Standard Practice for Marking Medical Devices and Other Items for Safety in the
Magnetic Resonance Environment (http://www.astm.org).

that they are performed at least once every three years. This does not mean, however, that they have to be performed together at the same time. Some organizations, often those that are smaller in size, may choose to combine competency assessments with performance evaluations. Others may choose to handle these activities separately. If an organization chooses to combine the activities, it needs to make sure that the performance evaluation contains specific competencies. However these two activities are conducted, feedback on performance is most useful to staff if it is given whenever an opportunity arises.

Standard HR.01.06.01

Staff are competent to perform their responsibilities.

Elements of Performance for HR.01.06.01

1. The organization defines the competencies it requires of its staff who provide patient care, treatment, or services.

3. An individual with the educational background, experience, or knowledge related to the skills being reviewed assesses competence. **R**

   Note: *When a suitable individual cannot be found to assess staff competence, the organization can utilize an outside individual for this task. If a suitable individual inside or outside the organization cannot be found, the organization may consult the competency guidelines from an appropriate professional organization to make its assessment.*

5. Ⓓ Staff competence is initially assessed and documented as part of orientation.

6. Ⓓ Staff competence is assessed and documented once every three years, or more frequently as required by organization policy or in accordance with law and regulation.

Standard HR.01.07.01

The organization evaluates staff performance.

Elements of Performance for HR.01.07.01

1. The organization evaluates staff based on performance expectations that reflect their job responsibilities.

2. Ⓓ The organization evaluates staff performance once every three years, or more frequently as required by organization policy or in accordance with law and regulation. This evaluation is documented.

5. When a licensed independent practitioner brings a nonemployee individual into the organization to provide care, treatment, or services, the organization reviews the individual's competencies and performance at the same frequency as individuals employed by the organization.

    Note: *This review can be accomplished either through the organization's regular process or with the licensed independent practitioner who brought staff into the organization.*

Introduction to Standard HR.02.01.03

One of the most important and difficult responsibilities of an organization is deciding whether licensed independent practitioners are competent to provide safe, quality patient care. Before the organization can grant privileges, it must ascertain that licensed independent practitioners have the necessary credentials to perform their privileges. To grant privileges to licensed independent practitioners, the organization must collect, verify, and assess information related to their credentials, including current licensure, relevant training, current competence, and the ability to perform the clinical privileges that they have requested.

Verifying current licensure tells the organization that licensed independent practitioners are appropriately licensed to practice as required by state and/or federal law. Before granting initial, renewed, or revised privileges and at the time of licensure expiration, the organization documents required current licensure of a licensed independent practitioner using primary sources, if available.

Verifying relevant training tells the organization about licensed independent practitioners' clinical knowledge and skills. This verification must be obtained from the primary source of each specific credential. Primary sources include the specialty certifying boards and letters from professional schools, and from postgraduate education or postdoctoral programs for completion of training. When it is not possible to obtain verification from the primary source, the organization may use reliable secondary sources, provided that the organization documents its attempt to contact the primary source. An example of a reliable secondary source would be another organization that has documented primary source verification of the applicant's credentials.

The organization is also responsible for evaluating current challenges to licensure or registration; voluntary and involuntary relinquishment of licensure and registration; voluntary and involuntary termination of medical staff membership at another organization; voluntary and involuntary limitation, reduction, or loss of clinical privilege; and any professional liability actions that resulted in a final judgment against the applicant. This kind of information can be obtained through self-reporting by the practitioner, the Federation of State Medical Boards, and queries to the National Practitioner Data Bank.

Standard HR.02.01.03

The organization grants initial, renewed, or revised clinical privileges to individuals who are permitted by law and the organization to practice independently.

Elements of Performance for HR.02.01.03

1. The organization follows a process, approved by its leaders, to grant initial, renewed, or revised privileges and to deny privileges.

2. Before granting initial privileges, the organization verifies the identity of the individual seeking privileges by viewing a valid picture identification issued by a state or federal agency (for example, a driver's license or passport).

3. Ⓓ Before granting initial or revised privileges, the organization uses primary sources when documenting training specific to the privileges requested.

   Note 1: *The verification of relevant training informs the organization of the licensed independent practitioner's clinical knowledge and skill set. Verification must be obtained from the primary source of the specific credential. Primary sources include the specialty certifying boards approved by the American Dental Association for a dentist's board certification, letters from professional schools (for example, medical, dental, nursing) and letters from postgraduate education or postdoctoral programs for completion of training. Designated equivalent sources may be used to verify certain credentials in lieu of using the primary source. See the Glossary for the list of designated equivalent sources.*

   Note 2: *A primary source of verified information may designate to an agency the role of communicating credentials information. The designated agency then becomes acceptable to be used as a primary source.*

   Note 3: *An external organization (for example, a credentials verification organization [CVO]) or a Joint Commission–accredited health care organization functioning as a CVO may be used to collect credentialing information. Both of these* *organizations must meet the CVO guidelines listed in the Glossary.*

Note 4: *When it is not possible to obtain information from the primary source, reliable secondary sources may be used. A reliable secondary source could be another health care organization that has documented primary source verification of the applicant's credentials.*

4. All licensed independent practitioners that provide care possess a current license, certification, or registration, as required by law and regulation. **R**

5. Ⓓ Before granting initial, renewed, or revised privileges and at the time of licensure expiration, the organization documents required current licensure of a licensed independent practitioner using primary sources, if available.

    Note 1: *A primary source of verified information may designate to an agency the role of communicating credentials information. The designated agency then becomes acceptable to be used as a primary source.*

    Note 2: *An external organization (for example, a credentials verification organization [CVO]) or a Joint Commission–accredited health care organization functioning as a CVO may be used to collect credentialing information. Both of these organizations must meet the CVO guidelines listed in the Glossary.*

    Note 3: *Verification of current licensure with the primary source through a secure electronic communication or by telephone is acceptable if this verification is documented.*

6. Ⓓ Before granting initial, renewed, or revised privileges to a licensed independent practitioner, the organization's leadership documents current evidence, which includes peer and/or faculty recommendations, of the individual's ability to perform the privileges requested.

7. Before granting renewed or revised privileges to a licensed independent practitioner, the organization does the following:
    - Reviews information from any of its performance improvement activities pertaining to professional performance, judgment, and clinical or technical skills.
    - Evaluates the results of any peer review of the individual's clinical performance.
    - Reviews any clinical performance in the organization that is outside acceptable standards.

Before granting initial, renewed, revised, or temporary privileges to a licensed independent practitioner, leadership evaluates the following:

10. Ⓓ The applicant's written statement that no health problems exist that could affect their ability to perform the requested privileges.

    Note: *Organizations should consider the applicability of the Americans with Disabilities Act to their credentialing and privileging activities, and, if applicable, review their policies and procedures. In addition, federal entities are required to comply with the Rehabilitation Act of 1974.*

11. Before granting initial, renewed, or revised privileges to a licensed independent practitioner, leadership evaluates the following:
    - Any challenges to licensure or registration

    Note: *The challenges addressed here are those that are in the process of an active investigation by the state licensing board.*
    - Any voluntary and involuntary relinquishment of license or registration
    - Any voluntary and involuntary termination of medical staff membership at another organization.
    - Any voluntary or involuntary limitation, reduction, or loss of clinical privileges
    - Any professional liability actions that resulted in a final judgment against the applicant
    - Information from the National Practitioner Data Bank
    - Whether the requested privileges are consistent with the population served by the organization
    - Whether the requested privileges are consistent with the site-specific care, treatment, or services provided by the organization

19. Before granting renewed or revised privileges to a licensed independent practitioner, the organization confirms the licensed independent practitioner's adherence to organization policies, procedures, rules, and regulations.

20. The organization uses current, written, privileging information as the basis for granting or denying all privileges for licensed independent practitioners.

21. The organization grants initial, renewed, or revised privileges for no longer than a two-year period.

24. Ⓓ The organization notifies the requesting practitioner about the decision to

grant, renew, or deny requested privileges. The notification may be in either written or electronic format.

25. The scope and content of patient services provided by a licensed independent practitioner is limited to the granted initial, renewed, or revised privileges. **R**

27. **For organizations providing telemedicine services to patients at a hospital:** Before granting renewed or revised privileges, leaders do the following:
    - Evaluate the comparison of relevant practitioner-specific data to aggregate data
    - Evaluate morbidity and mortality data

    Note: *Leaders chosen to evaluate credentialing and privileging information of a licensed independent practitioner who provides services through a telemedical link should, whenever possible, represent disciplines and expertise consistent with the privileges being sought.*

29. **For organizations providing telemedicine services to patients at a hospital:** The organization obtains peer recommendations from practitioners who are in the same professional discipline as the applicant requesting privileges and who have personal knowledge of the applicant's ability to practice.

30. **For organizations providing telemedicine services to patients at a hospital:** Peer recommendations for applicants requesting privileges include information on the applicant's relevant training and experience, current competence, and health status.

31. **For ambulatory surgical centers that elect to use The Joint Commission deemed status option:** Medical staff members are legally and professionally qualified for the positions to which they are appointed.

32. **For ambulatory surgical centers that elect to use The Joint Commission deemed status option:** Medical staff members are legally and professionally qualified to perform the privileges granted.

33. **For ambulatory surgical centers that elect to use The Joint Commission deemed status option:** Physicians who perform surgery in the ambulatory surgical center have been granted clinical privileges to do so by the ambulatory surgical center's governing body.

34. **For ambulatory surgical centers that elect to use The Joint Commission deemed status option:** Medical staff are accountable to the governing body.

35. Ⓓ Before granting initial or revised privileges to physicians responsible for interpreting sleep studies, the organization verifies that they have at least one of the following qualifications:

   - Certification in Sleep Medicine by the American Board of Sleep Medicine (ABSM) or by a member board of either the American Board of Medical Specialties (ABMS) or the American Osteopathic Association (AOA)
   - A completed fellowship in sleep medicine through an Accreditation Council for Graduate Medical Education (ACGME)–accredited program. Following the completed fellowship, certification in sleep medicine is completed within two examination cycles through the American Board of Sleep Medicine (ABSM) or a member board of either the American Board of Medical Specialties (ABMS) or the American Osteopathic Association (AOA).

Standard HR.02.01.05

The organization may grant temporary privileges.

Elements of Performance for HR.02.01.05

1. The organization follows a process for granting temporary privileges to licensed independent practitioners new to the organization or to meet important patient needs.

2. Ⓓ Before the organization grants temporary privileges either to a licensed independent practitioner new to the organization or to meet important patient needs, the organization does the following:

   - Uses primary source verification to document current licensure
   - Uses primary source verification to document current competency
   - Uses primary source verification to document the individual's training
   - Evaluates practitioner-specific information from the National Practitioner Data Bank
   - Evaluates any involuntary termination of medical staff membership at another organization
   - Evaluates any voluntary or involuntary limitation, reduction, or loss of clinical privileges

   Note 1: *A primary source of verified information may designate to an agency the role of communicating credentials information. The designated agency then becomes acceptable to be used as a primary source.*

   Note 2: *An external organization (for example, a credentials verification*

*organization [CVO]) or a Joint Commission–accredited health care organization
functioning as a CVO may be used to collect credentialing information. Both of these
organizations must meet the CVO guidelines listed in the Glossary.*

9. The administrator or the administrator's designee grants temporary privileges
    either to licensed independent practitioners new to the organization or to meet
    important patient needs upon recommendation of clinical leadership or the
    medical director.

10. Temporary privileges for licensed independent practitioners new to the organiza-
    tion do not exceed 120 days.

Standard HR.02.02.01

The organization provides orientation to licensed independent practitioners.

Elements of Performance for HR.02.02.01

1. Ⓓ The organization orients its licensed independent practitioners to key safety
    content it identifies before they provide care, treatment, or services. Completion
    of this orientation is documented.

    Note: *Key safety content may include specific processes and procedures related to the
    provision of care, the environment of care, and infection control.*

3. Ⓓ The organization orients licensed independent practitioners on the following:
    - Relevant policies and procedures
    - Their specific responsibilities, including those related to infection prevention
      and control and assessing and managing pain
    - Sensitivity to cultural diversity based on their specific responsibilities

    Completion of this orientation is documented.

Standard HR.02.03.01

The organization has a fair hearing and appeal process for addressing adverse
credentialing and privileging decisions.

Elements of Performance for HR.02.03.01

1. The organization has a fair hearing and appeal process that includes the
    following:
    - Allows the scheduling of hearings and appeals
    - Identifies the procedures for hearings and appeals
    - Defines the composition of the hearing committee

■ Allows adverse decisions to be appealed

6. The organization consistently applies its fair hearing and appeal process.

Standard HR.02.04.01

For organizations providing telemedicine services to patients at a hospital:
Leadership implements a process to identify and manage matters of individual health or impairment for licensed independent practitioners that is separate from actions taken for disciplinary purposes.

Elements of Performance for HR.02.04.01

1. **For organizations providing telemedicine services to patients at a hospital:** The organization educates staff and licensed independent practitioners about how to recognize risk criteria for illness and impairment in licensed independent practitioners.

2. **For organizations providing telemedicine services to patients at a hospital:** The organization has a process for licensed independent practitioners to refer themselves for evaluation, diagnosis, and treatment of illness or impairment.

3. **For organizations providing telemedicine services to patients at a hospital:** The organization has a process for staff and licensed independent practitioners to confidentially report concerns about a perceived illness or impairment of a licensed independent practitioner.

4. **For organizations providing telemedicine services to patients at a hospital:** The organization has a process to refer licensed independent practitioners who have an illness or impairment to internal or external professional resources for evaluation, diagnosis, and treatment of the concern or condition.

5. **For organizations providing telemedicine services to patients at a hospital:** The organization has a process to protect the confidentiality of a licensed independent practitioner who seeks a referral or who is referred for assistance, except as limited by applicable law, ethical obligation, or when the health and safety of a patient is threatened.

6. **For organizations providing telemedicine services to patients at a hospital:** The organization has a process to evaluate the credibility of a complaint, allegation, or concern about the possible illness or impairment of a licensed independent practitioner.

7. **For organizations providing telemedicine services to patients at a hospital:**
The organization has a process to monitor the licensed independent practitioner receiving treatment and the safety of their patients until treatment is completed and, if required, periodically thereafter.

8. **For organizations providing telemedicine services to patients at a hospital:**
The organization has a process for staff and licensed independent practitioners to report to leadership instances in which a licensed independent practitioner is providing unsafe care.

9. **For organizations providing telemedicine services to patients at a hospital:**
Leadership has a process to initiate appropriate action if a licensed independent practitioner fails to complete required treatment.

Standard HR.02.04.03

For organizations providing telemedicine services to patients at a hospital: The organization has a process for focused review of a licensed independent practitioner's performance.

Elements of Performance for HR.02.04.03

1. **For organizations providing telemedicine services to patients at a hospital:**
The organization defines the special circumstances requiring a focused review of a licensed independent practitioner's performance.

2. **For organizations providing telemedicine services to patients at a hospital:**
The organization's leaders are involved in the focused review process.

3. **For organizations providing telemedicine services to patients at a hospital:**
The focused review process includes a method for selecting focused review panels.

4. **For organizations providing telemedicine services to patients at a hospital:**
The focused review process includes time frames for conducting focused review activities.

5. **For organizations providing telemedicine services to patients at a hospital:**
The focused review process includes the circumstances that require external peer review.

6. **For organizations providing telemedicine services to patients at a hospital:**
The focused review process includes evaluation of clinical privileges for individuals whose performance is under review.

2022 Standards for Ambulatory Care

7. **For organizations providing telemedicine services to patients at a hospital:** The focused review process includes provisions for participation by the licensed independent practitioner whose performance is being reviewed.

8. **For organizations providing telemedicine services to patients at a hospital:** The focused review process includes communicating to the appropriate parties the findings, recommendations, and any actions taken to improve practitioner performance.

9. **For organizations providing telemedicine services to patients at a hospital:** The organization follows its focused review process.

Standard HR.03.01.01

For organizations that elect The Joint Commission Primary Care Medical Home option: Qualified individuals serve in the role of primary care clinician.

Elements of Performance for HR.03.01.01

1. **For organizations that elect The Joint Commission Primary Care Medical Home option:** Primary care clinicians have the educational background and broad-based knowledge and experience necessary to handle most medical and other health care needs of the patients who selected them. This includes resolving conflicting recommendations for care. A primary care clinician is a doctor of medicine or doctor of osteopathy, or an advanced practice nurse or physician assistant practicing in collaboration with a doctor of medicine or doctor of osteopathy. The term "collaboration" in this context means that health care providers work together to meet the needs of the patient. It is not the intent of this requirement to impose additional restrictions on the scope of practice of an advanced practice nurse, nor is it meant to preempt applicable state law. (For more information, refer to Standards HR.01.06.01 and HR.02.01.03)

Infection Prevention and Control (IC)

Overview

When most health care professionals think of infection prevention and control measures, they think of the need to prevent and control hospital–acquired infections. However, the ambulatory care setting has its own needs for infection prevention and control. Even though patients do not generally stay overnight at ambulatory care centers or undergo the kind of extensive care typically received in a hospital or nursing and rehabilitation center, ambulatory care staff do encounter health care–associated infections, sometimes received elsewhere, that need to be controlled.

Certainly, all ambulatory care centers, regardless of location, should be on the lookout for infections. The types of infections they are likely to encounter depend heavily on the specific risks faced by the organization's location, the population it serves, and the services it provides. For example, most ambulatory care centers know to be on the alert for cases of Methicillin-resistant *Staphylococcus aureus* (MRSA) and other multidrug-resistant infections. Ambulatory care centers that serve particular populations, such as those on college campuses, are likely to encounter other types of infections such as sexually transmitted diseases (STDs), while those working with prison populations are likely to encounter patients with acquired immunodeficiency syndrome (AIDS) and tuberculosis. Centers working in low income areas may encounter higher rates of patients with community-acquired infections, while ambulatory care centers working primarily with the elderly are likely to encounter higher rates of pneumonia. Because infection prevention and control is important to all ambulatory care centers, all staff, regardless of position, need to observe proper infection prevention and control techniques at all times.

To help reduce the possibility of acquiring and transmitting an infection, ambulatory care centers should establish a systematic infection prevention and control program. The activities the organization adopts need to be practical and reasonable to follow. No organization wants to jeopardize a patient's health because its infection prevention and control activities are obsolete or too confusing to practice daily. To create a successful program, leadership should have input and lend support. After an effective program is in place, the organization takes measures so that the program operates according to plan and is properly evaluated.

About This Chapter

The processes outlined in the "Infection Prevention and Control" (IC) chapter are applicable to all infections or potential sources of infection that an ambulatory health care practitioner might encounter, including a sudden influx of potentially infectious patients. The standards are designed to assist ambulatory care centers, both large and small, in developing and maintaining an effective program that covers a wide range of situations.

These standards address activities of planning, implementation, and evaluation and are based on the following conditions necessary to establish and operate an effective infection prevention and control program. Every ambulatory care center, regardless of its size or the services it provides, should do the following:

- Recognize that its infection prevention and control program plays a major role in its efforts to improve patient safety and quality of care
- Demonstrate leadership's commitment to infection prevention and control by endorsing and participating in the organization's efforts to control infection, provide resources, and encourage improvement
- See that staff collaborate with each other when designing and implementing the infection prevention and control program
- Regularly assess its infection prevention and control program by using an epidemiological approach that consists of surveillance, data collection, analysis, and trend identification
- Coordinate its program with the larger community
- Take into account that the potential exists for an infection outbreak so extensive that it overwhelms the ambulatory care center's resources

Chapter Outline

I. Planning
   A. Responsibility (IC.01.01.01)
   B. Resources (IC.01.02.01)
   C. Risks (IC.01.03.01)
   D. Goals (IC.01.04.01)
   E. Activities (IC.01.05.01)
   F. Influx (IC.01.06.01)

II. Implementation
   A. Activities (IC.02.01.01)
   B. Medical Equipment, Devices, and Supplies (IC.02.02.01)
   C. Transmission of Infections (IC.02.03.01)
   D. Influenza Vaccinations (IC.02.04.01)
   E. Health Care-Associated Infections (HAI) (IC.02.05.01)

III. Evaluation and Improvement (IC.03.01.01)

Standards, Rationales, and Elements of Performance

Introduction to Standards IC.01.01.01 Through IC.01.06.01 – Planning

For any of the infection prevention and control activities to be effective, they need to be well managed. Toward that end, the ambulatory care center assigns one or more people the responsibility for the development of the activities and their daily implementation. Large, complex ambulatory care centers may want to employ a contractor or consultant. Smaller organizations may do well by simply designating a current employee. Each organization should assess its own needs in this regard. After this person is in place, the work of planning the infection prevention and control activities can begin by gathering staff with knowledge in infection prevention and control and other staff members who can perform a risk assessment and then build activities based upon their risks. The individual responsible for infection prevention and control may want to consult with community leaders and other outside infection control experts who can provide important information about the ambulatory care center's population and associated health risks.

The results of the ambulatory care center's infection risk assessment should be prioritized, ideally in order of level of probability and potential for harm. The organization can then set goals for reducing the risks of the infections that pose the greatest threat to patients and the community. These goals should lead to focused activities, based on relevant professional guidelines and sound practices.

Standard IC.01.01.01 ▬▬▬▬▬▬▬▬▬▬▬▬▬▬▬▬▬▬

The organization identifies the individual(s) responsible for infection prevention and control.

Elements of Performance for IC.01.01.01

3. The organization assigns responsibility for the management of infection prevention and control activities.

   (*See also* HR.01.01.01, EP 1; LD.03.06.01, EP 2)

5. **For ambulatory surgical centers that elect to use The Joint Commission deemed status option:** The infection control program is under the direction of a designated and qualified professional who has training in infection control.

Standard IC.01.02.01

Organization leaders allocate needed resources for infection prevention and control activities.

Elements of Performance for IC.01.02.01

1. The organization provides access to information needed to support infection prevention and control activities.

    (*See also* IM.02.02.03, EP 2)

2. The organization provides for laboratory resources when needed to support infection prevention and control activities.

3. The organization provides equipment and supplies to support infection prevention and control activities.

Standard IC.01.03.01

The organization identifies risks for acquiring and transmitting infections.

Elements of Performance for IC.01.03.01

1. The organization identifies infection risks based on the following:
    - Its geographic location, community, and population served
    - The care, treatment, or services it provides
    - The analysis of its infection surveillance and control data

    (*See also* IC.02.05.01, EP 2)

3. Ⓓ The organization prioritizes the identified risks for acquiring and transmitting infections. These prioritized risks are documented.

    (*See also* IC.02.05.01, EP 2)

Standard IC.01.04.01

Based on the identified risks, the organization sets goals to minimize the possibility of transmitting infections.

Note: See *NPSG.07.01.01 for hand hygiene guidelines.*

Elements of Performance for IC.01.04.01

1. Ⓓ The organization's written infection prevention and control goals include the following:
   - Addressing its prioritized risks
   - Limiting unprotected exposure to pathogens
   - Limiting the transmission of infections associated with procedures
   - Limiting the transmission of infections associated with the use of medical equipment, devices, and supplies
   - Improving compliance with hand hygiene guidelines

   (*See also* NPSG.07.01.01, EP 1)

Standard IC.01.05.01 ━━━━━━━━━━━━━━━━━━━━━━━━━━━

The organization plans for preventing and controlling infections.

Elements of Performance for IC.01.05.01

1. When developing infection prevention and control activities, the organization uses evidence-based national guidelines or, in the absence of such guidelines, expert consensus.
   For ambulatory surgical centers that elect to use The Joint Commission deemed status option: The organization considers, selects, and implements nationally recognized infection control program guidelines. Ⓡ

2. Ⓓ The organization plans infection prevention and control activities, including surveillance, to minimize, reduce, or eliminate the risk of infection. These activities are documented.

5. Ⓓ The organization describes, in writing, the method for investigating outbreaks of infectious disease within the organization.

   (*See also* IC.02.01.01, EP 5)

6. Everyone who works in the organization has responsibilities for preventing and controlling infection.

9. Ⓓ **For ambulatory surgical centers that elect to use The Joint Commission deemed status option:** The organization plans infection prevention and control activities, including surveillance, to minimize, reduce, or eliminate the risk of infection and communicable diseases. These activities are documented.

11. **For ambulatory surgical centers that elect to use The Joint Commission deemed status option:** The infection control program includes a plan of action for preventing, identifying, and managing infections and communicable diseases and for immediately implementing corrective and preventive measures that result in improvement.

Standard IC.01.06.01 ━━━━━━━━━━━━━━━━━━━━━━━━━

The organization prepares to respond to an influx of potentially infectious patients.

Elements of Performance for IC.01.06.01

2. The organization obtains current clinical and epidemiological information from its resources regarding new infections that could cause an influx of potentially infectious patients.

3. The organization has a method for communicating critical information to licensed independent practitioners and staff about emerging infections that could cause an influx of potentially infectious patients.

4. ⒟ The organization describes, in writing, how it will respond to an influx of potentially infectious patients.

    Note: *One acceptable response is to decide not to accept patients.*

    (*See also* EM.01.01.01, EP 2)

Introduction to Standards IC.02.01.01 Through IC.02.03.01 – Implementation

Infection prevention and control activities should be practical and involve collaboration between staff. Everyone who works in the organization should have a role and hold each other accountable. Important infection prevention and control information should be available to both staff and patients. Standard and transmission-based precautions should be used, and any outbreak of infection within the organization should be investigated.

Standard IC.02.01.01

The organization implements infection prevention and control activities.

Elements of Performance for IC.02.01.01

1. The organization implements its planned infection prevention and control activities and practices, including surveillance, to reduce the risk of infection. **R**

2. The organization uses standard precautions,* including the use of personal protective equipment, to reduce the risk of infection. **R**

   Note: *Standard precautions are infection prevention and control measures to protect against possible exposure to infectious agents. These precautions are general and applicable to all patients.*

   (*See also* EC.02.02.01, EP 3)

3. The organization implements transmission-based precautions† in response to the pathogens that are suspected or identified within the organization's service setting and community. **R**

   Note: *Transmission-based precautions are infection prevention and control measures to protect against exposure to a suspected or identified pathogen. These precautions are specific and based on the way the pathogen is transmitted. Categories include contact, droplet, airborne, or a combination of these precautions.*

5. The organization investigates outbreaks of infectious disease within the organization. **R**

   (*See also* IC.01.05.01, EP 5)

6. The organization minimizes the risk of infection when storing and disposing of infectious waste.

   (*See also* EC.02.02.01, EP 12)

---

* For further information regarding standard precautions, refer to the website of the Centers for Disease Control and Prevention (CDC) at https://www.cdc.gov/hicpac/recommendations/core-practices.html (Infection Control in Healthcare Settings).
† For further information regarding transmission-based precautions, refer to the website of the Centers for Disease Control and Prevention (CDC) at http://www.cdc.gov/hai/ (Infection Control in Healthcare Settings).

7. The organization implements its methods to communicate responsibilities for preventing and controlling infection to licensed independent practitioners, staff, visitors, patients, and families. Information for visitors, patients, and families includes hand and respiratory hygiene practices. **R**

    Note: *Information may be provided via different forms of media, such as posters or pamphlets.*

8. The organization reports infection surveillance, prevention, and control information to the appropriate staff within the organization. **R**

9. The organization reports infection surveillance, prevention, and control information to local, state, and federal public health authorities in accordance with law and regulation. **R**

10. When the organization becomes aware that it transferred a patient who has an infection requiring monitoring, treatment, and/or isolation, it informs the receiving organization.

11. When the organization becomes aware that it received a patient from another organization who has an infection requiring action, and the infection was not communicated by the referring organization, it informs the referring organization.

    Note: *Infections requiring action include those that require isolation and/or public health reporting or those that may aid in the referring organization's surveillance.*

Standard IC.02.02.01 ━━━━━━━━━━━━━━━━

The organization reduces the risk of infections associated with medical equipment, devices, and supplies.

Rationale for IC.02.02.01

The Centers for Disease Control and Prevention (CDC) estimate that 46.5 million surgical procedures are performed in hospitals and ambulatory settings each year; this includes approximately 5 million gastrointestinal endoscopies.[‡] Each of these procedures involves contact with a medical device or surgical instrument. A major risk of all such procedures is the introduction of pathogens that can lead to infection. In addition, many more people are at risk of developing an infection from contact with medical equipment, devices, or supplies while seeking other health services. Failure to properly clean, disinfect, or sterilize, and use or store medical equipment, devices, and supplies, not only poses risks for the person seeking health services, but also carries the risk for person-to-person transmission of infections.

There are numerous steps involved in the cleaning, disinfecting, and sterilizing of medical equipment, devices, and supplies. It is critical that health care workers follow standardized practices to minimize infection risks related to medical equipment, devices, and supplies. In order to maintain a reliable system for controlling this process, organizations pay attention to the following:

- Orientation, training, and competency of health care workers who are processing medical equipment, devices, and supplies
- Levels of staffing and supervision of the health care workers who are processing medical equipment, devices, and supplies
- Standardization of process regardless of whether it is centralized or decentralized
- Reinforcing the process (for example, the use of placards which list the steps to be followed, according to manufacturer's guidelines)
- Ongoing quality monitoring

Elements of Performance for IC.02.02.01

The organization implements infection prevention and control activities when doing the following:

1. Cleaning and performing low-level disinfection of medical equipment, devices, and supplies.[§] **R**

[‡] https://www.cdc.gov/infectioncontrol/guidelines/disinfection/introduction.html
[§] For further information regarding cleaning and performing low-level disinfection of medical equipment, devices, and supplies, refer to the website of the Centers for Disease Control and Prevention (CDC) at https://www.cdc.gov/infectioncontrol/guidelines/disinfection/#r3.

Note: *Low-level disinfection is used for items such as stethoscopes and blood glucose meters. Additional cleaning and disinfecting is required for medical equipment, devices, and supplies used by patients who are isolated as part of implementing transmission-based precautions.*

2. Performing intermediate and high-level disinfection and sterilization of medical equipment, devices, and supplies.^{||} **R**

    Note: *Sterilization is used for items such as implants and surgical instruments. High-level disinfection may also be used if sterilization is not possible, as is the case with flexible endoscopes.*

(*See also* EC.02.04.03, EP 4)

3. Disposing of medical equipment, devices, and supplies. **R**

4. Storing medical equipment, devices, and supplies. **R**

5. When reprocessing single-use devices, the organization implements infection prevention and control activities that are consistent with regulatory and professional standards. **R**

Standard IC.02.03.01

The organization works to prevent the transmission of infectious disease among patients, licensed independent practitioners, and staff.

Elements of Performance for IC.02.03.01

1. The organization makes screening for exposure and/or immunity to infectious disease available to licensed independent practitioners and staff who may come in contact with infections at the workplace.

2. When licensed independent practitioners or staff have, are suspected of having, or have been occupationally exposed to an infectious disease that puts others at risk, the organization provides them with or refers them for assessment and potential testing, prophylaxis/treatment, or counseling.

---

^{||} For further information regarding performing intermediate and high-level disinfection of medical equipment, devices, and supplies, refer to the website of the Centers for Disease Control and Prevention (CDC) at https://www.cdc.gov/infectioncontrol/guidelines/disinfection/#r3 (Sterilization and Disinfection in Healthcare Settings).

4. When patients have been exposed to an infectious disease, the organization provides them with or refers them for assessment and potential testing, prophylaxis/treatment, or counseling.

Introduction to Standard IC.02.04.01

Influenza vaccination for staff and licensed independent practitioners is a major safety issue in the United States. Unvaccinated individuals who become infected are contagious at least one day before any signs or symptoms of influenza appear, and therefore these individuals can infect others without knowing they are contagious. Both government and professional organizations emphasize increasing safety to those receiving health care by decreasing their exposure to the influenza virus while receiving this care. One way to improve patient safety is for staff and licensed independent practitioners to receive the influenza vaccination annually. According to the Centers for Disease Control and Prevention, vaccination is an effective preventive measure against influenza and can prevent many illnesses, deaths, and losses in productivity. Health care staff are considered a high priority for expanding influenza vaccine use. Achieving and sustaining high influenza vaccination coverage among health care staff is intended to help protect staff and patients and reduce disease burden and health care costs (*see* https://www.cdc.gov/nhsn/acute-care-hospital/hcp-vaccination/index.html and https://www.cdc.gov/infectioncontrol/guidelines/healthcare-personnel/index.html).

The Joint Commission's Standard IC.02.04.01 reflects current science and the national focus on influenza vaccination. It requires that each organization has an influenza vaccination program and that the influenza vaccination is offered to staff and licensed independent practitioners. However, The Joint Commission does not mandate influenza vaccination for licensed independent practitioners and staff as a condition of Joint Commission accreditation. In addition, The Joint Commission does not require accredited organizations to pay for the influenza vaccination for its licensed independent practitioners and staff. The decision on whether to pay for the influenza vaccination for staff and licensed independent practitioners will need to be made independently by each accredited organization.

Standard IC.02.04.01 ━━━━━━━━━━━━━━━━━━━━━━━━━━━━━━━

The organization offers vaccination against influenza to licensed independent practitioners and staff.

Note: *This standard is applicable to staff and licensed independent practitioners only when care, treatment, or services are provided on site. When care, treatment, or services are provided off site, such as with telemedicine or telephone consultation, this standard is not applicable to off-site staff and licensed independent practitioners.*

Elements of Performance for IC.02.04.01

1. The organization establishes an annual influenza vaccination program that is offered to licensed independent practitioners and staff.

2. The organization educates licensed independent practitioners and staff about, at a minimum, the influenza vaccine; non-vaccine control and prevention measures; and the diagnosis, transmission, and impact of influenza.

3. The organization offers the influenza vaccination on site to licensed independent practitioners and staff or facilitates their obtaining the influenza vaccination off site.

4. Ⓓ The organization includes in its infection control plan the goal of improving influenza vaccination rates. (For more information, refer to Standard IC.01.04.01.)

6. Ⓓ The organization has a written description of the methodology used to determine influenza vaccination rates.

    Note: *The Centers for Disease Control and Prevention's National Healthcare Safety Network provides influenza vaccination reporting and protocol guidance at https:// www.cdc.gov/nhsn/faqs/vaccination/faq-influenza-vaccination-summary-reporting.html and https://www.cdc.gov/nhsn/pdfs/hps-manual/vaccination/hps-flu-vaccine-protocol.pdf.*

7. The organization collects and reviews the reasons given by staff and licensed independent practitioners for declining the influenza vaccination. This collection and review occur at least annually.

8. Ⓓ The organization improves its vaccination rates according to its established, internal goals at least annually. (For more information, refer to Standards PI.02.01.01 and PI.03.01.01.)

9. The organization provides influenza vaccination rate data to organization leaders at least annually.

Standard IC.02.05.01 ━━━━━━━━━━━━━

Implement evidence-based practices to prevent surgical site infections.

Elements of Performance for IC.02.05.01

1. The organization develops policies and practices based on evidence and implements these policies and practices aimed at reducing the risk for surgical site infections.

2. The organization implements processes as indicated by periodic risk assessments (in time frames defined by the organization) for prevention of surgical site infections.

    Note: *Surveillance may be targeted rather than organizationwide.*

    (*See also* IC.01.03.01, EPs 1, 3)

3. The organization measures and monitors its infection prevention processes, outcomes, and compliance using evidence-based guidelines or best practices for surgical site infections.

    Note: *Surveillance may be targeted rather than organizationwide.*

Introduction to Standard IC.03.01.01— Evaluation and Improvement

Evaluation and improvement of the infection prevention and control activities are important steps in the ambulatory care center's efforts to control and prevent infection. Infection prevention and control practices should become a routine part of the care, treatment, or services the ambulatory care center provides to patients. They expect and deserve hygienic and safe care even if their contact with the ambulatory care center does not extend beyond a single visit. Continuous review of the goals, activities, and outcomes of the organization's initiative are therefore followed by improvement activities that are realistic in expectation and, above all, effective.

Standard IC.03.01.01 ━━━━━━━━━━━━━━━━

The organization evaluates the effectiveness of its infection prevention and control activities.

Elements of Performance for IC.03.01.01

1. The organization evaluates its infection prevention and control activities annually and whenever risks significantly change. The evaluation includes a review of the following:

   ■ The infection prevention and control prioritized risks
   ■ The infection prevention and control goals
   ■ Implementation of infection prevention and control activities
   ■ Outcomes of infection prevention and control activities

   (*See also* NPSG.07.01.01, EP 2)

6. Findings from the evaluation are communicated at least annually to the individuals or interdisciplinary group that manages the patient safety program.

7. The organization uses the findings of the evaluation when revising the prioritized risks, goals, and activities for preventing and controlling infection.

Information Management (IM)

Overview

Every episode of care generates health information that must be managed systematically by the organization. All data and information used by the organization are categorized, filed, and maintained. The system should accurately capture health information generated by the delivery of care, treatment, or services. Health information should be accessed by authorized users who will use health information to provide safe, quality care. Unauthorized access can be limited by the adoption of policies that address the privacy, security, and integrity of health information.

Depending on the type of organization, the system used for information management may be basic or sophisticated. As technology develops, many organizations find their information management systems in a state of transition from paper to fully electronic or a combination of the two. Regardless of the type of system used, these standards are designed to be equally compatible with noncomputerized systems and evolving technologies.

About This Chapter

As with other chapters, planning is the initial focus of "Information Management" (IM). A well-planned system meets the internal and external information needs of the organization with efficiency and accuracy. Planning provides for continuity in the event that the organization's operations are disrupted or fail. The organization also plans to protect the privacy, security, and integrity of the data and information it collects, which results in preserving confidentiality. The chapter concludes with a standard on maintaining accurate health information.

Requirements in this chapter apply to all types of information managed by the organization, unless the requirement specifically limits the type of information to health information. Refer to the Glossary for a definition of health information.

Chapter Outline

Standards, Rationales, and Elements of Performance

Introduction to Standard IM.01.01.01

Planning is the most critical part of the organization's information management process and requires the collaborative involvement of all levels and areas of the organization. The organization's plan for information management considers the full spectrum of data generated and used by the organization; financial data, human resources data, supply inventories, and health information are examples of the different types of data that are considered in the information management planning process. Planning for the management of information does not necessarily result in a single, comprehensive written information management plan; however, planning does establish clear relationships between the organization's needs and its goals. In addition to the organization's goals, the organization's mission, services, staff, patient safety practices, modes of service delivery, resources, and technology are considered during the information management planning process.

The flow of information within the organization, as well as to and from external organizations, is another important consideration for information management planning. Planning takes into account the data and information required to support relationships with outside providers, services, contractors, purchasers, and payers. By identifying internal and external information needs, organizations can make information available when and where it is needed. Organizations that understand the flow of information can achieve efficient data collection and distribution, along with effective security of health information.

Standard IM.01.01.01 ━━━━━━━━━━━━━━━━━━━━━━━━━━━━━━━━━━━━━━

The organization plans for managing information.

Elements of Performance for IM.01.01.01

2.   The organization identifies how data and information enter, flow within, and leave the organization.

Introduction to Standard IM.01.01.03

The primary goal of the information continuity process is to return the organization to normal operations as soon as possible with minimal downtime and no data loss. The organization needs to be prepared for events that could impact the availability of data and information regardless of whether interruptions are scheduled or unscheduled (due to a local or regional disaster or an emergency). Interruptions to an organization's information system can potentially have a devastating impact on its ability to deliver quality care and continue its business operations. Planning for emergency situations helps the organization mitigate the impact that interruptions, emergencies, and disasters have on its ability to manage information. The organization plans for interruptions by training staff on alternative procedures, testing the organization's Emergency Management Plan, conducting regularly scheduled data backups, and testing data restoration procedures.

Regardless of whether an organization uses a paper-based system or an electronic system, a plan to address the process for information continuity, including knowledge-based information, should be in place. Organizations that plan for maintaining access to electronic information systems by using various electronic backup and restore procedures can quickly recover from interruptions with minimal downtime and data loss.

Standard IM.01.01.03

The organization plans for continuity of its information management processes.

Elements of Performance for IM.01.01.03

1. ⓓ The organization follows a written plan for managing interruptions to its information processes (paper-based, electronic, or a mix of paper-based and electronic).

   (*See also* EM.01.01.01, EP 6)

2. The organization's plan for managing interruptions to information processes addresses the following:
   - Scheduled and unscheduled interruptions of electronic information systems
   - Training for staff and licensed independent practitioners on alternative procedures to follow when electronic information systems are unavailable
   - Backup of electronic information systems

   (*See also* EM.01.01.01, EP 6; IM.03.01.01, EP 1)

5.   Ⓓ **For ambulatory surgical centers that elect to use The Joint Commission deemed status option:** The organization implements a system of medical documentation that preserves patient information during an emergency.

6.   Ⓓ **For rural health clinics and federally qualified health centers:** The organization implements a system of medical documentation that preserves patient information during an emergency.

Introduction to Standard IM.02.01.01

The privacy of health information is a critical information management concern. Privacy of health information applies to electronic, paper, and verbal communications. Protecting the privacy of health information is the responsibility of the entire organization. Organizations protect privacy by limiting the use of information to only what is needed to provide care, treatment, or services.

Privacy, along with security, results in the confidentiality of health information. Health information is kept confidential when the information is secure and its use is limited. The end result of protecting the privacy and security of health information is the preservation of confidentiality. To illustrate this relationship, confidentiality is violated in situations when a patient's health information is used, accessed, or disclosed to an individual who does not have permission to access the information or when an individual uses a patient's health information for purposes outside of delivering care, treatment, or services. A confidentiality violation occurs when an individual is able to bypass privacy and security measures to gain access to health information. The organization's written policy on the privacy of health information can assist the organization to maintain the confidentiality of health information while providing access to appropriate care providers.

Note: *For additional guidance about limiting the use of information, refer to 45 CFR 164.502(b) and 164.514(d) under "Minimum Necessary" within the Health Insurance Portability and Accountability Act of 1996 (HIPAA).*

Standard IM.02.01.01 ▬▬▬▬▬▬▬

The organization protects the privacy of health information.

Elements of Performance for IM.02.01.01

1.   Ⓓ The organization follows a written policy addressing the privacy of health

information.

Note: *For ambulatory surgical centers that elect to use The Joint Commission deemed status option: The organization must comply with Section 45 of the Code of Federal Regulations parts 160 and 164, generally known as the Health Insurance Portability and Accountability Act (HIPAA) Privacy and Security Rules.*

(*See also* RI.01.01.01, EP 7)

3. The organization uses health information only for purposes permitted by law and regulation or as further limited by its policy on privacy.

    Note: *For ambulatory surgical centers that elect to use The Joint Commission deemed status option: The organization must comply with Section 45 of the Code of Federal Regulations parts 160 and 164, generally known as the Health Insurance Portability and Accountability Act (HIPAA) Privacy and Security Rules.*

    (*See also* MM.01.01.01, EP 1; RI.01.01.01, EP 7)

4. The organization discloses health information only as authorized by the patient or as otherwise consistent with law and regulation.

    Note: *For ambulatory surgical centers that elect to use The Joint Commission deemed status option: The organization must comply with Section 45 of the Code of Federal Regulations parts 160 and 164, generally known as the Health Insurance Portability and Accountability Act (HIPAA) Privacy and Security Rules.*

    (*See also* RI.01.01.01, EP 7)

Introduction to Standard IM.02.01.03

The security and integrity of health information are closely related. Health information is collected and processed through various information sources and systems throughout the organization. As a result, breaches in security can lead to the unauthorized disclosure or alteration of health information. When this occurs, the integrity of the data and information is compromised. Even simple mistakes, such as writing the incorrect date of a service or diagnosis, can undermine data integrity just as easily as intentional breaches. For these reasons, an examination of the use of paper and electronic information systems is considered in the organization's approach to maintaining the security and integrity of health information. Regardless of the type of system, security measures should address the use of security levels, passwords, and other forms of controlled access. Because information technology and its associated security measures are continuously changing, the organization should do its best to stay informed about technological developments and best practices that can help it improve information security and therefore protect data integrity.

Monitoring access to health information systems can help organizations be vigilant about protecting health information security. Regular security audits can identify system vulnerabilities in addition to security policy violations. For example, as part of the process, the organization could identify system users who have altered, edited, or deleted information. The results from this audit process can be used to validate that user permissions are appropriately set. Conducting security audits can be particularly effective in identifying when employee turnover causes vulnerabilities in security because user access and permissions were not removed or updated.

Standard IM.02.01.03

The organization maintains the security and integrity of health information.

Elements of Performance for IM.02.01.03

1. Ⓓ The organization follows a written policy that addresses the security of health information, including access, use, and disclosure.

   Note: *For ambulatory surgical centers that elect to use The Joint Commission deemed status option: The organization must comply with Section 45 of the Code of Federal Regulations parts 160 and 164, generally known as the Health Insurance Portability and Accountability Act (HIPAA) Privacy and Security Rules.*

2. Ⓓ The organization implements a written policy addressing the following:
   - The integrity of health information against loss, damage, unauthorized alteration, unintentional change, and accidental destruction
   - The intentional destruction of health information
   - When and by whom the removal of health information is permitted

   Note: *Removal refers to those actions that place health information outside the organization's control.*

5. The organization protects against unauthorized access, use, and disclosure of health information.

   Note: *For ambulatory surgical centers that elect to use The Joint Commission deemed status option: The organization must comply with Section 45 of the Code*

of Federal Regulations parts 160 and 164, generally known as the Health Insurance
Portability and Accountability Act (HIPAA) Privacy and Security Rules.

6.   The organization protects health information against loss, damage, unauthorized
      alteration, unintentional change, and accidental destruction.

7.   The organization controls the intentional destruction of health information.

Standard IM.02.02.01

The organization effectively manages the collection of health information.

Rationale for IM.02.02.01

Within the organization, health information can come from multiple sources. The use
of standardized formats and terminology can help clarify information that is used by
different individuals for various purposes. Capturing data in standardized language can
lead to greater data integrity and reliability, as well as an increased potential for ease of
use by internal and external systems and users. The more consistent the organization's
efforts are to capture accurate data in standardized language, the more likely the
organization will be to rely on that data for patient-related purposes, including
reimbursement, risk management, performance improvement, and infection surveillance.

Elements of Performance for IM.02.02.01

2.   Ⓓ The organization uses standardized terminology, definitions, abbreviations,
      acronyms, symbols, and dose designations.

3.   The organization follows its list of prohibited abbreviations, acronyms, symbols,
      and dose designations, which includes the following:
      - U,u
      - IU
      - Q.D., QD, q.d., qd
      - Q.O.D., QOD, q.o.d, qod
      - Trailing zero (X.0 mg)
      - Lack of leading zero (.X mg)
      - MS
      - MSO_4
      - $MgSO_4$

      Note 1: *A trailing zero may be used only when required to demonstrate the level of
      precision of the value being reported, such as for laboratory results, imaging studies*

that report the size of lesions, or catheter/tube sizes. It may not be used in medication orders or other medication-related documentation.

Note 2: *The prohibited list applies to all orders, preprinted forms, and medication-related documentation. Medication-related documentation can be either handwritten or electronic.*

Introduction to Standard IM.02.02.03

Standardizing the collection of data, a concept that is supported by the requirements of Standard IM.02.02.03, helps with the effective dissemination of data and information. Consistency in data collection systems (paper-based, electronic, or a combination) creates the foundation for retrieving and disseminating data and information in the most useful format. For information about data collection and dissemination, visit the websites of the Office of the National Coordinator for Health Information Technology (ONC) (http://www.healthit.gov/) and the Certification Commission for Healthcare Information Technology (CCHIT) (http://www.cchit.org).

Standard IM.02.02.03 ▄▄▄▄▄▄▄▄▄▄▄▄▄▄▄▄▄▄▄▄▄▄▄▄▄▄▄▄▄▄▄▄▄

The organization retrieves, disseminates, and transmits health information in useful formats.

Rationale for IM.02.02.03

The ease of use of health information between systems and users contributes to its potential usefulness within the organization and for external reporting purposes. Data stored in different formats cannot easily be converted to a new format or transferred to other organizations or providers. For example, immediate access to infection control data can impact patient safety within the organization and outside of the organization. As more organizations automate various processes and activities, these systems need to allow for transmitting and receiving critical data while maintaining data integrity.

Elements of Performance for IM.02.02.03

2. The organization's storage and retrieval systems make health information accessible when needed for patient care, treatment, or services.

    (*See also* IC.01.02.01, EP 1)

3. The organization disseminates data and information in useful formats within

time frames that are defined by the organization and consistent with law and regulation.

13. **For organizations in California that provide computed tomography (CT) services:** The organization complies with radiation event reporting requirements specified in section 115113 of the California Health and Safety Code.

Standard IM.03.01.01

Knowledge-based information resources are available, current, and authoritative.

Elements of Performance for IM.03.01.01

1. The organization provides access to knowledge-based information resources during hours of operation.

   (*See also* IM.01.01.03, EP 2)

2022
SAC

Leadership (LD)

Leadership (LD)

Overview

The safety and quality of care, treatment, or services depend on many factors, including the following:

- A culture that fosters safety as a priority for everyone who works in the organization
- The planning and provision of services that meet the needs of patients
- The availability of resources—human, financial, and physical—for providing care, treatment, or services
- The recruitment and retention of competent staff and other care providers
- Ongoing evaluation of and improvement in performance

Management of these important functions is the direct responsibility of leaders; they are, in effect, responsible for the care, treatment, or services that the organization provides to its patients. In organizations with a governing body, governance has ultimate responsibility for this oversight. In larger organizations, different individuals or groups may be assigned different responsibilities, and they bring with them different skills, experience, and perspectives. In these situations, the way that the leaders interact with each other and manage their assigned accountabilities can affect overall organization performance. In smaller organizations, these responsibilities may be handled by just one or two individuals. This chapter addresses the role of leaders in managing their diverse and, at times complex, responsibilities.

Leaders shape the organization's culture, and the culture, in turn, affects how the organization accomplishes its work. A healthy, thriving culture is built around the organization's mission and vision, which reflect the core values and principles that the organization finds important. Leaders must ask some basic questions in order to provide this focus: How does the organization plan to meet the needs of its populations? By what ethical standards will the organization operate? What does the organization want to accomplish through its work? Once leaders answer these questions, the culture of the organization will begin to take shape. Leaders also have an obligation to set an example of how to work together to fulfill the organization's mission.

On a more practical level, leaders oversee operations and guide the organization on a day-to-day basis. They keep operations running smoothly so that the important work of the organization—serving its patients—can continue.

To meet their obligations effectively, leaders must collaborate, which means working together in a spirit of collegiality to achieve a common end. In smaller organizations, this may mean that a single leader or small group of leaders works closely with staff in order to meet the organization's managerial needs. In this case, key staff members share governance and decision making with senior leadership in order to direct the day-to-day operations, assess needs, secure resources, and plan for the future. Senior managers direct the day-to-day operations of the organization; governance determines what resources the organization needs and then secures those resources.

Proactive Risk Assessment

By undertaking a proactive risk assessment, an organization can correct process problems and reduce the likelihood of experiencing adverse events. An organization can use a proactive risk assessment to evaluate a process to see how it could fail, to understand the consequences of such a failure, and to identify parts of the process that need improvement. The term "process" applies broadly to processes that are integral to patient care, such as diagnostic procedures or physical therapy.

Proactive risk assessments are useful for analyzing new processes before they are implemented. Processes need to be designed with a focus on quality and reliability to achieve desired outcomes and protect patients. Proactive risk assessments are also used to evaluate existing processes that have the greatest potential for affecting patient safety. An organization's choice of which process it will assess may be based in part on information published periodically by The Joint Commission about frequently occurring sentinel events and processes that pose high risk to patients.

A proactive risk assessment increases understanding within the organization about the complexities of process design and management of circumstances if the process fails. If an adverse event occurs, the organization may be able to use the information gained from the prior risk assessment to minimize the consequences of the event—and to avoid simply reacting to it.

Although there are several methods that could be used to conduct a proactive risk assessment, the following steps make up one approach:
1. Describe the chosen process (for example, through a flowchart).
2. Identify ways in which the process could break down or fail to perform its desired functions, which is often referred to as failure mode.
3. Identify the possible effects that a breakdown or failure of the process could have on patients and the seriousness of the possible effects.

4. Prioritize the potential process breakdowns or failures.
5. Determine why the prioritized breakdowns or failures could occur, which may involve performing a hypothetical root cause analysis.
6. Design or redesign the process and/or underlying systems to minimize risk of the effects on patients.
7. Test and implement the newly designed or redesigned process.
8. Monitor the effectiveness of the newly designed or redesigned process.

About This Chapter

This chapter is divided into four sections: Leadership Structure, Leadership Relationships, Organization Culture and System Performance Expectations, and Operations. The organization's culture, systems, and leadership structure and relationships all come together to shape and drive its operations.

The standards in the Leadership Structure section identify and define the various leadership groups and their responsibilities. The standards in Leadership Relationships address the development of the organization's mission, vision, and goals, as well as communication among leaders. The standards in the Organization Culture and System Performance Expectations section focus on the framework for the organization's culture and systems. These standards also demonstrate how leaders help shape the culture of an organization and how culture, in turn, affects important systems within the organization (for example, data use, planning, communication, changing performance, staffing). The standards in the Operations section address the functions that are important to patient safety and high-quality care, treatment, or services. Some leaders may not be directly involved in the day-to-day operations of the organization, but the decisions they make and the initiatives they implement do affect operations.

Chapter Outline

I. Leadership Structure
    A. Leadership Structure (LD.01.01.01)
    B. Governance Accountabilities (LD.01.03.01)
    C. The Chief Executive Responsibilities (LD.01.04.01)
    D. Leaders' Knowledge (LD.01.07.01)

II. Leadership Relationships
    A. Mission, Vision, and Goals (LD.02.01.01)
    B. Communication Among Leaders (LD.02.03.01)

III. Organization Culture and System Performance Expectations
    A. Culture of Safety and Quality (LD.03.01.01)
    B. Using Data and Information (LD.03.02.01)
    C. Organizationwide Planning (LD.03.03.01)
    D. Communication (LD.03.04.01)
    E. Change Management and Performance Improvement (LD.03.05.01)
    F. Staffing (LD.03.06.01)
    G. Priorities for Performance Improvement (LD.03.07.01)
    H. Service/Process Design (LD.03.08.01)
    I. Safety Program (LD.03.09.01)
    J. Clinical Practice Guidelines (LD.03.10.01)

IV. Operations
    A. Administration (LD.04.01.01, LD.04.01.03, LD.04.01.05, LD.04.01.07, LD.04.01.11)
    B. Ethical Issues (LD.04.02.01, LD.04.02.03)
    C. Meeting Patient Needs (LD.04.03.01, LD.04.03.07, LD.04.03.09, LD.04.03.13)

Standards, Rationales, and Elements of Performance

Introduction to Leadership Structure, Standards LD.01.01.01 Through LD.01.07.01

Each organization, regardless of its complexity, has a structured leadership. Many leadership responsibilities directly affect the provision of care, treatment, or services, as well as the day-to-day operations of the organization. In some cases, these responsibilities will be shared among leaders, and in other cases, a particular leader has primary responsibility. Individual leaders may have several different roles. Regardless of the organization's structure, it is important that leaders carry out all their responsibilities.

A variety of individuals may work in the organization, including licensed independent practitioners, staff, volunteers, students, and independent contractors. These standards describe the overall responsibility of governance for the safety and quality of care, treatment, or services provided by all of these individuals.

How well leaders work together is key to effective organization performance, and the standards emphasize this. Leaders with different responsibilities—governance, management, and the clinical staff—bring different skills, experiences, and perspectives to the organization. Working together means that leaders have the opportunity to participate in discussions and have their opinions heard. Depending on the topic and the organization, individuals may participate in decision making, and the governing body may delegate decision making to certain leaders. Final decisions, however, are always the ultimate responsibility of governance; this key principle is assumed in any standard that describes how leaders work together.

Standard LD.01.01.01 ▬▬▬▬▬▬▬▬▬▬▬▬▬▬▬▬▬▬▬▬▬

The organization has a leadership structure.

Rationale for LD.01.01.01

Every organization has a leadership structure to support operations. Many functions need to be carried out, including governance, administration, and oversight of care, treatment, or services. In some organizations, leaders have distinct roles in carrying out these functions; in others a single individual may perform all leadership functions.

Elements of Performance for LD.01.01.01

1. The organization identifies those responsible for governance.

2. Governance identifies those responsible for planning, management, and operational activities.

3. Governance identifies those responsible for the provision of care, treatment, or services.

Standard LD.01.03.01 ━━━━━━━━━━━━━━━━━━━━━━━━━━

Governance is ultimately accountable for the safety and quality of care, treatment, or services.

Rationale for LD.01.03.01

Governance's ultimate responsibility for safety and quality derives from its legal responsibility and operational authority for organization performance. In this context, governance provides for internal structures and resources, including staff, that support safety and quality.

Elements of Performance for LD.01.03.01

1. Ⓓ Governance defines in writing its responsibilities.

2. Governance provides for organization management and planning.

3. Ⓓ Governance approves the organization's written scope of services.

4. Governance selects the chief executive.

5. Governance provides for the resources needed to maintain safe, quality care, treatment, or services.

6. Governance works with other leaders to annually evaluate the organization's performance in relation to its mission, vision, and goals.

12. **For ambulatory surgical centers that elect to use The Joint Commission deemed status option:** The ambulatory surgical center has a governing body that assumes full legal responsibility for the operation of the ambulatory surgical center.

22. **For ambulatory surgical centers that elect to use The Joint Commission deemed status option:** The governing body is responsible for the following:

- Determining, implementing, and monitoring policies governing the organization's total operation and establishing expectations for safety throughout the organization
- Defining, implementing, monitoring, and maintaining quality assurance and performance improvement activities
- Addressing identified priorities for quality assurance and performance improvement activities
- Evaluating the effectiveness of quality assurance and performance improvement activities

Standard LD.01.04.01

A chief executive manages the organization.

Elements of Performance for LD.01.04.01

1. The chief executive provides for the following:
   - Information and support systems
   - Physical and financial assets

Standard LD.01.07.01

Individual leaders have the knowledge needed for their roles in the organization or they seek guidance to fulfill their roles.

Elements of Performance for LD.01.07.01

2. Leaders are oriented to all of the following:
   - The organization's mission and vision
   - The organization's safety and quality goals
   - The organization's structure and the decision-making process
   - The development of the budget as well as the interpretation of the organization's financial statements
   - The population(s) served by the organization and any issues related to that population(s)
   - The individual and interdependent responsibilities and accountabilities of leaders as they relate to supporting the mission of the organization and to providing safe and quality care
   - Applicable law and regulation

3. Governance provides leaders with access to information and training in areas where they need additional skills or expertise.

Introduction to Leadership Relationships, Standards LD.02.01.01 and LD.02.03.01

How well leaders work together and manage conflict affects an organization's performance. In fulfilling its role, governance involves senior managers and leaders of the clinical staff in governance and management functions.

Good relationships thrive when leaders work together to develop the mission, vision, and goals of the organization; encourage honest and open communication; and address conflicts of interest.

Standard LD.02.01.01 ━━━━━━━━━━━━━━━━━━━━━━━

The mission, vision, and goals of the organization support the safety and quality of care, treatment, or services.

Rationale for LD.02.01.01

The primary responsibility of leaders is to provide for the safety and quality of care, treatment, or services. The purpose of the organization's mission, vision, and goals is to define how the organization will achieve safety and quality. The leaders are more likely to be aligned with the mission, vision, and goals when they create them together. The common purpose of the organization is most likely achieved when it is understood by all who work in or are served by the organization.

Elements of Performance for LD.02.01.01

1. Leaders work together to create the organization's mission, vision, and goals.

2. The organization's mission, vision, and goals guide the actions of leaders.

3. Leaders communicate the mission, vision, and goals to staff and the population(s) the organization serves.

Standard LD.02.03.01 ━━━━━━━━━━━━━━━━━━━━━━━

Leaders regularly communicate with each other on issues of safety and quality.

Rationale for LD.02.03.01

Leaders, who provide for safety and quality, must communicate with each other on matters affecting the organization and those it serves. The safety and quality of care, treatment, or services depend on open communication. Ideally, this will result in trust and mutual respect among those who work in the organization.

Elements of Performance for LD.02.03.01

1. Leaders discuss issues that affect the organization and the population(s) it serves, including the following:
    - Performance improvement activities
    - Reported safety and quality issues
    - Proposed solutions and their impact on the organization's resources
    - Reports on key quality measures and safety indicators
    - Safety and quality issues specific to the population served
    - Input from the population(s) served

2. The organization establishes time frames for the discussion of issues that affect the organization and the population(s) it serves.

Introduction to Organization Culture and System Performance Expectations, Standards LD.03.01.01 Through LD.03.06.01

An organization's culture reflects the beliefs, attitudes, and priorities of its members, and it influences the effectiveness of performance. Although there may be a dominant culture, in many larger organizations, diverse cultures exist that may or may not share the same values. In fact, diverse cultures can exist even in smaller organizations. Organization performance can be effective in either case. Successful organizations will work to develop a culture of safety and quality.

In a culture of safety and quality, all individuals are focused on maintaining excellence in performance. They accept the safety and quality of patient care, treatment, or services as personal responsibilities and work together to minimize any harm that might result from unsafe or poor quality of care, treatment, or services. Leaders create this culture by demonstrating their commitment to safety and quality and by taking actions to achieve the desired state. In a culture of this kind, one finds teamwork, open discussions of concerns about safety and quality, and the encouragement of and reward for internal and external reporting of safety and quality issues. Attention is focused on the performance of systems and processes instead of the individual, although reckless behavior and a blatant disregard for safety are not tolerated. Organizations are committed to ongoing learning and have the flexibility to accommodate changes in technology, science, and the environment.

The leaders provide for the effective functioning of the organization with a focus on safety and quality. Leaders plan, support, and implement key systems critical to this effort. The Joint Commission has identified five key systems that influence the effective performance of an organization:

1. Using data
2. Planning
3. Communicating
4. Changing performance
5. Staffing

The following diagram illustrates the role of leadership in the performance of these systems.

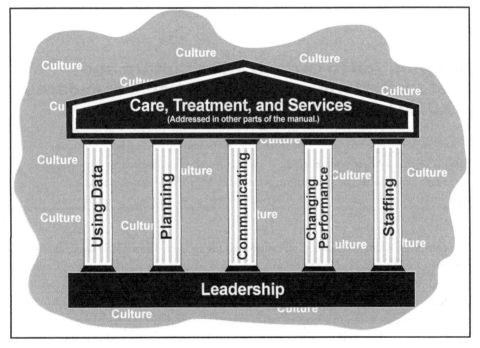

Leadership provides the foundation for effective performance. The five key systems serve as pillars that are based on the foundation set by leadership and, in turn, support the many organizationwide processes (such as medication management) that are important to individual care, treatment, or services. Culture permeates the entire structure.

The five key systems are interrelated and need to function well together. The integration of these systems throughout the organization will facilitate the effective performance of the organization as a whole. Leaders develop a vision and goals for the performance of these systems and then evaluate their performance. Leaders use results to develop strategies for future improvements.

Performance of many aspects of these systems may be directly observable. But in many cases, organizations demonstrate compliance through performance in standards located in other sections of this manual. These Leadership standards are cited when patterns of performance suggest organizationwide issues.

The effective performance of these systems results in a culture in which safety and quality are priorities. The organization demonstrates this through a proactive, nonpunitive culture that is monitored and sustained by related reporting systems and improvement initiatives.

Many of the concepts in the following section have long existed in the standards.

Standard LD.03.01.01

Leaders create and maintain a culture of safety and quality throughout the organization.

Rationale for LD.03.01.01

Safety and quality thrive in an environment that supports teamwork and respect for other people, regardless of their position in the organization. Leaders demonstrate their commitment to quality and set expectations for those who work in the organization. Leaders evaluate the culture on a regular basis using a variety of methods, such as formal surveys, focus groups, staff interviews, and data analysis.

Leaders encourage teamwork and create structures, processes, and programs that allow this positive culture to flourish. Behavior that intimidates others and affects morale or staff turnover undermines a culture of safety and can be harmful to patient care. Leaders must address such behavior in individuals working at all levels of the organization, including management, clinical and administrative staff, licensed independent practitioners, and governing body members.

Elements of Performance for LD.03.01.01

1. Leaders regularly evaluate the culture of safety and quality.

2. Leaders prioritize and implement changes identified by the evaluation.

4. Ⓓ Leaders develop a code of conduct that defines acceptable behavior and behaviors that undermine a culture of safety.

5. Leaders create and implement a process for managing behaviors that undermine a culture of safety.

Standard LD.03.02.01 ▬▬▬▬▬▬▬▬▬▬▬▬▬▬▬▬▬▬▬▬▬

The organization uses data and information to guide decisions and to understand variation in the performance of processes supporting safety and quality.

Rationale for LD.03.02.01

Data help organizations make the right decisions. When decisions are supported by data, organizations are more likely to move in directions that help them achieve their goals. Successful organizations measure and analyze their performance. When data are analyzed and turned into information, this process helps organizations see patterns and trends and understand the reasons for their performance. Many types of data are used to evaluate performance, including data on outcomes of care, performance on safety and quality initiatives, patient satisfaction, process variation, and staff perceptions.

Elements of Performance for LD.03.02.01

1. Leaders set expectations for using data and information for the following:
    - Improving the safety and quality of care, treatment, or services
    - Creating a culture of safety and quality
    - Decision making that supports the safety and quality of care, treatment, or services
    - Identifying and responding to internal and external changes in the environment

2. Leaders evaluate how effectively data and information are used throughout the organization.

Standard LD.03.03.01 ▬▬▬▬▬▬▬▬▬▬▬▬▬▬▬▬▬▬▬▬▬

Leaders use organizationwide planning to establish structures and processes that focus on safety and quality.

Rationale for LD.03.03.01

Planning is essential to the following:
- The achievement of short- and long-term goals
- Meeting the challenge of external changes
- The design of services and work processes

- The creation of communication channels
- The improvement of performance
- The introduction of innovation

Planning includes contributions from the populations served, those who work for the organization, and other interested groups or individuals.

Elements of Performance for LD.03.03.01

1. Planning activities focus on the following:
   - Improving patient safety and health care quality
   - Supporting a culture of safety and quality
   - Adapting to changes in the environment

2. Planning is organizationwide, systematic, and involves designated individuals and information sources.

3. Leaders evaluate the effectiveness of planning activities.

Standard LD.03.04.01

The organization communicates information related to safety and quality to those who need it, including staff, licensed independent practitioners, patients, families, and external interested parties.

Rationale for LD.03.04.01

Effective communication is essential among individuals and groups within the organization and between the organization and external parties. Poor communication often contributes to adverse events and can compromise safety and quality of care, treatment, or services. Effective communication is timely, accurate, and usable by the audience.

Elements of Performance for LD.03.04.01

1. Communication processes are effective in doing the following:
   - Fostering the safety of the patient and their quality of care
   - Supporting a culture of safety and quality
   - Meeting the needs of internal and external users
   - Informing those who work in the organization of changes in the environment

2. Leaders evaluate the effectiveness of communication methods.

Standard LD.03.05.01 ▬▬▬▬▬▬▬▬▬▬▬▬▬

Leaders manage change to improve the performance of the organization.

Rationale for LD.03.05.01

Change is inevitable, and agile organizations are able to manage change and rapidly execute new plans. The ability of leaders to manage change is necessary for performance improvement, for successful innovation, and to meet environmental challenges. The organization integrates change into all relevant processes so that its effectiveness can be sustained, assessed, and measured.

Elements of Performance for LD.03.05.01

1. The organization has a systematic approach to change and performance improvement.

2. Structures for managing change and performance improvement do the following:
    - Foster the safety of the patient and the quality of care, treatment, or services
    - Support a culture of safety and quality
    - Adapt to changes in the environment

3. Leaders evaluate the effectiveness of processes for the management of change and performance improvement.

Standard LD.03.06.01 ▬▬▬▬▬▬▬▬▬▬▬▬▬

Those who work in the organization are focused on improving safety and quality.

Rationale for LD.03.06.01

The safety and quality of care, treatment, or services are highly dependent on the people who work in the organization. The mission, scope, and complexity of services define the design of work processes and the skills and number of individuals needed. In a successful organization, work processes and the environment make safety and quality paramount. This standard, therefore, applies to all those who work in or for the organization, including staff and licensed independent practitioners.

Elements of Performance for LD.03.06.01

1. Leaders design work processes to focus individuals on safety and quality issues.

2. Leaders provide for a sufficient number and mix of individuals to support safe, quality care, treatment, or services.

    (*See also* IC.01.01.01, EP 3)

3. Those who work in the organization are competent to complete their assigned responsibilities.

4. Leaders evaluate the effectiveness of those who work in the organization to promote safety and quality.

5. Those who work in the organization adapt to changes in the environment.

Introduction to Operations, Standards LD.03.07.01 Through LD.04.03.09

Although some leaders may not be involved in the day-to-day, hands-on operations of the organization, their decisions and work affect, either directly or indirectly, every aspect of operations. They are the driving force behind the culture of the organization. Leaders establish the ethical framework in which the organization operates, create policies and procedures, and secure resources or services that support patient safety and quality care, treatment, or services. Policies, procedures, resources, or services are all influenced by the culture of the organization and, in turn, influence the culture.

Standard LD.03.07.01

Leaders establish priorities for performance improvement. (Refer to the "Performance Improvement" [PI] chapter.)

Elements of Performance for LD.03.07.01

1. Performance improvement occurs organizationwide.

2. As part of performance improvement, leaders do the following:
   - Set priorities for performance improvement activities and patient health outcomes
   - Give priority to high-volume, high-risk, or problem-prone processes for performance improvement activities
   - Identify the frequency of data collection for performance improvement activities
   - Reprioritize performance improvement activities in response to changes in the internal or external environment

(*See also* PI.01.01.01, EPs 2, 3, 5, 6, 7, 12, 13; PI.02.01.01, EP 1)

4. **For organizations that elect The Joint Commission Primary Care Medical Home option:** The interdisciplinary team actively participates in performance improvement activities.

13. **For ambulatory surgical centers that elect to use The Joint Commission deemed status option:** The infection control program is an integral part of the ambulatory surgical center's quality assessment and performance improvement program.

14. **For ambulatory surgical centers that elect to use The Joint Commission deemed status option:** The governing body makes certain that the quality assessment and performance improvement program is defined, implemented, and maintained.

15. **For ambulatory surgical centers that elect to use The Joint Commission deemed status option:** The governing body makes certain that adequate staff, time, information systems, and training are allocated to the quality assessment and performance improvement program.

16. **For ambulatory surgical centers that elect to use The Joint Commission deemed status option:** The governing body makes certain that the performance improvement data collection methods, frequency, and details are appropriate.

17. **For ambulatory surgical centers that elect to use The Joint Commission deemed status option:** The ambulatory surgical center sets priorities for its performance improvement activities that affect health outcomes, patient safety, and quality of care.

18. **For ambulatory surgical centers that elect to use The Joint Commission deemed status option:** The ambulatory surgical center develops an ongoing, data-driven quality assessment and performance improvement program.

19. **For ambulatory surgical centers that elect to use The Joint Commission deemed status option:** The ambulatory surgical center implements its quality assessment and performance improvement program.

20. **For ambulatory surgical centers that elect to use The Joint Commission deemed status option:** The ambulatory surgical center maintains its quality assessment and performance improvement program.

21. **For organizations that elect The Joint Commission Primary Care Medical Home option:** Leaders use qualitative data collection methods to involve patients in performance improvement activities.

    Note: *Qualitative data collection methods are used to provide insight into patients' opinions, along with underlying reasons, and motivations. Examples of qualitative methods include focus groups, telephonic or in-person patient interviews or patient rounding, and patient participation on performance improvement committees.*

23. **For ambulatory surgical centers that elect to use The Joint Commission deemed status option:** Leaders establish priorities that consider the incidence, prevalence, and severity of high-volume, high-risk, or problem-prone areas found in performance improvement activities.

Standard LD.03.08.01

New or modified services or processes are well designed.

Elements of Performance for LD.03.08.01

1. The organization's design of new or modified services or processes incorporates the following:
   - The needs of patients, staff, and others
   - The results of performance improvement activities
   - Information about potential risks to patients
   - Evidence-based information in the decision-making process
   - Information about sentinel events

   Note 1: *A proactive risk assessment is one of several ways to assess potential risks to patients. For suggested components, refer to the "Proactive Risk Assessment" section at the beginning of this chapter.*

   Note 2: *Evidence-based information could include practice guidelines, successful practices, information from current literature, and clinical standards.*

   (*See also* LD.03.09.01, EPs 3, 8)

2. Leaders involve staff and patients in the design of new or modified services or processes.

Introduction to Standard LD.03.09.01

This standard describes a safety program that integrates safety priorities into all processes, functions, or services within the organization, including patient care, support, and contract services. It addresses the responsibility of leaders to establish an organizationwide safety program; to proactively explore potential system failures; to analyze and take action on problems that have occurred; and to encourage the reporting of adverse events and close calls ("near misses"), both internally and externally. The organization's culture of safety and quality supports the safety program (refer to Standard LD.03.01.01).

This standard does not require the creation of a new structure or office in the organization. It only emphasizes the need to integrate patient safety activities, both existing and newly created, with the organization's leadership, which is ultimately responsible for this integration.

Standard LD.03.09.01

The organization has an organizationwide, integrated patient safety program.

Elements of Performance for LD.03.09.01

1. The leaders implement an organizationwide patient safety program as follows:
   - One or more qualified individuals manage the safety program.
   - All departments, programs, and services within the organization participate in the safety program.
   - The scope of the safety program includes the full range of safety issues, from potential or no-harm errors (sometimes referred to as close calls ["near misses"] or good catches) to hazardous conditions and sentinel events.

2. As part of the safety program, the leaders create procedures for responding to system or process failures.

   Note: *Responses might include continuing to provide care, treatment, or services to those affected, containing the risk, and preserving factual information for subsequent analysis.*

   (*See also* PI.04.01.01, EP 10)

3. The leaders provide and encourage the use of systems for blame-free internal reporting of a system or process failure, or the results of a proactive risk assessment.

Note: *This EP is intended to minimize staff reluctance to report errors in order to help an organization understand the source and results of system and process failures. The EP does not conflict with holding individuals accountable for their blameworthy errors.*

(*See also* LD.03.08.01, EP 1; PI.04.01.01, EP 10)

4.　The leaders define patient safety event and communicate this definition throughout the organization.

Note: *At a minimum, the organization's definition includes those events subject to review as described in the "Sentinel Event Policy" (SE) chapter of the* CAMAC.

(*See also* PI.04.01.01, EP 10)

5.　The organization conducts thorough and credible comprehensive systematic analyses (for example, root cause analyses) in response to sentinel events as described in the "Sentinel Event Policy" (SE) chapter of the *CAMAC*.

6.　The leaders make support systems available for staff who have been involved in an adverse or sentinel event.

Note: *Support systems recognize that conscientious health care workers who are involved in sentinel events are themselves victims of the event and require support. Support systems provide staff with additional help and support as well as additional resources through the human resources function or an employee assistance program. Support systems also focus on the process rather than blaming the involved individuals.*

8.　To improve safety, the organization analyzes and uses information about system or process failures and, when conducted, the results of proactive risk assessments.

(*See also* LD.03.08.01, EP 1)

9.　The leaders disseminate lessons learned from comprehensive systematic analyses (for example, root cause analyses), system or process failures, and the results of proactive risk assessments to all staff who provide services for the specific situation.

(*See also* PI.04.01.01, EP 10)

10.　Ⓓ At least once a year, the leaders provide governance with written reports on the following:
- All system or process failures
- The number and type of sentinel events

- Whether the patients and the families were informed of the event
- All actions taken to improve safety, both proactively and in response to actual occurrences

11. The leaders encourage external reporting of significant adverse events, including voluntary reporting programs in addition to mandatory programs.

   Note: *Examples of voluntary programs include The Joint Commission Sentinel Event Database and the US Food and Drug Administration (FDA) MedWatch. Mandatory programs are often state initiated.*

13. Ⓓ **For ambulatory surgical centers that elect to use The Joint Commission deemed status option:** The organization tracks adverse patient events, examines their causes, implements needed improvements, and makes certain improvements are sustained over time.

Standard LD.03.10.01

The organization uses clinical practice guidelines to design or to improve processes that evaluate and treat specific diagnoses, conditions, or symptoms.

Rationale for LD.03.10.01

Clinical practice guidelines can improve the quality, utilization, and value of health care services. Clinical practice guidelines help practitioners and patients make decisions about preventing, diagnosing, treating, and managing selected conditions. These guidelines can also be used in designing clinical processes or in checking the design of existing processes. The organization identifies criteria that guide the selection and implementation of clinical practice guidelines so that they are consistent with its mission and priorities. Sources of clinical practice guidelines include the Agency for Healthcare Research and Quality and professional organizations.

Elements of Performance for LD.03.10.01

1. The organization uses clinical practice guidelines to design or improve processes that evaluate and treat specific diagnoses, conditions, or symptoms.

2. The organization identifies criteria that guide the selection and implementation of guidelines to design or improve processes that evaluate and treat specific diagnoses, conditions, or symptoms.

3. Leaders do the following related to the use of clinical practice guidelines:
   - Review and approve the clinical practice guidelines that have been selected
   - Manage and evaluate the implementation of the guidelines

- Monitor and review clinical practice guidelines for their effectiveness and modify them as needed

Standard LD.04.01.01

The organization complies with law and regulation.

Elements of Performance for LD.04.01.01

1. ⑩ The organization is licensed, is certified, or has a permit, in accordance with law and regulation, to provide the care, treatment, or services for which the organization is seeking accreditation from The Joint Commission.

    Note 1: *Each service location that performs laboratory testing (waived or nonwaived) must have a Clinical Laboratory Improvement Amendments of 1988 (CLIA '88) certificate as specified by the federal CLIA regulations (42 CFR 493.55 and 493.3) and applicable state law.*

    Note 2: *For more information on how to obtain a CLIA certificate, see http:// www.cms.gov/Regulations-and-Guidance/Legislation/CLIA/ How_to_Apply_for_a_CLIA_Certificate_International_Laboratories.html.*

    (See also WT.01.01.01, EP 1; WT.04.01.01, EP 1)

2. The organization provides care, treatment, or services in accordance with licensure requirements, laws, and rules and regulations.

3. Leaders act on or comply with reports or recommendations from external authorized agencies, such as accreditation, certification, or regulatory bodies.

15. **For ambulatory surgical centers that elect to use The Joint Commission deemed status option:** The organization complies with part 493 of the Code of Federal Regulations.

    Note: *Part 493 of the Code of Federal Regulations requires organizations who perform laboratory testing to maintain compliance with the Clinical Laboratory Improvement Amendments of 1988 (CLIA '88).*

19. **For ambulatory surgical centers that elect to use The Joint Commission deemed status option:** Organizations that do not provide their own laboratory services have procedures for obtaining routine and emergency laboratory services from a certified laboratory in accordance with part 493 of the Code of Federal Regulations. The referral laboratory is certified in the associated specialties and subspecialties needed to perform tests ordered.

21. **For ambulatory surgical centers that elect to use The Joint Commission deemed status option:** The organization meets the definition of an ambulatory surgical center as described in the Glossary.

Standard LD.04.01.03

The organization develops an annual operating budget and, when needed, a long-term capital expenditure plan.

Elements of Performance for LD.04.01.03

1. Leaders solicit comments from those who work in the organization when developing the operational and capital budgets.

3. The operating budget reflects the organization's goals and objectives.

4. Ⓓ Governance approves an annual operating budget and, when needed, a long-term capital expenditure plan.

Standard LD.04.01.05

The organization effectively manages its programs, services, or sites.

Rationale for LD.04.01.05

Leaders at the program, service, site, or department level create a culture that enables the organization to fulfill its mission and meet its goals. They support staff and instill in them a sense of ownership of their work processes. Leaders may delegate work to qualified staff, but the leaders are responsible for the care, treatment, or services provided in their areas.

Elements of Performance for LD.04.01.05

2. Programs, services, or sites providing patient care are directed by one or more qualified professionals or by a qualified licensed independent practitioner with clinical privileges.

3. Ⓓ The organization defines, in writing, the responsibility of those with administrative and clinical direction of its programs, services, or sites.

4. Staff are held accountable for their responsibilities.

5. Leaders provide for the coordination of care, treatment, or services among the organization's different programs, services, or sites.

11. **For organizations that elect The Joint Commission Primary Care Medical Home option:** The organization evaluates how effectively the primary care clinician and the interdisciplinary team work in partnership with the patient to support the continuity of care and the provision of comprehensive and coordinated care, treatment, or services.

13. **For ambulatory surgical centers that elect to use The Joint Commission deemed status option:** If radiologic services are provided by the ambulatory surgical center, the governing body must appoint an individual qualified in accordance with state law and organizational policies who is responsible for making certain that all radiologic services are provided in accordance with law and regulation.

    Note: *The Joint Commission elements of performance that relate to laws and regulations for radiologic services are outlined in the ambulatory surgical center crosswalk on E-dition.*

25. The organization designates an individual to serve as the radiation safety officer who is responsible for making certain that radiologic services are provided in accordance with law, regulation, and organizational policy. This individual has the necessary authority and leadership support to do the following:
    - Monitor and verify compliance with established radiation safety practices (including oversight of dosimetry monitoring)
    - Provide recommendations for improved radiation safety
    - Intervene as needed to stop unsafe practices
    - Implement corrective action

Standard LD.04.01.07

The organization has policies and procedures that guide and support patient care, treatment, or services.

Elements of Performance for LD.04.01.07

1. Leaders review, approve, and manage the implementation of policies and procedures that guide and support patient care, treatment, or services.

10. **For ambulatory surgical centers that elect to use The Joint Commission deemed status option:** The organization establishes policies and procedures approved by the governing body for overseeing and evaluating the clinical activities of nonphysician practitioners who are assigned patient care responsibilities.

Standard LD.04.01.11

The organization makes space and equipment available as needed for the provision of care, treatment, or services.

Rationale for LD.04.01.11

The resources allocated to services provided by the organization have a direct effect on patient outcomes. Leaders should place highest priority on high-risk or problem-prone processes that can affect patient safety. Examples include infection control, medication management, use of anesthesia, and others defined by the organization.

Elements of Performance for LD.04.01.11

3. The interior and exterior space provided for care, treatment, or services meets the needs of patients.

4. The grounds, equipment, and special activity areas are safe, maintained, and supervised.

5. The leaders provide for equipment, information systems, supplies, and other resources.

8. Ⓓ **For ambulatory surgical centers that elect to use The Joint Commission deemed status option:** The organization's medical staff and governing body coordinate, develop, and revise policies and procedures that identify the types of emergency equipment required for use in operating rooms.

    (*See also* PC.02.01.09, EP 10)

Standard LD.04.02.01

The leaders address any conflict of interest involving licensed independent practitioners and/or staff that affects or has the potential to affect the safety or quality of care, treatment, or services.

Elements of Performance for LD.04.02.01

2. Ⓓ The leaders follow a written policy that defines situations that represent a conflict of interest involving licensed independent practitioners and/or staff and how the organization will address these conflicts of interest.

3. Existing or potential conflicts of interest involving licensed independent practitioners and/or staff, as defined by the organization, are disclosed.

4. The organization reviews its relationships with other care providers, educational institutions, manufacturers, and payers to determine whether conflicts of interest exist and whether they are within law and regulation.

5. Policies, procedures, and information about the relationship between care, treatment, or services and financial incentives are available upon request to all patients, and those individuals who work in the organization, including staff and licensed independent practitioners.

6. Ⓓ **For ambulatory surgical centers that elect to use The Joint Commission deemed status option:** The ambulatory surgical center discloses, where applicable, physician financial interests or ownership in the facility in accordance with 42 CFR Part 420. This disclosure information is in writing.

Standard LD.04.02.03

Ethical principles guide the organization's business practices.

Elements of Performance for LD.04.02.03

1. The organization follows a process that allows staff, patients, and families to address ethical issues or issues prone to conflict.

5. Care, treatment, or services are provided based on patient needs, regardless of compensation or financial risk-sharing with those who work in the organization, including staff and licensed independent practitioners.

7. Patients receive information about charges for which they will be responsible.

10. The safety and quality of care, treatment, or services do not depend on the patient's ability to pay.

Standard LD.04.03.01

The organization provides services that meet patient needs.

Elements of Performance for LD.04.03.01

1. The needs of the population(s) served guide decisions about which services will be provided directly or through referral, consultation, contractual arrangements, or other agreements.

25. **For ambulatory surgical centers that elect to use The Joint Commission deemed status option:** The ambulatory surgical center reviews and amends the scope of procedures that the organization can perform, according to a time frame determined by the organization.

Standard LD.04.03.07

Patients with comparable needs receive the same standard of care, treatment, or services throughout the organization.

Rationale for LD.04.03.07

Comparable standards of care means that the organization can provide the services that patients need within established time frames and that those providing care, treatment, or services have the required competence. Organizations may provide different services to patients with similar needs as long as individual outcomes are not affected. For example, some patients may receive equipment with enhanced features because of insurance situations. This does not ordinarily lead to different outcomes. Different settings, processes, or payment sources should not result in different standards of care.

Elements of Performance for LD.04.03.07

1. Variances in staff, setting, or payment source do not affect outcomes of care, treatment, or services in a negative way.

Introduction to Oversight of Care, Treatment, or Services Provided Through Contractual Agreement, Standard LD.04.03.09

The same level of care should be delivered to patients regardless of whether services are provided directly by the organization or through contractual agreement. Leaders provide oversight to make sure that care, treatment, or services provided directly are safe and effective. Likewise, leaders must also oversee contracted services to make sure that they are provided safely and effectively. Standard LD.04.03.09 outlines the requirements for leadership oversight of care, treatment, or services provided through contractual agreement.

The only contractual agreements subject to the requirements in Standard LD.04.03.09 are those for the provision of care, treatment, or services provided to the organization's patients. This standard does not apply to contracted services that are not directly related to patient care. In addition, contracts for consultation or referrals are not subject to the requirements in Standard LD.04.03.09. However, regardless of whether a contract is subject to this standard, the actual performance of any contracted service is evaluated at the other standards in this manual appropriate to the nature of the contracted service.

Monitoring Contracted Services

The expectations that leaders set for the performance of contracted services should reflect basic principles of risk reduction, safety, staff competence, and performance improvement. The requirements outlined in Standards HR.01.06.01, EC.01.01.01, EC.02.01.01, and PI.01.01.01 can provide ideas for setting expectations related to these topics. Additional ideas for expectations can also come from the elements of performance (EPs) found in specific standards applicable to the contracted service. Although leaders have the same responsibility for oversight of contracted services outside the organization's expertise as they do for contracted services within the organization's expertise, it may be more difficult to determine how to monitor such services.

The EPs do not prescribe the methods for evaluating contracted services; leaders are expected to select the best methods in which their organization oversees the quality and safety of services provided through contractual agreement. Examples of sources of information that may be used for evaluating contracted services include the following:

- Review of information about the contractor's Joint Commission accreditation or certification status
- Direct observation of the provision of care
- Audit of documentation, including medical records
- Review of incident reports
- Review of periodic reports submitted by the individual or organization providing services under contractual agreement
- Collection of data that address the efficacy of the contracted service
- Review of performance reports based on indicators required in the contractual agreement
- Input from staff and patients
- Review of patient satisfaction studies
- Review of results of risk management activities

If contracted services do not meet expectations, leaders take steps to improve care, treatment, or services. In some cases, it may be best to work with the contractor to make improvements, whereas in other cases it may be best to renegotiate or terminate the contractual relationship. When leaders anticipate the renegotiation or termination of a contractual agreement, planning needs to occur so that the continuity of care, treatment, or services is not disrupted.

Credentialing and Privileging

In most cases, each licensed independent practitioner providing services through a contractual agreement must be credentialed and privileged by the organization using the practitioner's services, following the process described in the "Human Resources" (HR) chapter.

However, there is one special circumstance when this is not required:
- Services provided by a pathologist through a contracted reference laboratory compliant with CLIA (Clinical Laboratory Improvement Amendments) regulations

Standard LD.04.03.09
Care, treatment, or services provided through contractual agreement are provided safely and effectively.

Elements of Performance for LD.04.03.09

1. Clinical leaders have an opportunity to provide advice about the sources of clinical services to be provided through contractual agreement.

2. Ⓓ The organization describes, in writing, the nature and scope of services provided through contractual agreements.

3. Ⓓ Designated leaders approve contractual agreements.

4. Leaders monitor contracted services by establishing expectations for the performance of the contracted services.

   Note: *When the organization contracts with another accredited organization for patient care, treatment, or services to be provided off site, it can do the following:*
   - *Verify that all licensed independent practitioners who will be providing patient care, treatment, or services have appropriate privileges by obtaining, for example, a copy of the list of privileges.*

- *Specify in the written agreement that the contracted organization will ensure that all contracted services provided by licensed independent practitioners will be within the scope of their privileges.*

5. Ⓓ Leaders monitor contracted services by communicating the expectations in writing to the provider of the contracted services.

   Note: *A written description of the expectations can be provided either as part of the written agreement or in addition to it.*

6. Leaders monitor contracted services by evaluating these services in relation to the organization's expectations.

7. Leaders take steps to improve contracted services that do not meet expectations.

   Note: *Examples of improvement efforts to consider include the following:*
   - *Increase monitoring of the contracted services*
   - *Provide consultation or training to the contractor*
   - *Renegotiate the contract terms*
   - *Apply defined penalties*
   - *Terminate the contract*

8. When contractual agreements are renegotiated or terminated, the organization maintains the continuity of patient care.

10. Ⓓ Reference and contract laboratory services meet the federal regulations for clinical laboratories and maintain evidence of the same.

Introduction to Standard LD.04.03.13

Gaps in the evidence on optimal pain management, combined with a substantial rise in opioid use and associated harms over the past two decades, are of great concern for health care organizations and the public. Solutions to these safety and quality problems require the coordination of administrative and physician leadership to promote quality initiatives and allocate resources for safe pain management. Organization leaders are required to support pain management and safe opioid prescribing by providing clinicians and staff with relevant education, resources, and tools, and monitoring performance improvement activities related to opioid prescribing to increase safety and quality for patients.

Standard LD.04.03.13 ━━━━━━━━━━━━━━━━━━━━━━

Pain assessment and pain management, including safe opioid prescribing, are identified as an organizational priority.

Elements of Performance for LD.04.03.13

1. The organization has a leader or leadership team that is responsible for pain management and opioid prescribing, as well as developing and monitoring performance improvement activities.

   (*See also* PI.03.01.01, EP 19)

3. The organization provides staff and licensed independent practitioners with educational resources to improve pain assessment, pain management, and the safe use of opioid medications based on the identified needs of its patient population.

4. The organization provides information to staff and licensed independent practitioners on available services for consultation and referral of patients with complex pain management needs.

6. The organization facilitates practitioner and pharmacist access to the Prescription Drug Monitoring Program databases.

   Note: *This element of performance is applicable in any state that has a Prescription Drug Monitoring Program database, whether querying is voluntary or is mandated by state regulations for all patients prescribed opioids.*

Life Safety (LS)

Overview

This chapter applies to sites of care that are considered ambulatory care occupancies. The National Fire Protection Agency's (NFPA) *Life Safety Code** (101-2012) defines an ambulatory care occupancy as a building or part of a building in which anesthesia or outpatient services are provided to four or more outpatients at the same time, making them incapable of saving themselves in emergencies. This chapter also applies to all ambulatory surgical centers seeking accreditation for Medicare certification purposes, regardless of the number of patients who are incapable of saving themselves in the event of an emergency within the organization.

When the ambulatory care organization occupies space in a building that it does not own, The Joint Commission will assess that space and all exits from that space to the outside at grade level. The Joint Commission will also expect to see that the ambulatory care organization works with the landlord to make sure that supporting building systems comply with the *Life Safety Code*. Examples of such systems include fire alarms and automatic sprinklers.

About This Chapter

Fire is a concern for everyone, but it is of special concern in ambulatory care organizations because patients are often unable to move to safety by themselves. The *Life Safety Code* considers several options for fire protection, whether it be an evacuation or defend-in-place strategy; for example, creating safe areas (smoke compartments) that allow people to remain in the building; moving people to protected areas within the building; and, as a last resort, moving people out of a building. Health care facility design and related features help prevent, detect, and suppress fires. The measures that organizations must take to protect occupants from the dangers of fire constitutes the content of this chapter. These standards focus on the importance of a fire-safe environment and buildings; however, The Joint Commission recognizes that people are equally important in reducing the risk of fire. The responsibilities of managing a safe

---

* *Life Safety Code*® is a registered trademark of the National Fire Protection Association, Quincy, MA.

environment (for example, identifying fire risks, conducting fire drills, maintaining fire protection equipment) by those who work in the organization are addressed in the "Environment of Care" (EC) chapter.

From time to time, building codes are updated to incorporate new technology that often cannot easily be introduced into older buildings. These settings tend to rely more on passive systems (such as doors and walls) for fire protection. In new buildings, fire protection is more often provided by active systems, such as fire alarms and automatic sprinkler systems. This chapter addresses both existing and new health care occupancies. Existing ambulatory care occupancy requirements are found in Chapter 21 of the *Life Safety Code* (101-2000). New ambulatory care occupancy requirements are found in Chapter 20 of the *Life Safety Code.*

The Joint Commission uses the 2012 edition of the NFPA's *Life Safety Code* as the source for the key structural components that help protect people during a fire. Each element of performance (EP) contains a reference to the *Life Safety Code.* A reference is also provided in those rare cases when a different edition or NFPA code is used as a source. The *Life Safety Code* may contain provisions to the requirements in this chapter. Compliance with these provisions is considered as meeting the *Life Safety Code* and is acceptable to The Joint Commission.

This chapter addresses a number of topics contained in the *Life Safety Code,* including the following:

- General life safety design and building construction
- Means of egress, including design of space, travel distances, illumination, and signage
- Protection provided by door features, fire windows, stairs, and other vertical openings; corridors; smoke barriers; and interior finishes
- Fire alarm notification, including audible and coded alarms
- Suppression of fires, including sprinkler systems
- Building services, including elevators and chutes
- Decorations, furnishings, and portable heaters

Chapter Outline

I. Administrative Activities
    A. Statement of Conditions (LS.01.01.01)
    B. Interim Life Safety Measures (LS.01.02.01)

II. Health Care Occupancy — Not applicable to ambulatory care

III. Ambulatory Health Care Occupancy
    A. All Ambulatory Health Care Occupancy Buildings
        1. General Building Requirements (LS.03.01.10)
        2. Means of Egress Requirements (LS.03.01.20)
        3. Protection (LS.03.01.30)
            a. Fire Alarm (LS.03.01.34)
            b. Extinguishment (LS.03.01.35)
        4. Special Provisions (LS.03.01.40)
        5. Building Services (LS.03.01.50)
        6. Operating Features (LS.03.01.70)

Standards, Rationales, and Elements of Performance

Introduction to Standard LS.01.01.01

Organizations must be vigilant about fire safety. An ongoing assessment of compliance with the *Life Safety Code* is an effective way to identify and minimize risks. The electronic Statement of Conditions™ (SOC) is used in a management process that continually identifies, assesses, and resolves *Life Safety Code* deficiencies. The SOC includes two main sections: Basic Building Information (BBI) and a Plan for Improvement (PFI). The organization uses the BBI to identify the life safety features of its building(s). When an organization has multiple sites, one BBI form is prepared for each site; however, a single BBI form may cover multiple buildings at that site if they are physically connected. Alternatively, the organization may prepare a separate BBI form for each building. In either case, the organization must address specific risks and the unique conditions at each of its sites and buildings.

The organization should establish the qualifications of the individual(s) it selects to assess compliance with the *Life Safety Code*. This individual(s) is not required to have any specific education or experience, although knowledge of the *Life Safety Code* and its application in unique occupancies is important. Qualifications should be based on the scope of the *Life Safety Code* assessment activities and the complexity of the building and occupancy being assessed.

Standard LS.01.01.01

The organization designs and manages the physical environment to comply with the *Life Safety Code*.

Note 1: *This standard applies to sites of care where four or more patients at the same time are provided either anesthesia or outpatient services that render patients incapable of saving themselves in the event of an emergency in the organization.*

Note 2: *This standard applies to all ambulatory surgical centers and outpatient surgical departments seeking accreditation for Medicare certification purposes, regardless of the number of patients rendered incapable.*

Elements of Performance for LS.01.01.01

1. The organization assigns an individual(s) to assess compliance with the *Life Safety Code* and manage the Statement of Conditions (SOC) when addressing survey-related deficiencies.

   Note 1: *For ambulatory surgical centers that elect to use The Joint Commission deemed status option:* *The organization complies with the 2012* Life Safety Code.

   Note 2: *The provisions of the* Life Safety Code *do not apply in a state where the Centers for Medicare & Medicaid Services finds that a fire and safety code imposed by state law adequately protects patients in an ambulatory surgical center.*

2. Ⓓ In time frames defined by the organization, the organization performs a building assessment to determine compliance with the "Life Safety" (LS) chapter. **R**

3. Ⓓ The organization maintains current and accurate drawings denoting features of fire safety and related square footage. Fire safety features include the following:
   - Areas of the building that are fully sprinklered (if the building is partially sprinklered)
   - Locations of all hazardous storage areas
   - Locations of all fire-rated barriers
   - Locations of all smoke-rated barriers
   - Sleeping and non-sleeping suite boundaries, including the size of the identified suites
   - Locations of designated smoke compartments
   - Locations of chutes and shafts
   - Any approved equivalencies or waivers

4. When the organization plans to resolve a deficiency through a Survey-Related Plan for Improvement (SPFI), the organization meets the 60-day time frame.

   Note 1: *If the corrective action will exceed the 60-day time frame, the organization must request a time-limited waiver within 30 days from the end of survey.*

Note 2: *If there are alternative systems, methods, or devices considered equivalent, the organization may submit an equivalency request using its Statement of Conditions (SOC).*

Note 3: *For further information on waiver and equivalency requests, see https:// www.jointcommission.org/resources/patient-safety-topics/the-physical-environment/ life-safety-code-information-and-resources/ and NFPA 101-2012: 1.4.*

6. The organization does not remove or minimize an existing life safety feature when such feature is a requirement for new construction. Existing life safety features, if not required by the *Life Safety Code*, can be either maintained or removed. (For full text, refer to NFPA 101-2012: 4.6.12.2; 4.6.12.3; 20/21.7.9)

7. Ⓓ The organization maintains current Basic Building Information (BBI) within the Statement of Conditions (SOC).

Standard LS.01.02.01

The organization protects occupants during periods when the *Life Safety Code* is not met or during periods of construction.

Note 1: *This standard applies to sites of care where four or more patients at the same time are provided either anesthesia or outpatient services that render patients incapable of saving themselves in the event of an emergency in the organization.*

Note 2: *This standard applies to all ambulatory surgical centers and outpatient surgical departments seeking accreditation for Medicare certification purposes, regardless of the number of patients rendered incapable.*

Elements of Performance for LS.01.02.01

2. Ⓓ When the organization identifies *Life Safety Code* deficiencies that cannot be immediately corrected or during periods of construction, the organization evacuates the building or notifies the fire department (or other emergency response group) and initiates a fire watch when a fire alarm system is out of service more than 4 out of 24 hours or a sprinkler system is out of service more than 10 hours in a 24-hour period in an occupied building. Notification and fire watch times are documented. (For full text, refer to NFPA 101-2012: 9.6.1.6; 9.7.6; NFPA 25-2011: 15.5.2) **R**

When the organization identifies *Life Safety Code* deficiencies that cannot be immediately corrected or during periods of construction, the organization does the following:

3. Posts signage identifying the location of alternative exits to everyone affected. **R**

4. Inspects exits in affected areas on a daily basis. The organization determines when these inspections are needed. **R**

5. Provides temporary but equivalent fire alarm and detection systems for use when a fire system is impaired. The organization determines when these systems are needed. **R**

6. Provides additional firefighting equipment. The organization determines when to provide this equipment. **R**

7. Uses temporary construction partitions that are smoke-tight, or made of noncombustible or limited-combustible material that will not contribute to the development or spread of fire. The organization determines when to use these partitions.

8. Increases surveillance of buildings, grounds, and equipment, giving special attention to construction areas and storage, excavation, and field offices. The organization determines when to increase surveillance.

9. Enforces storage, housekeeping, and debris-removal practices that reduce the building's flammable and combustible fire load to the lowest feasible level. The organization determines when these practices are needed.

10. Provides additional training to those who work in the organization on the use of firefighting equipment. The organization determines when to provide additional training.

11. Conducts one additional fire drill per quarter. The organization determines when these additional fire drills are needed.

(*See also* EC.02.03.03, EP 1)

12. Ⓓ Inspects and tests temporary systems monthly. The completion date of the tests is documented. The organization determines when these inspections and tests are needed.

13. The organization conducts education to promote awareness of building deficiencies, construction hazards, and temporary measures implemented to maintain fire safety. The organization determines when this education is needed. **R**

14. The organization trains those who work in the organization to compensate for impaired structural or compartmental fire safety features. The organization determines when this training is needed. **R**

   Note: *Compartmentalization is the concept of using various building components (for example, fire-rated walls and doors, smoke barriers, fire-rated floor slabs) to prevent the spread of fire and the products of combustion so as to provide a safe means of egress to an approved exit. The presence of these features varies, depending on the building occupancy classification.*

15. The organization's policy allows the use of other ILSMs not addressed in EPs 2–14.

   Note 1: *The organization's ILSM policy addresses* Life Safety Code *Requirements for Improvement (RFI) that are not immediately corrected during survey.*

   Note 2: *The "other" ILSMs used are documented by selecting "other" and annotating the associated text box in the organization's Survey-Related Plan for Improvement (SPFI) within the Statement of Conditions™ (SOC).*

Standard LS.03.01.10

Building and fire protection features are designed and maintained to minimize the effects of fire, smoke, and heat.

Note 1: *This standard applies to sites of care where four or more patients at the same time are provided either anesthesia or outpatient services that render patients incapable of saving themselves in an emergency in the organization.*

Note 2: *This standard applies to all ambulatory surgical centers seeking accreditation for Medicare certification purposes, regardless of the number of patients rendered incapable.*

Note 3: *In leased facilities, the elements of performance of this standard apply only to the space in which the accredited organization is located; all exits from the space to the outside at grade level; and any* Life Safety Code *building systems that support the space (for example, fire alarm system, automatic sprinkler system).*

Rationale for LS.03.01.10

Space should be designed, constructed, and maintained in order to minimize danger from the effects of fire, including smoke, heat, and toxic gases. The structural characteristics of the building, as well as its age, determine the types of fire protection features that are needed. The features covered in this standard include the structure, automatic sprinkler systems, building separations, and doors.

When remodeling or designing a new building or space, the organization should also satisfy any requirements of other codes and standards (local, state, or federal) that may be more stringent than the *Life Safety Code*.

Elements of Performance for LS.03.01.10

1. Buildings meet requirements for construction type and height. In Types I and II construction, alternative protection measures are permitted to be substituted for sprinkler protection in specific areas where state or local regulations prohibit sprinklers. All new buildings contain approved automatic sprinkler systems. Existing buildings contain approved automatic sprinkler systems as required by the construction type. (For full text, refer to NFPA 101-2012: 20/21.1.6.1–20/ 21.1.6.6; 20/21.3.5)

2. Interior nonbearing walls in Types I or II construction are constructed of noncombustible or limited-combustible materials. Interior nonbearing walls that are required to have a minimum of two-hour fire resistance rating are made with fire retardant–treated wood and enclosed within noncombustible or limited-combustible materials, provided they are not used as shaft enclosures. (For full text, refer to NFPA 101-2012: 20.1.6.3; 20.1.6.4; 21.1.6.3; 21.1.6.4)

3. When building rehabilitation occurs, the organization incorporates NFPA 101-2012: Chapters 20, 21, and 43. (For full text, refer to NFPA 101-2012: Chapter 43; 20/21.1.1.4; 4.6.7)

4. Ambulatory occupancies located in multioccupancy buildings are separated from health care occupancies by two-hour fire-rated walls and from business occupancies by one-hour fire-rated walls. (For full text, refer to NFPA 101-2012: 20/21.1.3; 20/21.3.7.1) **R**

    Note: *Per Centers for Medicare & Medicaid Services' regulation, ambulatory surgical centers are classified as ambulatory health care occupancies, regardless of the number of patients served. (For full text, refer to NFPA 101-2012: 20/21.1.3.2; 20/21.3.7.1)*

5. Fire barriers are continuous from outside wall to outside wall or from one fire barrier to another, or a combination thereof, including continuity through all concealed spaces, such as those found above a ceiling, including interstitial spaces. For those fire barriers terminating at the bottom side of an interstitial space, the construction assembly forming the bottom of the interstitial space must have a fire resistance rating not less than that of the fire barrier. (For full text, refer to NFPA 101-2012: 8.3.1.2)

6. The fire protection rating for opening protectives in fire barriers, fire-rated smoke barriers, and fire-rated smoke partitions is as follows:
    - Three hours in three-hour barriers and partitions
    - Ninety minutes in two-hour barriers and partitions
    - Forty-five minutes in one-hour barriers and partitions
    - Twenty minutes in ½-hour barriers and partitions

    Labels on fire door assemblies must be maintained in legible condition. (For full text, refer to NFPA 101-2012: 8.3.4.2; Table 8.3.4.2; 8.3.3.2.3; NFPA 80-2010: 5.2.13.3)

    Note: ***For ambulatory surgical centers that elect to use The Joint Commission deemed status option:*** *The organization meets the applicable provisions of the* Life Safety Code *Tentative Interim Amendment (TIA) 12-1.*

7. Doors within walls and floors that are required to be fire rated have functioning hardware, including positive latching devices and self-closing or automatic-closing devices. Gaps between meeting edges of door pairs are no more than ⅛-inch wide, and undercuts are no larger than ¾ of an inch. Blocking or wedging open fire-rated doors is prohibited. Doors required to be fire rated in the walls do not have unapproved protective plates greater than 16 inches from the bottom of the door. (For full text, refer to NFPA 101-2012: 8.3.3.1; NFPA 80-2010: 4.8.4.1; 5.2.13.3; 6.3.1.7; 6.4.5)

8. Doors requiring a minimum fire rating of ¾ of an hour are free of coverings, decorations, or other objects applied to the door face. Informational signs, which are applied with adhesive only, are allowed provided that the informational signage does not exceed 5% of the door face area. (For full text, refer to NFPA 80-2010: 4.1.4)

9. Ducts penetrating the walls and floors with a fire-resistance rating of less than three hours are protected by dampers that are fire rated for 1½ hours; penetrations of three hours or greater are protected by fire dampers that are fire rated for three hours. (For full text, refer to NFPA 101-2012: 8.3.5.7; 9.2.1; NFPA 90A-2012: 5.4)

10. The space around pipes, conduits, bus ducts, cables, wires, air ducts, or pneumatic tubes penetrating the walls or floors are protected with an approved fire-rated material.

Note: *Non-approved polyurethane expanding foam is not an accepted fire-rated material for this purpose. (For full text, refer to NFPA 101-2012: 8.3.5)*

11. The organization meets all other *Life Safety Code* requirements related to NFPA 101-2012: 20/21.1.

Standard LS.03.01.20

The organization maintains the integrity of the means of egress.

Note 1: *This standard applies to sites of care where four or more patients at the same time are provided either anesthesia or outpatient services that render patients incapable of saving themselves in an emergency in the organization.*

Note 2: *This standard applies to all ambulatory surgical centers seeking accreditation for Medicare certification purposes, regardless of the number of patients rendered incapable.*

Note 3: *In leased facilities, the elements of performance of this standard apply only to the space in which the accredited organization is located; all exits from the space to the outside at grade level; and any* Life Safety Code *building systems that support the space (for example, fire alarm system, automatic sprinkler system).*

Rationale for LS.03.01.20

Because patients are ill and in many cases cannot escape the danger of fire on their own, buildings in which patients are cared for must be designed and maintained so that patients can be moved to safe places in the building (instead of evacuated to a place outside the building).

Means of egress are corridors, stairways, and doors that allow individuals to leave a building or to move between specific spaces in a building. They allow individuals to escape from fire and smoke, and, therefore, are an integral part of a fire protection strategy. The organization should make sure that a sufficient number of exits exist and that they are configured to provide protection from fire. It is important that egress doors are not locked in a way that restricts passage to safety.

Elements of Performance for LS.03.01.20

1. Doors in a means of egress are not equipped with a latch or lock that requires the use of a tool or key from the egress side, unless a compliant locking configuration is used, such as a delayed-egress locking system as defined in NFPA 101-2012: 7.2.1.6.1 or access-controlled egress door assemblies as defined in NFPA 101-2012: 7.2.1.6.2. Elevator lobby exit access door locking is allowed if compliant with 7.2.1.6.3. (For full text, refer to NFPA 101-2012: 20/21.2.2)

2. Any door required to be self-closing, including those in an exit stair enclosure, may be held open provided there is an automatic release device that closes the door in response to the manual fire alarm system, loss of power, and smoke detectors. (For full text, refer to NFPA 101-2012: 20/21.2.2.4; 20/21.2.2.5; 7.2.1.8.2)

3. Exits discharge to the outside at grade level or through an approved exit passageway that is continuous and provides a level walking surface. The exit discharge is a hard-packed, all-weather travel surface that is free from obstructions and terminates at a public way or at an exterior exit discharge. (For full text, refer to NFPA 101-2012: 20/21.2.1; 20/21.2.7; 38/39.2.7; 7.1.7; 7.1.10.1; 7.2.6; 7.7) **R**

4. The capacity of the means of egress complies with NFPA 101-2012: 7.3. (For full text, refer to NFPA 101-2012: 20/21.2.3.1)

5. Exit corridors or passageways serving as a means of egress are 44 (or more) inches wide. Doors opening in the means of egress from diagnostic or treatment areas are 32 inches wide (unless the existing door opening is 34 inches). (For full text, refer to NFPA 101-2012: 20/21.2.3.2; 2.3.4)

6. Exits, exit accesses, and exit discharges are clear of obstructions or impediments to the public way, such as clutter (for example, equipment, carts, furniture), construction material, and snow and ice. (For full text, refer to NFPA 101-2012: 7.1.10.1)

7. Exit access doors and exit doors are free of mirrors, hangings, or draperies that might conceal, obscure, or confuse the direction of exit. (For full text, refer to NFPA 101-2012: 20/21.2.1; 7.5.2.2.1)

8. Each floor of a building has at least two exits that are remote from each other and accessible from every part of the floor. Each smoke compartment has two distinct egress paths to exits that do not require entry into the same adjacent smoke compartment. Patient care suites larger than 2,500 square feet have two exits remotely located from each other. (For full text, refer to NFPA 101-2012: 20/21.2.4.2; 7.4; 38/39.2.4)

9. In new buildings protected throughout by an approved automatic sprinkler system, dead-end corridors are no longer than 50 feet. In new buildings not provided with automatic sprinklers throughout, dead-end corridors are no longer than 20 feet. In existing buildings, dead-end corridors are no longer than 50 feet. (For full text, refer to NFPA 101-2012: 20/21.2.5; 38/39.2.5.2)

10. The travel distance from any point in a room to an exit is 150 feet or less; the travel distance is 200 feet or less in buildings protected throughout by an approved automatic sprinkler system. (For full text, refer to NFPA 101-2012: 20/21.2.6)

11. Nothing is stored in any exit enclosure. (For full text, refer to NFPA 101-2012: 20/21.2.1; 7.2.2.5) **R**

12. Means of egress are automatically and adequately illuminated at all points, including angles and intersections of corridors and passageways, stairways, stairway landings, exit doors, and exit discharges. (For full text, refer to NFPA 101-2012: 20/21.2.8; 7.8)

13. Illumination in the means of egress, including exit discharge, is arranged so that failure of any single lighting unit will not result in darkness (less than 0.2 footcandles of illumination). Emergency lighting of at least 1½-hours duration is provided automatically in accordance with NFPA 101-2012: 7.9. (For full text, refer to NFPA 101-2012: 20/21.2.8; 7.8.1.4)

14. Signs reading "NO EXIT" are posted on doors to stairs in areas that are not conforming exits and that may be mistaken for exits. (For full text, refer to NFPA 101-2012: 20/21.2.10; 7.10.8.3)

15. Exit signs are visible when the path to the exit is not readily apparent. Signs are adequately lit and have letters that are 4 or more inches high or 6 inches high if externally lit. (*See* NFPA 101-2012: 20/21.2.10; 7.10.5)

16. New buildings equipped with or requiring the use of life support systems (electromechanical or inhalation anesthetics) have illumination for the following: means of egress, emergency lighting equipment, exit, and directional signs supplied by the life safety branch of the electrical system described in NFPA 99-2012. (For full text, refer to NFPA 101-2012: 20.2.9.2; NFPA 99-2012: 6.4.2.2.3)

17. The organization meets all other *Life Safety Code* means of egress requirements related to NFPA 101-2012: 20/21.2.

Standard LS.03.01.30 ━━━━━━━━━━━━━━━━━━━━━━━━━━

The organization provides and maintains building features to protect individuals from the hazards of fire and smoke.

Note 1: *This standard applies to sites of care where four or more patients at the same time are provided either anesthesia or outpatient services that render patients incapable of saving themselves in an emergency in the organization.*

Note 2: *This standard applies to all ambulatory surgical centers seeking accreditation for Medicare certification purposes, regardless of the number of patients rendered incapable.*

Note 3: *In leased facilities, the elements of performance of this standard apply only to the space in which the accredited organization is located; all exits from the space to the outside at grade level; and any* Life Safety Code *building systems that support the space (for example, fire alarm system, automatic sprinkler system).*

Rationale for LS.03.01.30

Fire and smoke are concerns in organizations because of the inability of some patients to evacuate. The effects of fire and smoke can be contained when sections of a building are separated into multiple compartments and when interior finishes are controlled. Smoke and fire can travel through openings in a building. Necessary openings may include heating, ventilating, and air conditioning (HVAC) systems and elevator shafts, and organizations should design and maintain these openings to contain smoke and fire.

Elements of Performance for LS.03.01.30

1. In new construction, vertical openings, including exit stairs, are enclosed by one-hour fire-rated walls when connecting three or fewer floors and two-hour fire-rated walls when connecting four or more floors. Existing vertical openings, including exit stairs, are enclosed with a minimum of one-hour fire-rated construction. (For full text, refer to NFPA 101-2012: 20/21.3.1; 8.6; 8.6.5; 38/39.3.1) **R**

    Note: *These vertical openings include, but are not limited to, shafts (including elevator, light, and ventilation), communicating stairs, ramps, trash chutes, linen chutes, and utility chases.*

2. In buildings, exit stairs connecting three or fewer floors are fire rated for one hour; exit stairs connecting four or more floors are fire rated for two hours. (For full text, refer to NFPA 101-2012: 20/21.3.1; 38/39.3.1; 8.6.5)

3. All hazardous areas are enclosed with one-hour fire-rated walls with ¾-hour fire-rated doors; or hazardous areas have sprinkler systems and are constructed to resist the passage of smoke with doors equipped with self-closing or automatic-closing devices. (For full text, refer to NFPA 101-2012: 20/21.3.2; 38/39.3.2; 8.7; NFPA 80-2010: 4.8.4.1; 6.3.1.7; 6.5)

4. Laboratories using quantities of flammable, combustible, or hazardous materials that are considered as a severe hazard are protected in accordance with NFPA 101-2012: 8.7 and NFPA 99-2012 requirements. (For full text, refer to NFPA 101-2012: 20/21.3.2.2)

5. Alcohol-based hand rubs (ABHR) are stored and handled in accordance with NFPA 101-2012: 8.7.3.1, unless all of the following conditions are met:
    - Corridor is at least six feet wide.
    - ABHR does not exceed 95% alcohol.
    - Maximum individual dispenser capacity is 0.32 gallons of fluid (0.53 gallons in suites) or 18 ounces of NFPA Level 1–classified aerosols.
    - Dispensers have a minimum of four feet of horizontal spacing between them.
    - Dispensers are not installed within one inch of an ignition source.
    - If floor is carpeted, the building is fully sprinkler protected.
    - Operation of the dispenser complies with NFPA 101-2012: 20/21.3.2.6(11).
    - ABHR is protected against inappropriate access.
    - Not more than an aggregate of 10 gallons of fluid or 1135 ounces of aerosol are used in a single smoke compartment outside a storage cabinet, excluding one individual dispenser per room.
    - Storing more than five gallons of fluid in a single smoke compartment complies with NFPA 30.

6. Commercial cooking equipment is installed per NFPA 96-2011, unless only used for food warming or limited cooking. (For full text, refer to NFPA 101-2012: 20/21.3.2.4; 20/21.3.2.5; 9.2.3)

7. Wall and ceiling interior finishes of exits and enclosed corridors are rated Class A or B for limiting smoke development and the spread of flames. (For full text, refer to NFPA 101-2012: 20/21.3.3; 38/39.3.3.2; 10.2.3)

8. Newly installed interior floor finishes in exits and enclosed corridors have a Class I or II radiant flux rating. (For full text, refer to NFPA 101-2012: 20/21.3.3; 10.2.7)

9. In new construction, openings in vision panels or doors are permitted without protection provided the openings are installed at or below one half the distance from the floor to the room ceiling and do not exceed 20 square inches. In rooms protected throughout by an approved automatic sprinkler system, the aggregate area of openings is limited to 80 square inches. In existing construction, openings are not limited. (For full text, refer to NFPA 101-2012: 20.3.6.2)

   Note: *Openings may include, but are not limited to, mail slots and pass-through windows in areas such as laboratory, pharmacy, and cashier stations.*

10. In new construction, corridors that provide access to exits are separated from other areas by one-hour fire-rated barriers unless otherwise permitted by NFPA 101-2012: 38.3.6.1.

    Note: *For existing construction, there are no requirements. (For full text, refer to NFPA 101-2012: 20.3.6.2; 38.3.6.1)*

11. Ambulatory health care space must be separated from other tenants with a one-hour fire resistance–rated barrier, constructed from the floor slab below to the floor or roof above. Doors in the barrier are 1¾ inch thick, solid bonded (or equivalent), self-closing, and have positive latching. Doors are kept in the closed position except when in use. Windows in the barrier comply with NFPA 101-2012: 8.3. (For full text, refer to NFPA 101-2012: 20/21.3.7.1; 8.3)

12. At least two smoke compartments are provided for every story unless one of the following conditions are met:
    - Facility is less than 5,000 square feet and protected by an approved smoke detection system
    - Facility is less than 10,000 square feet and protected by an approved, supervised sprinkler system per NFPA 101-2012: 9.7
    - Adjoining occupancy is used as a smoke compartment if all of the following conditions are met:
      - ❑ Separating wall has a fire-resistive rating of one hour
      - ❑ Doors in the one-hour fire-rated wall are 1¾-inch thick
      - ❑ Doors in the one-hour fire-rated wall are self-closing
      - ❑ Windows in the one-hour fire-rated wall are fixed fire window assemblies per NFPA 101-2012: 8.3
      - ❑ The ambulatory health care facility is less than 22,500 square feet
      - ❑ Access from the ambulatory health care facility is unrestricted to another occupancy

(For full text, refer to NFPA 101-2012: 20/21.3.7.2)

13. Smoke barriers extend from the floor slab to the upper floor or roof slab above, through any concealed spaces (such as those above suspended ceilings and interstitial spaces), continuously from exterior wall to exterior wall. All penetrations are sealed. New smoke barriers are constructed of one-hour fire-rated materials. (For full text, refer to NFPA 101-2012: 20/21.3.7.5; 20/21.3.7.6)

14. Ducts that penetrate smoke barriers, are protected by approved smoke dampers that close when a local smoke detector is activated. The detector is located either within the duct system or in the corridor.

    Note: *In buildings with a fully ducted HVAC system and protected throughout by an approved automatic sprinkler system, dampers are not required. (For full text, refer to NFPA 101-2012: 20/21.3.7.6; 8.5.5)*

15. Fixed fire window assemblies in smoke barrier walls or doors are fire rated for 20 minutes and are 25% or less of the size of the fire barrier in which they are installed.

    Note: *Existing window installations that have wired glass or fire-rated glazing, are 1,296 square inches in size or smaller, and are set in approved metal frames are acceptable. (For full text, refer to NFPA 101-2012: 20/21.3.7.7, 8.3.3)*

16. Doors in smoke barriers are constructed of 1¾ inch or thicker solid-bonded wood core (or equivalent) and are self-closing or automatic-closing. For new buildings, doors are required to swing in the direction of egress travel; rabbets, bevels, or astragals are at meeting edges; and stops are at the head and sides of door frames. Center mullions are prohibited in smoke barrier door openings. (For full text, refer to NFPA 101-2012: 20/21.3.7.9; 20/21.2.2.4; 20.3.7.9; 20.3.7.10; 3.7.13; 3.7.14)

17. The organization meets all other *Life Safety Code* fire and smoke protection requirements related to NFPA 101-2012: 20/21.3.

Standard LS.03.01.34 ▬▬▬▬▬▬▬

The organization provides and maintains fire alarm systems.

Note 1: *This standard applies to sites of care where four or more patients at the same time are provided either anesthesia or outpatient services that render patients incapable of saving themselves in an emergency in the organization.*

Note 2: *This standard applies to all ambulatory surgical centers seeking accreditation for Medicare certification purposes, regardless of the number of patients rendered incapable.*

Note 3: *In leased facilities, the elements of performance of this standard apply only to the space in which the accredited organization is located; all exits from the space to the outside at grade level; and any* Life Safety Code *building systems that support the space (for example, fire alarm system, automatic sprinkler system).*

Elements of Performance for LS.03.01.34

1. A fire alarm system is installed with systems and components to provide effective warning of fire in any part of the building in accordance with NFPA 70-2012, National Electric Code, and NFPA 72-2010, National Fire Alarm Code.

2. The master fire alarm control panel is located in an area with a smoke detector or in an area that is continuously occupied and protected, which is an area enclosed with one-hour fire-rated walls and ¾-hour fire-rated doors. In areas not continuously occupied and protected, a smoke detector is installed at each fire alarm control unit. In a new building, detection is also installed at notification appliance circuit power extenders and supervising station transmitting equipment. Fire alarm system wiring or other transmission paths are monitored for integrity. (For full text, refer to NFPA 101-2012: 20/21.3.4.1; 9.6)

3. Initiation of the fire alarm system is by manual means and by any required sprinkler system alarm, detection device, or detection system. Manual alarm boxes are provided in the path of egress near each required exit and 200 feet of travel distance is not exceeded. (For full text, refer to NFPA 101-2012: 20/21.3.4.2.1; 20/21.3.4.2.2; 9.6.2.5)

4. For new buildings, occupant notification is provided automatically in accordance with NFPA 101-2012: 9.6.3 by audible and visual signals. Positive alarm sequence in accordance with 9.6.3.4 is permitted in buildings protected throughout by a sprinkler system. In critical care areas, visual alarms are sufficient. The fire alarm system transmits the alarm automatically to notify emergency forces in the event of a fire. Annunciation zoning for the fire alarm and sprinklers is provided by audible and visual indicators; zones are not larger than 22,500 square feet per zone. (For full text, refer to NFPA 101-2012: 20.3.4.3–20.3.4.4; 9.6.4)

5. For existing buildings, occupant notification is provided automatically in accordance with NFPA 101-2012: 9.6.3 by audible and visual signals. Positive alarm sequence in accordance with 9.6.3.4 is permitted in buildings protected throughout by a sprinkler system. In critical care areas, visual alarms are sufficient. The fire alarm system transmits the alarm automatically to notify emergency forces in the event of a fire. (For full text, refer to NFPA 101-2012: 21.3.4.3; 9.6.4; 9.7.1.1(1))

6. Activation of the required fire alarm control functions occurs automatically and is provided with an alternative power supply in accordance with NFPA 72-2010. (For full text, refer to NFPA 101-2012: 20/21.3.4.4; 9.6.1; 9.6.5)

7. The fire alarm signal automatically transmits to one of the following: **R**
    - An auxiliary fire alarm system
    - Central station fire alarm system
    - A proprietary supervising station fire alarm system
    - A remote supervising station fire alarm system

    (For full text, refer to NFPA 101-2012: 20/21.3.4.3.2; NFPA 101-2012: 9.6.4)

8. The remote ancillary annunciator panel is in a location approved by the local fire department or its equivalent. (For full text, refer to NFPA 101-2012: 20/21.3.4.3, 9.6.3)

9. The fire alarm system contains an audible and visual evacuation signal throughout the building and provides occupant notification without delay. (For full text, refer to NFPA 101-2012: 20/21.3.4.3, 9.6.3) **R**

10. The organization meets all other *Life Safety Code* fire alarm requirements related to NFPA 101-2012: 20.3.4/21.3.4.

Standard LS.03.01.35 ▬▬▬▬▬▬▬

The organization provides and maintains equipment for extinguishing fires.

Note 1: *This standard applies to sites of care where four or more patients at the same time are provided either anesthesia or outpatient services that render patients incapable of saving themselves in an emergency in the organization.*

Note 2: *This standard applies to all ambulatory surgical centers seeking accreditation for Medicare certification purposes, regardless of the number of patients rendered incapable.*

Note 3: *In leased facilities, the elements of performance of this standard apply only to the space in which the accredited organization is located; all exits from the space to the outside at grade level; and any* Life Safety Code *building systems that support the space (for example, fire alarm system, automatic sprinkler system).*

Elements of Performance for LS.03.01.35

1. For new construction, the fire alarm system monitors the components of any required approved automatic sprinkler system. (For full text, refer to NFPA 101-2012: 20/21.3.5.2; 9.7.1.1) **R**

2. The fire alarm system is connected to water flow alarms of any required automatic sprinkler system. (For full text, refer to NFPA 101-2012: 20/21.3.4.4; 20/21.3.5; 9.7.1.1) **R**

3. Piping supports for approved automatic sprinkler systems are not damaged or loose. (For full text, refer to NFPA 101-2012: 20/21.3.4.4; NFPA 25-2011: 5.2.1; 5.2.2; 5.2.3)

4. Approved automatic sprinkler systems piping is not used to support any other item. (For full text, refer to NFPA 101-2012: 20/21.3.4.4; NFPA 25-2011: 5.2.2; NFPA 13-2010: 8.5.5.2; 8.5.5.3)

5. Sprinkler heads are not damaged and are free from corrosion, foreign materials, and paint. (For full text, refer to NFPA 101-2012: 20/21.3.4.4; NFPA 25-2011: 5.2.1; 5.2.2; NFPA 13-2010: 6.2.6.2; 6.2.7.1)

6. There is 18 inches or more of open space maintained below a sprinkler deflector to the top of storage.

    Note: *Perimeter wall shelving may extend up to the ceiling when not located directly below a sprinkler head. (For full text, refer to NFPA 101-2012: 20/21.3.4.4; NFPA 25-2011: 5.2.1; 5.2.2; NFPA 13-2010: 8.5.5; 8.5.6)*

7. At least six spare sprinkler heads that correspond to the types and temperature rating of the organization's sprinkler heads, with associated wrenches, are kept in a cabinet that will not exceed 100°F. (For full text, refer to NFPA 101-2012: 9.7.1.1; NFPA 13-2010: 6.2.9; 6.2.9.1; 6.2.9.3; 6.2.9.6)

    Note: *If the organization has more than 300 sprinklers, the minimum spare sprinkler head requirement incrementally increases. (For full text, refer to NFPA 13-2010: 6.2.9.5)*

10. The travel distance from any point to the nearest portable fire extinguisher is 75 feet or less. Portable fire extinguishers have appropriate signage, are installed in a cabinet or secured on a hanger made for the extinguisher, and are at least four inches off the floor. Those fire extinguishers that are 40 pounds or less are installed so the top is not more than 5 feet above the floor. (For full text, refer to NFPA 101-2012: 20/21.3.5.3; 9.7.4.1; NFPA 10-2010: 6.1.3; 6.2.1)

11. The organization meets all other *Life Safety Code* extinguishing requirements related to NFPA 101-2012: 20/21.3.5.

Standard LS.03.01.40 ▬▬▬▬▬▬▬▬▬▬▬▬▬▬▬▬▬▬▬▬▬▬▬▬▬▬▬▬▬▬

The organization provides and maintains special features to protect individuals from the hazards of fire and smoke.

Note 1: *This standard applies to sites of care where four or more patients at the same time are provided either anesthesia or outpatient services that render patients incapable of saving themselves in an emergency in the organization.*

Note 2: *This standard applies to all ambulatory surgical centers seeking accreditation for Medicare certification purposes, regardless of the number of patients rendered incapable.*

Note 3: *In leased facilities, the elements of performance of this standard apply only to the space in which the accredited organization is located; all exits from the space to the outside at grade level; and any* Life Safety Code *building systems that support the space (for example, fire alarm system, automatic sprinkler system).*

Elements of Performance for LS.03.01.40

1. Windowless buildings or portions of windowless buildings meet the requirements of NFPA 101-2012: 20/21.4; 11.7.

2. Existing high-rise buildings have approved automatic sprinkler systems that meet the requirements of NFPA 101-2012: 20/21.4; 11.8; 9.7.1.1(1), or they have an engineered life safety system complying with NFPA 101-2012: 39.4.2.1(2). New high-rise buildings comply with NFPA 101-2012: 11.8. (For full text, refer to NFPA 101-2012: 20/21.4; 11.8; 39.4.2.1)

3. The organization meets all other *Life Safety Code* extinguishing requirements related to NFPA 101-2012: 20/21.3.5.

Standard LS.03.01.50 ▬▬▬▬▬▬▬

The organization provides and maintains building services to protect individuals from the hazards of fire and smoke.

Note 1: *This standard applies to sites of care where four or more patients at the same time are provided either anesthesia or outpatient services that render patients incapable of saving themselves in an emergency in the organization.*

Note 2: *This standard applies to all ambulatory surgical centers seeking accreditation for Medicare certification purposes, regardless of the number of patients rendered incapable.*

Note 3: *In leased facilities, the elements of performance of this standard apply only to the space in which the accredited organization is located; all exits from the space to the outside at grade level; and any* Life Safety Code *building systems that support the space (for example, fire alarm system, automatic sprinkler system).*

Elements of Performance for LS.03.01.50

1. Equipment using gas or related gas piping complies with NFPA 54-2012, National Fuel Gas Code; electrical wiring and equipment complies with NFPA 70-2012, National Electric Code. Existing installations can continue in service provided there are no life-threatening hazards. (For full text, refer to NFPA 101-2012: 20/21.5.1; 9.1.1)

2. Heating, ventilation, and air conditioning comply with NFPA 101-2012: 9.2 and are installed in accordance with the manufacturers' specifications. (For full text, refer to NFPA 101-2012: 20/21.5.2.1; 9.2)

3. Any heating device (other than a central heating plant) is designed and installed so combustible materials cannot be ignited by the device, and safety features stop fuel and shut down equipment if it experiences excessive temperature or ignition failure. (For full text, refer to NFPA 101-2012: 20/21.5.2.2)

    Note: *If fuel fired, the heating device is designed as follows:*
    - *Chimney or vent connected*
    - *Takes air for combustion from outside*
    - *Combustion system that is separate from occupied area atmosphere*

4. A suspended unit heater(s) is permitted provided the following conditions are met:
    - Not located in means of egress or in patient rooms
    - Located high enough to be out of reach of people in the area

- Has a safety feature to stop fuel and shut down equipment if it experiences excessive temperature or ignition failure

(For full text, refer to NFPA 101-2012: 20/21.5.2.2)

5. New elevators are equipped with all of the following: **R**
   - Firefighters service key recall and smoke detector automatic recall
   - Firefighters service emergency in-car key operation
   - Machine room smoke detectors
   - Elevator lobby smoke detectors

   Existing elevators meet these requirements when they have a travel distance of 25 feet or more above or below the level that best serves the needs of firefighters. (For full text, refer to NFPA 101-2012: 20/21.5.3; 9.4)

6. Escalators, dumbwaiters, and moving walks comply with the provisions of 9.4. All existing escalators, dumbwaiters, and moving walks (including escalator emergency stop buttons and automatic skirt obstruction stop) conform to the requirements of ASME/ANSI A17.3, Safety Code for Existing Elevators and Escalators. (For full text, refer to NFPA 101-2012: 20/21.5.3; 9.4.2)

7. The organization does not allow unvented fuel-fired heaters. (For full text, refer to NFPA 101-2012: 20/21.5.2.2) **R**

8. All heating appliances are provided with safety features to stop the flow of fuel and turn off the appliance during times of excessive temperatures or ignition failure. (For full text, refer to NFPA 101-2012: 20/21.5.2.2) **R**

9. Waste chutes are installed per NFPA 101-2012: 9.5 and meet the following requirements:
   - Walls, partitions, and inlet openings meet the requirements of NFPA 101-2012: 8.3.
   - Doors of chutes open to a room designed exclusively for accessing the chute opening.
   - Rooms used for accessing the chute opening(s) are separated from other spaces per NFPA 101-2012: 8.7.
   - Chutes are permitted to open into rooms not exceeding 400 cubic feet in size if the room is sprinkler protected and not used for storage.

(For full text, refer to NFPA 101-2012: 20/21.5.4; 9.5; NFPA 82-2009)

Note: *Existing installations having properly enclosed and maintained chute openings are permitted to have inlets open to a corridor or normally occupied space.*

10. The organization meets all other *Life Safety Code* building service requirements related to NFPA 101-2012: 20/21.5.

Standard LS.03.01.70 ━━━━━━━━━━━━━━━━━━━━━━━━━━━━

The organization provides and maintains operating features that conform to fire and smoke prevention requirements.

Note 1: *This standard applies to sites of care where four or more patients at the same time are provided either anesthesia or outpatient services that render patients incapable of saving themselves in an emergency in the organization.*

Note 2: *This standard applies to all ambulatory surgical centers departments seeking accreditation for Medicare certification purposes, regardless of the number of patients rendered incapable.*

Note 3: *In leased facilities, the elements of performance of this standard apply only to the space in which the accredited organization is located; all exits from the space to the outside at grade level; and any* Life Safety Code *building systems that support the space (for example, fire alarm system, automatic sprinkler system).*

Elements of Performance for LS.03.01.70

1. In areas where smoking is permitted, ashtrays are safely designed and made of noncombustible material. Metal containers with self-closing cover devices in which ashtrays can be emptied are readily available to all areas where smoking is permitted. (For full text, refer to NFPA 101-2012: 20/21.7.4)

2. Smoking is prohibited in any room, ward, or compartment where flammable liquids, combustible gases, or oxygen is used or stored; these areas have signs that read "NO SMOKING" or display the international symbol for no smoking. In facilities where smoking is prohibited and signs are prominently placed at all major entrances, secondary signs that prohibit smoking in hazardous areas are not required. (For full text, refer to NFPA 101-2012: 18/19.7.4)

   Note: *The secondary sign exception is not applicable to medical gas storage areas.*

3. Draperies, curtains (including cubicle curtains) and loosely hanging fabric comply with NFPA 101-2012: 10.3.1. (For full text, refer to NFPA 101-2012: 18/19.7.5.1; 18/19.3.5.11; 10.3.1)

Note: *Exceptions include shower/bath curtains in addition to window coverings in patient sleeping rooms and in non-patient sleeping rooms located in sprinklered compartments where individual drapery or curtain panels do not exceed 48 square feet or total area does not exceed 20% of the wall.*

4. In buildings without sprinkler protection, upholstered furniture purchased on or after July 5, 2016, meets Class I or char length and heat release criteria in accordance with NFPA 101-2012: 10.3.2.1 and 10.3.3. Mattresses purchased on or after July 5, 2016, meet char length and heat release criteria in accordance with NFPA 101-2012: 10.3.2.2 and 10.3.4. (For full text, refer to NFPA 101-2012: 20/21.7.5.2; 20/21.7.5.4)

5. The organization prohibits all combustible decorations unless they meet the criteria of NFPA 101-2012: 20/21.7.5.4.

6. Soiled linen and trash receptacles larger than 32 gallons (including recycling containers) are located in a room protected as a hazardous area. (For full text, refer to NFPA 101-2012: 20/21.7.5.5)

7. When installed, new engineered smoke control systems are tested in accordance with NFPA 92-2012, Standard for Smoke Control Systems. Existing engineered smoke control systems are tested in accordance with established engineering principles. (For full text, refer to NFPA 101-2012: 20/21.7.7)

8. Portable space heaters are prohibited in smoke compartments containing staff sleeping rooms and patient treatment areas. Non-sleeping rooms occupied by staff and employee areas separated from the corridor are permitted to have portable space heaters that contain heating elements not exceeding 212°F. (For full text, refer to NFPA 101-2012: 20/21.7.8)

9. The organization meets all other *Life Safety Code* operating feature requirements related to NFPA 101-2012: 20/21.7.

Medication Management (MM)

Overview

Medication management is an important component in the palliative, symptomatic, and curative treatment of many diseases and conditions. However, medications are also capable of causing great harm if the incorrect dose or medication is inadvertently administered to a patient. To eliminate any potential harm that could be caused by medications, organizations need to develop an effective and safe medication management system.

A safe medication management system addresses an organization's medication processes, which in many organizations include the following (as applicable):
- Planning
- Selection and procurement
- Storage
- Ordering
- Preparing and dispensing
- Administration
- Monitoring
- Evaluation

The "Medication Management" (MM) chapter addresses these critical processes, including those undertaken by the organization and those provided through contracted pharmacy services. However, the specifics of the medication management system used by the organization can vary depending on the care, treatment, or services it provides. Not all organizations will implement all of the medication processes. For example, organizations without pharmacy services will conduct the medication ordering process and will provide patients with prescriptions.

Effective and safe medication management also involves multiple services and disciplines working closely together. The medication management standards address activities involving various individuals, such as licensed independent practitioners and staff, within an organization's medication management system.

In addition, an effective medication management system includes mechanisms for reporting potential and actual medication-related errors and a process to improve medication management processes and patient safety based on this information.

In essence, a well-planned and implemented medication management system supports patient safety and improves the quality of care by doing the following:

- Reducing variation, errors, and misuse
- Using evidence-based practices to develop medication management processes
- Managing critical processes to promote safe medication management throughout the organization
- Standardizing equipment and handling processes, including those for sample medications, across the organization to improve the medication management system
- Monitoring the medication management process for efficiency, quality, and safety

About This Chapter

The goal of the medication management standards is to provide a framework for an effective and safe medication management system. Effective and safe medication management is dependent on carefully implementing medication management processes based on the care, treatment, or services provided by the organization. Planning provides the groundwork for the following critical areas of performance outlined in this chapter:

- Managing high-alert and hazardous medications
- Selecting and procuring medications
- Storing medications
- Managing emergency medications
- Controlling medications brought into the organization by patients, their families, and licensed independent practitioners
- Managing medication orders
- Preparing medications
- Labeling medications
- Dispensing medications
- Retrieving recalled or discontinued medications
- Administering medications
- Managing investigational medications
- Monitoring patients' reactions to medications
- Responding to real or potential adverse drug events, adverse drug reactions, and medication errors

Selected elements of performance (EPs) that are applicable to sample medications include a note that states, "This element of performance is also applicable to sample medications." The Joint Commission is not endorsing the use of sample medications.

The note is only intended to identify which Medication Management EPs are applicable to sample medications for organizations that permit their use. Medication Management EPs that do not include this note are not applicable to sample medications.

Chapter Outline

I.   Planning
    A. Medication Planning (MM.01.01.01, MM.01.01.03)
    B. Look-alike/Sound-alike Medications (MM.01.02.01)

II. Selection and Procurement (MM.02.01.01)

III. Storage (MM.03.01.01, MM.03.01.03, MM.03.01.05)

IV. Ordering and Transcribing (MM.04.01.01)

V.   Preparing and Dispensing (MM.05.01.01, MM.05.01.07, MM.05.01.09, MM.05.01.11, MM.05.01.15, MM.05.01.17, MM.05.01.19)

VI. Administration (MM.06.01.01, MM.06.01.05)

VII. Monitoring (MM.07.01.01, MM.07.01.03)

VIII. Evaluation (MM.08.01.01)

IX. Antimicrobial Stewardship (MM.09.01.03)

Standards, Rationales, and Elements of Performance

Standard MM.01.01.01 ━━━━━━━━━━━━━━━

The organization plans its medication management processes.

Rationale for MM.01.01.01

Medication management is often complicated, involving many people and processes. For this reason, the organization plans each part of the process with care so that safety and quality are maintained. This planning may involve the coordinated efforts of multiple services and disciplines.

Elements of Performance for MM.01.01.01

1.   Ⓓ The organization follows a written policy that describes that the following information about the patient is accessible to licensed independent practitioners and staff who participate in the management of the patient's medications:
   ■ Age
   ■ Sex
   ■ Diagnoses
   ■ Allergies
   ■ Sensitivities
   ■ Current medications
   ■ Height and weight (when necessary)
   ■ Pregnancy and lactation information (when necessary)
   ■ Laboratory results (when necessary)
   ■ Any additional information required by the organization

   Note 1: *This element of performance does not apply in emergency situations.*

   Note 2: *This element of performance is also applicable to sample medications.*

   (*See also* IM.02.01.01, EP 3)

3.   **For ambulatory surgical centers that elect to use The Joint Commission deemed status option:** One individual is designated as responsible for pharmaceutical services.

4.   **For ambulatory surgical centers that elect to use The Joint Commission deemed status option:** Medications are prepared and administered in accordance with organizational policies and established standards of practice.

Standard MM.01.01.03

The organization safely manages high-alert and hazardous medications.

Rationale for MM.01.01.03

High-alert medications are those medications that bear a heightened risk of causing significant patient harm and/or sentinel events when they are used in error and, as a result, require special safeguards to reduce the risk of errors. Examples of high-alert medications include opioids, insulin, anticoagulants, and neuromuscular blocking agents. Lists of high-alert medications are available from organizations such as the Institute for Safe Medication Practices (ISMP).

Hazardous drugs and medications are those in which studies in animals or humans indicate that exposure to them has a potential for causing cancer, developmental or reproductive toxicity, genotoxicity, or harm to organs. An example of a hazardous drug is one that contains antineoplastic agents or other ingredients that cause the aforementioned risks. Lists of hazardous drugs are available from the National Institute for Occupational Safety and Health (NIOSH).

For safe management, the organization needs to develop its own lists of both high-alert medications and hazardous drugs. These should be based on the organization's unique utilization patterns, its own internal data about medication errors and sentinel events, and known safety issues published in professional literature. It is up to the organization to determine whether medications that are new to the market are high alert or hazardous. In addition, the organization may separately choose to include other drugs that require special precautions such as investigational medications, controlled substances, and psychotherapeutic medications.

Note: *For a list of high-alert medications, see https://www.ismp.org/recommendations. For a list of hazardous drugs, see https://www.cdc.gov/niosh/docs/2016-161/pdfs/2016-161.pdf.*

Elements of Performance for MM.01.01.03

1. Ⓓ The organization identifies, in writing, its high-alert and hazardous medications.* **R**

   Note: *This element of performance is also applicable to sample medications.*

   (*See also* EC.02.02.01, EP 1)

---

* For a list of high-alert medications, *see* https://www.ismp.org/recommendations. For a list of hazardous drugs, *see* https://www.cdc.gov/niosh/docs/2016-161/pdfs/2016-161.pdf.

2. The organization follows a process for managing high-alert and hazardous medications. **R**

   Note: *This element of performance is also applicable to sample medications.*

   (*See also* EC.02.02.01, EP 8; MM.03.01.01, EP 9)

Standard MM.01.02.01

The organization addresses the safe use of look-alike/sound-alike medications.

Elements of Performance for MM.01.02.01

1. Ⓓ The organization develops a list of look-alike/sound-alike medications it stores, dispenses, or administers. **R**

   Note 1: *One source of look-alike/sound-alike medication name pairs is the Institute for Safe Medication Practices (https://www.ismp.org/recommendations/confused-drug-names-list).*

   Note 2: *This element of performance is also applicable to sample medications.*

2. The organization takes action to prevent errors involving the interchange of the medications on its list of look-alike/sound-alike medications. **R**

   Note: *This element of performance is also applicable to sample medications.*

3. The organization annually reviews and, as necessary, revises its list of look-alike/sound-alike medications.

   Note: *This element of performance is also applicable to sample medications.*

Standard MM.02.01.01

The organization selects and procures medications.

Elements of Performance for MM.02.01.01

1. The organization develops criteria for determining which medications are available for dispensing or administering to patients.

   Note: *This element of performance is also applicable to sample medications.*

2. The criteria for selecting medications are approved by the organization and include indications for use, effectiveness, and risks.

   Note: *This element of performance is also applicable to sample medications.*

3. Before using a medication new to the organization, the organization determines a method to monitor the response of the patient.

    Note: *This element of performance is also applicable to sample medications.*

    (*See also* MM.07.01.01, EP 2)

4. Ⓓ The organization maintains a written list of medications, including strength and dosage, for dispensing and administering. The list is readily available to those involved in medication management.

    Note: *Sample medications are not required to be on this list.*

6. The organization standardizes and limits the number of drug concentrations available in the organization.

7. The organization follows a process to select and procure medications that are not on its list of medications.

    Note: *This element of performance is also applicable to sample medications.*

9. Medications designated as available for dispensing or administration are reviewed at least annually based on emerging safety and efficacy information.

10. The organization follows a process to communicate medication shortages and outages to licensed independent practitioners and staff who participate in medication management.

12. Ⓓ The organization follows written medication substitution protocols to be used in the event of a medication shortage or outage.

14. The organization follows a process to communicate the medication substitution protocols for shortages or outages to licensed independent practitioners and staff who participate in medication management.

Standard MM.03.01.01 ▬▬▬▬▬▬▬▬▬▬▬▬▬▬▬▬▬▬▬▬▬▬▬▬▬▬▬▬▬
The organization safely stores medications.

Rationale for MM.03.01.01
Medication storage is designed to assist in maintaining medication integrity, promote the availability of medications when needed, minimize the risk of medication diversion, and reduce potential dispensing errors. Law and regulation and manufacturers' guidelines further define the organization's approach to medication storage.

Elements of Performance for MM.03.01.01

2. The organization stores medications according to the manufacturers' recommendations. **R**

    Note: *This element of performance is also applicable to sample medications.*

3. The organization stores controlled (scheduled) medications to prevent diversion, in accordance with law and regulation.

    Note: *This element of performance is also applicable to sample medications.*

4. The organization safely handles medications between receipt by licensed independent practitioners or staff and administration of the medications.

    Note: *This element of performance is also applicable to sample medications.*

6. The organization prevents unauthorized individuals from obtaining medications in accordance with its policy and law and regulation.

    Note: *This element of performance is also applicable to sample medications.*

7. All stored medications and the components used in their preparation are labeled with the contents, expiration date, and any applicable warnings.

    Note: *This element of performance is also applicable to sample medications.*

8. The organization removes all expired, damaged, and/or contaminated medications and stores them separately from medications available for administration.

    Note: *This element of performance is also applicable to sample medications.*

9. The organization keeps concentrated electrolytes present in patient care areas only when patient safety necessitates their immediate use, and precautions are used to prevent inadvertent administration. **R**

    (*See also* MM.01.01.03, EP 2)

18. The organization periodically inspects all medication storage areas.

    Note: *This element of performance is also applicable to sample medications.*

Standard MM.03.01.03 ▬▬▬▬▬▬▬▬▬▬▬▬▬▬▬▬▬▬▬▬▬▬

The organization safely manages emergency medications.

Rationale for MM.03.01.03

Patient emergencies occur frequently in health care settings. The organization, therefore, needs to plan how it will address patient emergencies and what medications and supplies it will need. Although the processes may be different, the organization treats emergency medications with the same care for safety as it does medications in nonemergency settings.

Elements of Performance for MM.03.01.03

1. Organization leaders decide which, if any, emergency medications and their associated supplies will be readily accessible in patient care areas based on the population served. Whenever possible, emergency medications are available in unit-dose, age-specific, and ready-to-administer forms.

6. When emergency medications or supplies are used or expired, the organization replaces them as soon as possible to maintain a full stock.

Standard MM.03.01.05

The organization safely controls medications brought into the organization by patients, their families, or licensed independent practitioners.

Rationale for MM.03.01.05

A number of valid reasons exist for allowing the patient to use their own medications in an organization. The organization needs to control the use of these medications in order to protect the safety of the patient and the quality of care provided. Therefore, the organization needs to define its responsibilities for the safe use of these medications.

Elements of Performance for MM.03.01.05

1. The organization defines when medications brought into the organization by patients, their families, or licensed independent practitioners can be administered.

    Note: *This element of performance is also applicable to sample medications.*

2. Before use or administration of a medication brought into the organization by a patient, their family, or a licensed independent practitioner, the organization identifies the medication and visually evaluates the medication's integrity.

    Note: *This element of performance is also applicable to sample medications.*

    (*See also* MM.06.01.01, EP 3)

Introduction to Standard MM.04.01.01

Medication errors may occur when staff are communicating or transcribing medication orders. Verbal and telephone orders are particularly susceptible to error. The organization is responsible for reducing the potential for medication errors and the misinterpretation of these medication orders. As part of this process, the organization determines the required elements of a medication order, the type of medication orders that are deemed acceptable for use, and the actions to take when medication orders are incomplete, illegible, or unclear. Clear understanding and communication between staff and licensed independent practitioners involved in the medication process are essential.

Standard MM.04.01.01 ▬▬▬▬▬▬▬▬▬▬▬▬▬▬▬▬▬▬▬▬▬

Medication orders are clear and accurate.

Elements of Performance for MM.04.01.01

1. Ⓓ The organization follows a written policy that identifies the specific types of medication orders that it deems acceptable for use.

    Note: *There are several different types of medication orders. Medication orders commonly used include the following:*

    - *As needed (PRN) orders: Orders acted on based on the occurrence of a specific indication or symptom*
    - *Standing orders: A prewritten medication order and specific instructions from the licensed independent practitioner to administer a medication to a person in clearly defined circumstances*
    - *Automatic stop orders: Orders that include a date or time to discontinue a medication*
    - *Titrating orders: Orders in which the dose is either progressively increased or decreased in response to the patient's status*
    - *Taper orders: Orders in which the dose is decreased by a particular amount with each dosing interval*
    - *Range orders: Orders in which the dose or dosing interval varies over a prescribed range, depending on the situation or patient's status*
    - *Signed and held orders: New prewritten (held) medication orders and specific instructions from a licensed independent practitioner to administer medication(s) to a patient in clearly defined circumstances that become active upon the release of the orders on a specific date(s) and time(s)*
    - *Orders for compounded drugs or drug mixtures not commercially available*
    - *Orders for medication-related devices (for example, nebulizers, catheters)*

- *Orders for investigational medications*
- *Orders for herbal products*
- *Orders for medications at the end of an episode of care, or at discharge or transfer*

2. Ⓓ The organization follows a written policy that defines the following:
   - The minimum required elements of a complete medication order, which must include medication name, medication dose, medication route, and medication frequency
   - When indication for use is required on a medication order
   - The precautions for ordering medications with look-alike or sound-alike names
   - Actions to take when medication orders are incomplete, illegible, or unclear
   - For medication titration orders, required elements include the medication name, medication route, initial rate of infusion (dose/unit of time), incremental units to which the rate or dose can be increased or decreased, how often the rate or dose can be changed, the maximum rate or dose of infusion, and the objective clinical measure to be used to guide changes

   Note: *Examples of objective clinical measures to be used to guide titration changes include blood pressure, Richmond Agitation–Sedation Scale (RASS), and the Confusion Assessment Method (CAM).*

7. If the organization uses preprinted medication order sheets, it updates them based on current evidence and practice.

8. The organization prohibits summary (blanket) orders to resume previous medications.

12. Ⓓ **For ambulatory surgical centers that elect to use The Joint Commission deemed status option:** Orders given verbally for medications and biologicals are followed by a written order signed by the prescribing physician.

14. The organization requires an order from a doctor of medicine or osteopathy or, as permitted by law and regulation, organization-specific protocol(s) approved by a doctor of medicine or osteopathy to administer influenza and pneumococcal polysaccharide vaccines.

21. **For organizations that elect The Joint Commission Primary Care Medical Home option:** The primary care medical home has an electronic prescribing process.

Standard MM.05.01.01 ━━━━━━━━━━━━━━━━━━━━━━

The organization reviews the appropriateness of all medication orders for medications to be dispensed in the organization.

Elements of Performance for MM.05.01.01

1. The organization defines who can review medication orders or prescriptions for dispensed medications, and under what conditions this occurs, in accordance with law and regulation.

4. All medication orders are reviewed for the following: **R**
   - Patient allergies or potential sensitivities
   - Existing or potential interactions between the medication ordered and food and medications the patient is currently taking
   - The appropriateness of the medication, dose, frequency, and route of administration
   - Current or potential impact as indicated by laboratory values
   - Therapeutic duplication
   - Other contraindications

11. After the medication order has been reviewed, all concerns, issues, or questions are clarified with the individual prescriber before dispensing.

Standard MM.05.01.07 ━━━━━━━━━━━━━━━━━━━━━━

The organization safely prepares medications.

Note: *This standard is applicable to all organizations that prepare medications for administration.*

Elements of Performance for MM.05.01.07

1. When an on-site licensed pharmacy is available, a pharmacist, or pharmacy staff under the supervision of a pharmacist, compounds or admixes all compounded sterile preparations except in urgent situations in which a delay could harm the patient or when the product's stability is short.

2. Staff use clean or sterile techniques and maintain clean, uncluttered, and functionally separate areas for product preparation to avoid contamination of medications. **R**

3. During preparation, staff visually inspect the medication for particulates, discoloration, or other loss of integrity. **R**

4. The organization uses a laminar airflow hood or other ISO Class 5 environment in the pharmacy for preparing intravenous (IV) admixture or any sterile product that will not be used within 24 hours.

Standard MM.05.01.09 ▬▬▬▬▬▬▬▬▬▬▬▬▬▬▬▬▬▬▬▬

Medications are labeled.

Note: *This standard is applicable to all organizations that prepare and administer medications.*

Rationale for MM.05.01.09

A label on every medication and medication container has long been a standard of practice by the pharmacy profession and is required by law and regulation. A standardized method to label medications and containers promotes medication safety.

Elements of Performance for MM.05.01.09

1. Medication containers are labeled whenever medications are prepared but not immediately administered. **R**

   Note 1: *An organization that exclusively uses a single medication in a patient care area can draw up or prepare multiple doses for later use as long as the medication is segregated and secured from all other medications in the organization (for example, a vaccine, flu shot) and the container holding the individual doses is labeled.*

   Note 2: *An immediately administered medication is one that an authorized staff member prepares or obtains, takes directly to a patient, and administers to that patient without any break in the process.*

   Note 3: *This element of performance is also applicable to sample medications.*

2. Information on medication labels is displayed in a standardized format, in accordance with law and regulation and standards of practice.

   Note: *This element of performance is also applicable to sample medications.*

3. All medications prepared in the organization are correctly labeled with the following: **R**
   - Medication name, strength, and amount (if not apparent from the container)

   Note: *This is also applicable to sample medications.*
   - Expiration date when not used within 24 hours
   - Expiration date and time when expiration occurs in less than 24 hours

- The date prepared and the diluent for all compounded intravenous admixtures and parenteral nutrition formulas

7. When preparing individualized medications for multiple patients, the label also includes the following: **R**
   - The patient's name
   - The location where the medication is to be delivered
   - Directions for use and applicable accessory and cautionary instructions

   (*See also* NPSG.01.01.01, EP 1)

10. When an individualized medication(s) is prepared by someone other than the person administering the medication, the label includes the following: **R**
    - The patient's name
    - The location where the medication is to be delivered
    - Directions for use and applicable accessory and cautionary instructions

    (*See also* NPSG.01.01.01, EP 1)

Standard MM.05.01.11
The organization safely dispenses medications.

Elements of Performance for MM.05.01.11

2. The organization dispenses medications and maintains clinical records in accordance with law and regulation, licensure, and professional standards of practice.

   Note 1: *Dispensing practices and recordkeeping include antidiversion strategies.*

   Note 2: *This element of performance is also applicable to sample medications.*

Standard MM.05.01.15
The organization safely obtains medications when it does not operate a pharmacy.

Elements of Performance for MM.05.01.15

1. If the organization does not operate a pharmacy, the organization follows a process for obtaining medications from a pharmacy or licensed pharmaceutical supplier to meet patient needs.

Standard MM.05.01.17
The organization follows a process to retrieve recalled or discontinued medications.

Note: *This standard is applicable to all organizations that dispense medications, including sample medications.*

Elements of Performance for MM.05.01.17

1. ⓓ The organization follows a written policy describing how it will retrieve and handle medications within the organization that are recalled or discontinued for safety reasons by the manufacturer or the US Food and Drug Administration (FDA).

   Note: *This element of performance is also applicable to sample medications.*

   (*See also* EC.02.01.01, EP 11)

3. When a medication is recalled or discontinued for safety reasons by the manufacturer or the US Food and Drug Administration (FDA), the organization notifies the prescribers and those who dispense or administer the medication.

   Note: *This element of performance is also applicable to sample medications.*

   (*See also* EC.02.01.01, EP 11)

4. When required by law and regulation or organization policy, the organization informs patients that their medication has been recalled or discontinued for safety reasons by the manufacturer or the US Food and Drug Administration (FDA).

   Note: *This element of performance is also applicable to sample medications.*

   (*See also* EC.02.01.01, EP 11)

Standard MM.05.01.19
The organization safely manages returned medications.

Rationale for MM.05.01.19
Medications may be returned to the organization when allowed by law or regulation and organization policy. Previously dispensed but unused, expired, or returned medications in the organization must be accounted for, controlled, and disposed of in order to keep patients safe and prevent diversion.

Elements of Performance for MM.05.01.19

1. The organization determines under what circumstances unused, expired, or returned medications will be managed by the pharmacy or the organization.

   Note: *This element of performance is also applicable to sample medications.*

2. When the organization accepts unused, expired, or returned medications, it follows a process for returning medications to the pharmacy's or organization's control which includes procedures for preventing diversion.

   Note: *This element of performance is also applicable to sample medications.*

3. The organization determines if and when outside sources are used for destruction of medications.

   Note: *This element of performance is also applicable to sample medications.*

Standard MM.06.01.01

The organization safely administers medications.

Elements of Performance for MM.06.01.01

1. Ⓓ Only authorized licensed independent practitioners and clinical staff administer medications. The organization defines, in writing, those who are authorized to administer medication, with or without supervision, in accordance with law and regulation.

   Note: *This does not prohibit self-administration of medications by patients, when indicated.*

3. Before administration, the individual administering the medication does the following:
   - Verifies that the medication selected matches the medication order and product label
   - Visually inspects the medication for particulates, discoloration, or other loss of integrity
   - Verifies that the medication has not expired
   - Verifies that no contraindications exist
   - Verifies that the medication is being administered at the proper time, in the prescribed dose, and by the correct route
   - Discusses any unresolved concerns about the medication with the patient's licensed independent practitioner, prescriber (if different from the licensed independent practitioner), and/or staff involved with the patient's care, treatment, or services

Note 1: **For ambulatory surgical centers that elect to use The Joint Commission deemed status option:** *The Centers for Medicare & Medicaid Services require ambulatory surgical centers to use single dose (single-use) medication vials for only one patient.*

Note 2: **For ambulatory surgical centers that elect to use The Joint Commission deemed status option:** *The Centers for Medicare & Medicaid Services require ambulatory surgical centers to date multi-dose injectable medications that are used for more than one patient when they are opened, and discard them within 28 days of opening or according to the manufacturer's recommendations, whichever is more stringent.*

(*See also* MM.03.01.05, EP 2)

9. Before administering a new medication, the patient or family is informed about any potential clinically significant adverse drug reactions or other concerns regarding administration of a new medication.

(*See also* PC.02.03.01, EP 10)

13. Before administering a radioactive pharmaceutical for diagnostic purposes, staff verify that the dose to be administered is within 20% of the prescribed dose, or, if the dose is prescribed as a range, staff verify that the dose to be administered is within the prescribed range.

Standard MM.06.01.05
The organization safely manages investigational medications.

Rationale for MM.06.01.05
Investigational medications can be of great help to the patient. In some cases, investigational medications may represent one of a few options in the patient's plan of care. The organization contributes to the safety of patients participating in investigational or clinical medication studies by controlling and monitoring the use of these medications.

Note: *For a discussion of patient rights regarding the use of investigational medications,* see *Standard RI.01.03.05.*

Elements of Performance for MM.06.01.05

1. Ⓓ The organization follows a written process addressing the use of investigational medications that includes review, approval, supervision, and monitoring.

2. If the organization operates a pharmacy, the process for the use of investigational medications specifies that the pharmacy controls the storage, dispensing, labeling, and distribution of investigational medications.

3. The written process for the use of investigational medications specifies that when a patient is involved in an investigational protocol that is independent of the organization, the organization evaluates and accommodates the patient's continued participation in the protocol.

Standard MM.07.01.01

The organization monitors patients to determine the effects of their medication(s).

Elements of Performance for MM.07.01.01

1. The organization monitors the patient's perception of side effects and the effectiveness of the patient's medication(s).

   Note: *This element of performance is also applicable to sample medications.*

2. The organization monitors the patient's response to medication(s) by taking into account clinical information from the clinical record, relevant lab values, clinical response, and medication profile.

   Note 1: *Monitoring the patient's response to medications is an important assessment activity for nurses, physicians, and pharmacists. In particular, monitoring the patient's response to the first dose of a new medication is essential to the safety of the patient because any adverse reactions, including serious ones, are more unpredictable if the medication has never been used before with the patient.*

   Note 2: *This element of performance is also applicable to sample medications.*

   (*See also* MM.02.01.01, EP 3)

Standard MM.07.01.03

The organization responds to actual or potential adverse drug events, significant adverse drug reactions, and medication errors.

Rationale for MM.07.01.03

Adverse drug reactions and medication errors place patients at considerable risk. For safe, quality care, organizations must have systems in place to respond to and monitor a patient in the event of an adverse drug reaction or medication error.

Elements of Performance for MM.07.01.03

1. Ⓓ The organization follows a written process to respond to actual or potential adverse drug events, significant adverse drug reactions, and medication errors.

    Note: *This element of performance is also applicable to sample medications.*

2. Ⓓ The organization follows a written process addressing prescriber notification in the event of an adverse drug event, significant adverse drug reaction, or medication error.

    Note: *This element of performance is also applicable to sample medications.*

3. The organization complies with internal and external reporting requirements for actual or potential adverse drug events, significant adverse drug reactions, and medication errors.

    Note: *This element of performance is also applicable to sample medications.*

4. **For ambulatory surgical centers that elect to use The Joint Commission deemed status option:** All adverse drug events are reported to the physician (as defined in section 1861(r) of the Social Security Act) responsible for the patient and are documented in the clinical record.

Standard MM.08.01.01

The organization evaluates the effectiveness of its medication management system.

Note: *This evaluation includes reconciling medication information. (Refer to NPSG.03.06.01 for more information)*

Elements of Performance for MM.08.01.01

1. As part of its evaluation of the effectiveness of medication management, the organization does the following:
    - Collects data on the performance of its medication management system
    - Analyzes data on its medication management system
    - Compares data over time to identify risk points, levels of performance, patterns, trends, and variations of its medication management system

    Note: *This element of performance is also applicable to sample medications.*

    (*See also* PI.01.01.01, EPs 12, 13)

5. Based on analysis of its data, as well as review of the literature for new technologies and best practices, the organization identifies opportunities for improvement in its medication management system.

6. When opportunities are identified for improvement of the medication management system, the organization does the following:
   - Takes action on improvement opportunities identified as priorities for its medication management system
   - Evaluates its actions to confirm that they resulted in improvements

   Note: *This element of performance is also applicable to sample medications.*

   (*See also* PI.04.01.01, EP 2)

8. The organization takes additional action when planned improvements for its medication management processes are either not achieved or not sustained.

16. ⒟ When automatic dispensing cabinets (ADCs) are used, the organization has a policy that describes the types of medication overrides that will be reviewed for appropriateness and the frequency of the reviews. A 100% review of overrides is not required.

Standard MM.09.01.03 ━━━━━━━━━━━━━━━━━━━━━━━

Antimicrobial stewardship is identified as an organizational priority.

Elements of Performance for MM.09.01.03

1. The organization identifies an individual(s) responsible for developing, implementing, and monitoring activities to promote appropriate antimicrobial medication prescribing practices.

2. The organization sets at least one annual antimicrobial stewardship goal.

   Note: *Examples of antimicrobial stewardship goals may include decreasing the use of antibiotics to treat viral infections or addressing overuse of a specific medication.*

3. The organization uses evidence-based practice guidelines related to its annual antimicrobial stewardship goal(s).

   Note: *Guidelines may include diagnostic criteria and treatment recommendations to use when prescribing antimicrobial medications.*

4. The organization provides all clinical staff and licensed independent practitioners with educational resources related to its antimicrobial stewardship goal(s) and strategies that promote appropriate antimicrobial medication prescribing practices.

5. The organization collects, analyzes, and reports data pertaining to the antimicrobial stewardship goal(s) to organizational leadership and prescribers.

   Note: *Data may include antimicrobial medication prescribing patterns, antimicrobial resistance patterns, or an evaluation of the antimicrobial stewardship activities implemented.*

   (*See also* PI.04.01.01, EP 5)

National Patient Safety Goals (NPSG)

Chapter Outline

National Patient Safety Goals

I.   Goal 1—Improve the accuracy of patient identification.
     A. Use of Two Patient Identifiers (NPSG.01.01.01)

II. Goal 3—Improve the safety of using medications.
     A. Labeling Medications (NPSG.03.04.01)
     B. Reducing Harm from Anticoagulation Therapy (NPSG.03.05.01)
     C. Reconciling Medication Information (NPSG.03.06.01)

III. Goal 7—Reduce the risk of health care–associated infections.
     A. Meeting Hand Hygiene Guidelines (NPSG.07.01.01)

Universal Protocol for Preventing Wrong Site, Wrong Procedure, and Wrong Person Surgery ™

I.   Universal Protocol
     A. Conducting a Preprocedure Verification Process (UP.01.01.01)
     B. Marking the Procedure Site (UP.01.02.01)
     C. Performing a Time-Out (UP.01.03.01)

Requirements, Rationales, and Elements of Performance

Goal 1
Improve the accuracy of patient identification.

NPSG.01.01.01 ▬▬▬▬▬▬▬▬▬▬▬▬▬▬▬▬▬▬▬▬
Use at least two patient identifiers when providing care, treatment, or services.

Rationale for NPSG.01.01.01
Wrong-patient errors occur in virtually all stages of diagnosis and treatment. The intent for this goal is two-fold: first, to reliably identify the individual as the person for whom the service or treatment is intended; second, to match the service or treatment to that individual. Acceptable identifiers may be the individual's name, an assigned identification number, telephone number, or other person-specific identifier.

Elements of Performance for NPSG.01.01.01

1. Use at least two patient identifiers when administering medications, blood, or blood components; when collecting blood samples and other specimens for clinical testing; and when providing treatments or procedures. The patient's room number or physical location is not used as an identifier. **R**

   (*See also* MM.05.01.09, EPs 7, 10; PC.02.01.01, EP 10)

2. Label containers used for blood and other specimens in the presence of the patient. **R**

   (*See also* PC.02.01.01, EP 10)

Goal 3
Improve the safety of using medications.

NPSG.03.04.01 ▬▬▬▬▬▬▬▬▬▬▬▬▬▬▬▬▬▬▬▬
Label all medications, medication containers, and other solutions on and off the sterile field in perioperative and other procedural settings.

Note: *Medication containers include syringes, medicine cups, and basins.*

Rationale for NPSG.03.04.01

Medications or other solutions in unlabeled containers are unidentifiable. Errors, sometimes tragic, have resulted from medications and other solutions removed from their original containers and placed into unlabeled containers. This unsafe practice neglects basic principles of safe medication management, yet it is routine in many organizations.

The labeling of all medications, medication containers, and other solutions is a risk-reduction activity consistent with safe medication management. This practice addresses a recognized risk point in the administration of medications in perioperative and other procedural settings. Labels for medications and medication containers are also addressed at Standard MM.05.01.09.

Elements of Performance for NPSG.03.04.01

1. In perioperative and other procedural settings both on and off the sterile field, label medications and solutions that are not immediately administered. This applies even if there is only one medication being used. **R**

   Note: *An immediately administered medication is one that an authorized staff member prepares or obtains, takes directly to a patient, and administers to that patient without any break in the process.*

2. In perioperative and other procedural settings both on and off the sterile field, labeling occurs when any medication or solution is transferred from the original packaging to another container. **R**

3. In perioperative and other procedural settings both on and off the sterile field, medication or solution labels include the following: **R**
   - Medication or solution name
   - Strength
   - Amount of medication or solution containing medication (if not apparent from the container)
   - Diluent name and volume (if not apparent from the container)
   - Expiration date when not used within 24 hours
   - Expiration time when expiration occurs in less than 24 hours

   Note: *The date and time are not necessary for short procedures, as defined by the organization.*

4. Verify all medication or solution labels both verbally and visually. Verification is

done by two individuals qualified to participate in the procedure whenever the person preparing the medication or solution is not the person who will be administering it. **R**

5. Label each medication or solution as soon as it is prepared, unless it is immediately administered. **R**

   Note: *An immediately administered medication is one that an authorized staff member prepares or obtains, takes directly to a patient, and administers to that patient without any break in the process.*

6. Immediately discard any medication or solution found unlabeled. **R**

7. Remove all labeled containers on the sterile field and discard their contents at the conclusion of the procedure. **R**

   Note: *This does not apply to multiuse vials that are handled according to infection control practices.*

8. All medications and solutions both on and off the sterile field and their labels are reviewed by entering and exiting staff responsible for the management of medications. **R**

NPSG.03.05.01 ━━━━━━━━━━━━━━━━━━━━━━━━━━

Reduce the likelihood of patient harm associated with the use of anticoagulant therapy.

Note: *This requirement does not apply to routine situations in which short-term prophylactic anticoagulation is used for preventing venous thromboembolism (for example, related to procedures or hospitalization).*

Rationale for NPSG.03.05.01

Anticoagulation therapy can be used as therapeutic treatment for several conditions, the most common of which are atrial fibrillation, deep vein thrombosis, pulmonary embolism, and mechanical heart valve implant. However, it is important to note that anticoagulant medications are more likely than others to cause harm due to complex dosing, insufficient monitoring, and inconsistent patient compliance. This National Patient Safety Goal has great potential to positively impact the safety of patients on this class of medications, including improving patient outcomes.

To achieve better patient outcomes, patient education is a vital component of an anticoagulation therapy program. Effective anticoagulation education includes face-to-face interaction with a trained professional who works closely with patients to be sure that they understand the risks involved with anticoagulation therapy and the precautions they need to take. The use of standardized practices for anticoagulation therapy that include patient involvement can reduce the risk of adverse drug events associated with heparin (unfractionated), low molecular weight heparin, warfarin, and direct oral anticoagulants (DOACs).

Elements of Performance for NPSG.03.05.01

1. The organization uses approved protocols and evidence-based practice guidelines for the initiation and maintenance of anticoagulant therapy that address medication selection; dosing, including adjustments for age and renal or liver function; drug–drug and drug–food interactions; and other risk factors as applicable. **R**

2. The organization uses approved protocols and evidence-based practice guidelines for reversal of anticoagulation and management of bleeding events related to each anticoagulant medication. **R**

4. ⒹThe organization has a written policy addressing the need for baseline and ongoing laboratory tests to monitor and adjust anticoagulant therapy. **R**

   Note: *For all patients receiving warfarin therapy, use a current international normalized ratio (INR) to monitor and adjust dosage. For patients on a direct oral anticoagulant (DOAC), follow evidence-based practice guidelines regarding the need for laboratory testing.*

5. The organization addresses anticoagulation safety practices through the following: **R**
   - Establishing a process to identify, respond to, and report adverse drug events, including adverse drug event outcomes
   - Evaluating anticoagulation safety practices, taking actions to improve safety practices, and measuring the effectiveness of those actions in a time frame determined by the organization

6. The organization provides education to patients and families specific to the anticoagulant medication prescribed, including the following: **R**
   - Adherence to medication dose and schedule
   - Importance of follow-up appointments and laboratory testing (if applicable)
   - Potential drug–drug and drug–food interactions
   - The potential for adverse drug reactions

Introduction to Reconciling Medication Information

The large number of people receiving health care who take multiple medications and the complexity of managing those medications make medication reconciliation an important safety issue. In medication reconciliation, a clinician compares the medications a patient should be using (and is actually using) to the new medications that are ordered for the patient and resolves any discrepancies.

The Joint Commission recognizes that organizations face challenges with medication reconciliation. The best medication reconciliation requires a complete understanding of what the patient was prescribed and what medications the patient is actually taking. It can be difficult to obtain a complete list from every patient in an encounter, and accuracy is dependent on the patient's ability and willingness to provide this information. A good faith effort to collect this information is recognized as meeting the intent of the requirement. As health care evolves with the adoption of more sophisticated systems (such as centralized databases for prescribing and collecting medication information), the effectiveness of these processes will grow.

This National Patient Safety Goal (NPSG) focuses on the risk points of medication reconciliation. The elements of performance in this NPSG are designed to help organizations reduce negative patient outcomes associated with medication discrepancies. Some aspects of the care process that involve the management of medications are addressed in the standards rather than in this goal. These include coordinating information during transitions in care both within and outside of the organization (PC.02.02.01), patient education on safe medication use (PC.02.03.01), and communications with other providers (PC.04.02.01).

In settings where medications are not routinely prescribed or administered, this NPSG provides organizations with the flexibility to decide what medication information they need to collect based on the services they provide to patients. It is often important for clinicians to know what medications the patient is taking when planning care, treatment, or services, even in situations where medications are not used.

NPSG.03.06.01 ▬▬▬▬▬▬▬▬▬▬▬▬▬▬▬▬▬▬▬▬▬▬▬

Maintain and communicate accurate patient medication information.

Rationale for NPSG.03.06.01

There is evidence that medication discrepancies can affect patient outcomes. Medication reconciliation is intended to identify and resolve discrepancies—it is a process of comparing the medications a patient is taking (or should be taking) with newly ordered medications. The comparison addresses duplications, omissions, and interactions, and the need to continue current medications. The types of information that clinicians use to reconcile medications include (among others) medication name, dose, frequency, route, and purpose. Organizations should identify the information that needs to be collected in order to reconcile current and newly ordered medications and to safely prescribe medications in the future.

Elements of Performance for NPSG.03.06.01

1. Ⓓ Obtain and/or update information on the medications the patient is currently taking. This information is documented in a list or other format that is useful to those who manage medications. **R**

   Note 1: *The organization obtains the patient's medication information at the beginning of an episode of care. The information is updated when the patient's medications change.*

   Note 2: *Current medications include those taken at scheduled times and those taken on an as-needed basis. See the Glossary for a definition of medications.*

   Note 3: *It is often difficult to obtain complete information on current medications from the patient. A good faith effort to obtain this information from the patient and/ or other sources will be considered as meeting the intent of the EP.*

2. Define the types of medication information (for example, name, dose, route, frequency, purpose) to be collected in different settings. **R**

   Note: *Examples of such settings include primary care, urgent and emergent care, ambulatory surgery, convenient care, outpatient radiology, and diagnostic settings.*

3. **For organizations that prescribe medications:** Compare the medication information the patient brought to the organization with the medications ordered for the patient by the organization in order to identify and resolve discrepancies. **R**

   Note: *Discrepancies include omissions, duplications, contraindications, unclear information, and changes. A qualified individual, identified by the organization, does the comparison.*

4. Ⓓ **For organizations that prescribe medications:** Provide the patient (or family as needed) with written information on the medications the patient should be

taking at the end of the episode of care (for example, name, dose, route, frequency, purpose). **R**

5. **For organizations that prescribe medications:** Explain the importance of managing medication information to the patient at the end of the episode of care. **R**

   Note: Examples include instructing the patient to give a list to their primary care physician; to update the information when medications are discontinued, doses are changed, or new medications (including over-the-counter products) are added; and to carry medication information at all times in the event of emergency situations. (For information on patient education on medications, refer to Standards PC.02.03.01 and PC.04.01.05.)

Goal 7

Reduce the risk of health care–associated infections.

NPSG.07.01.01

Comply with either the current Centers for Disease Control and Prevention (CDC) hand hygiene guidelines and/or the current World Health Organization (WHO) hand hygiene guidelines.

Rationale for NPSG.07.01.01

According to the Centers for Disease Control and Prevention, each year, millions of people acquire an infection while receiving care, treatment, or services in a health care organization. Consequently, health care–associated infections (HAIs) are a patient safety issue affecting all types of health care organizations. One of the most important ways to address HAIs is by improving the hand hygiene of health care staff. Compliance with the World Health Organization (WHO) and/or Centers for Disease Control and Prevention (CDC) hand hygiene guidelines will reduce the transmission of infectious agents by staff to patients, thereby decreasing the incidence of HAIs. To ensure compliance with this National Patient Safety Goal, an organization should assess its compliance with the CDC and/or WHO guidelines through a comprehensive program that provides a hand hygiene policy, fosters a culture of hand hygiene, monitors compliance, and provides feedback.

Elements of Performance for NPSG.07.01.01

1. Implement a program that follows categories IA, IB, and IC of either the current

Centers for Disease Control and Prevention (CDC) and/or the current World Health Organization (WHO) hand hygiene guidelines. **R**

(*See also* IC.01.04.01, EP 1)

2. Set goals for improving compliance with hand hygiene guidelines. **R**

    (*See also* IC.03.01.01, EP 1)

3. Improve compliance with hand hygiene guidelines based on established goals. **R**

Introduction to the Universal Protocol for Preventing Wrong Site, Wrong Procedure, and Wrong Person Surgery™

The Universal Protocol applies to all surgical and nonsurgical invasive procedures. Evidence indicates that procedures that place the patient at the most risk include those that involve general anesthesia or deep sedation, although other procedures may also affect patient safety. Organizations can enhance safety by correctly identifying the patient, the appropriate procedure, and the correct site of the procedure.

The Universal Protocol is based on the following principles:

■ Wrong-person, wrong-site, and wrong-procedure surgery can and must be prevented.

■ A robust approach using multiple, complementary strategies is necessary to achieve the goal of always conducting the correct procedure on the correct person, at the correct site.

■ Active involvement and use of effective methods to improve communication among all members of the procedure team are important for success.

■ To the extent possible, the patient and, as needed, the family are involved in the process.

■ Consistent implementation of a standardized protocol is most effective in achieving safety.

The Universal Protocol is implemented most successfully in organizations with a culture that promotes teamwork and where all individuals feel empowered to protect patient safety. An organization should consider its culture when designing processes to meet the Universal Protocol. In some organizations, it may be necessary to be more prescriptive on certain elements of the Universal Protocol or to create processes that are not specifically addressed within these requirements.

Organizations should identify the timing and location of the preprocedure verification and site marking based on what works best for their own unique circumstances. The frequency and scope of the preprocedure verification will depend on the type and complexity of the procedure. The three components of the Universal Protocol are not necessarily presented in chronological order (although the preprocedure verification and site marking precede the final verification in the time-out). Preprocedure verification, site marking, and the time-out procedures should be as consistent as possible throughout the organization.

Note: *Site marking is not required when the individual doing the procedure is continuously with the patient from the time of the decision to do the procedure through to the performance of the procedure.*

UP.01.01.01 ▬▬▬▬▬▬▬▬▬▬▬▬▬▬▬▬▬▬▬▬▬

Conduct a preprocedure verification process.

Rationale for UP.01.01.01

Organizations should always make sure that any procedure is what the patient needs and is performed on the right person. The frequency and scope of the verification process will depend on the type and complexity of the procedure.

The preprocedure verification is an ongoing process of information gathering and confirmation. The purpose of the preprocedure verification process is to make sure that all relevant documents and related information or equipment are as follows:

- Available prior to the start of the procedure
- Correctly identified, labeled, and matched to the patient's identifiers
- Reviewed and are consistent with the patient's expectations and with the team's understanding of the intended patient, procedure, and site

Preprocedure verification may occur at more than one time and place before the procedure. It is up to the organization to decide when this information is collected and by which team member, but it is best to do it when the patient can be involved. Possibilities include the following:

- When the procedure is scheduled
- At the time of preadmission testing and assessment
- At the time of admission or entry into the facility for a procedure
- Before the patient leaves the preprocedure area or enters the procedure room

Missing information or discrepancies are addressed before starting the procedure.

Elements of Performance for UP.01.01.01

1. Implement a preprocedure process to verify the correct procedure, for the correct patient, at the correct site. **R**

    Note: *The patient is involved in the verification process when possible.*

2. Ⓓ Identify the items that must be available for the procedure and use a standardized list to verify their availability. At a minimum, these items include the following: **R**
    - Relevant documentation (for example, history and physical, signed procedure consent form, nursing assessment, and preanesthesia assessment)
    - Labeled diagnostic and radiology test results (for example, radiology images and scans, or pathology and biopsy reports) that are properly displayed
    - Any required blood products, implants, devices, and/or special equipment for the procedure

    Note: *The expectation of this element of performance is that the standardized list is available and is used consistently during the preprocedure verification. It is not necessary to document that the standardized list was used for each patient.*

3. Match the items that are to be available in the procedure area to the patient. **R**

Introduction to UP.01.02.01

Wrong-site surgery should never happen, yet it is an ongoing problem in health care that compromises patient safety. Marking the procedure site is one way to protect patients; patient safety is enhanced when a consistent marking process is used throughout the organization. Site marking is done to prevent errors when there is more than one possible location for a procedure. Examples include different limbs, fingers and toes, lesions, level of the spine, and organs. In cases where bilateral structures are removed (such as tonsils or ovaries) the site does not need to be marked.

Responsibility for marking the procedure site is a hotly debated topic. One position is that since the licensed independent practitioner is accountable for the procedure, they should mark the site. Another position is that other individuals should be able to mark the site in the interests of work flow and efficiency.

There is no evidence that patient safety is affected by the job function of the individual who marks the site. The incidence of wrong-site surgery is low enough that it is unlikely that valid data on this subject will ever be available. Furthermore, there is no clear consensus in the field on who should mark the site. Rather than remaining silent on the subject of site marking, The Joint Commission sought a solution that supports the purpose of the site mark. The mark is a communication tool about the patient for members of the team. Therefore, the individual who knows the most about the patient should mark the site. In most cases, that will be the person performing the procedure.

Recognizing the complexities of the work processes supporting invasive procedures, The Joint Commission believes that delegation of site marking to another individual is acceptable in limited situations as long as the individual is familiar with the patient and involved in the procedure. These individuals would include the following:

- Individuals who are permitted through a postgraduate education program to participate in the procedure.
- A licensed individual who performs duties requiring collaborative or supervisory agreements with a licensed independent practitioner. These individuals include advanced practice registered nurses (APRNs) and physician assistants (PAs).

The licensed independent practitioner remains fully accountable for all aspects of the procedure even when site marking is delegated.

UP.01.02.01
Mark the procedure site.

Elements of Performance for UP.01.02.01

1. Identify those procedures that require marking of the incision or insertion site. At a minimum, sites are marked when there is more than one possible location for the procedure and when performing the procedure in a different location would negatively affect quality or safety. **R**

   Note: *For spinal procedures, in addition to preoperative skin marking of the general spinal region, special intraoperative imaging techniques may be used for locating and marking the exact vertebral level.*

2. Mark the procedure site before the procedure is performed and, if possible, with the patient involved. **R**

3. The procedure site is marked by a licensed independent practitioner who is ultimately accountable for the procedure and will be present when the procedure is performed. In limited circumstances, the licensed independent practitioner may delegate site marking to an individual who is permitted by the organization to participate in the procedure and has the following qualifications: **R**

- An individual in a medical postgraduate education program who is being supervised by the licensed independent practitioner performing the procedure; who is familiar with the patient; and who will be present when the procedure is performed
- A licensed individual who performs duties requiring a collaborative agreement or supervisory agreement with the licensed independent practitioner performing the procedure (that is, an advanced practice registered nurse [APRN] or physician assistant [PA]); who is familiar with the patient; and who will be present when the procedure is performed.

Note: *The organization's leaders define the limited circumstances (if any) in which site marking may be delegated to an individual meeting these qualifications.*

4. The method of marking the site and the type of mark is unambiguous and is used consistently throughout the organization. **R**

   Note: *The mark is made at or near the procedure site and is sufficiently permanent to be visible after skin preparation and draping. Adhesive markers are not the sole means of marking the site.*

5. Ⓓ A written, alternative process is in place for patients who refuse site marking or when it is technically or anatomically impossible or impractical to mark the site (for example, mucosal surfaces or perineum). **R**

   Note: *Examples of other situations that involve alternative processes include:*
   - *Minimal access procedures treating a lateralized internal organ, whether percutaneous or through a natural orifice*
   - *Teeth*
   - *Premature infants, for whom the mark may cause a permanent tattoo*

UP.01.03.01

A time-out is performed before the procedure.

Rationale for UP.01.03.01

The purpose of the time-out is to conduct a final assessment that the correct patient, site, and procedure are identified. This requirement focuses on those minimum features of the time-out. Some believe that it is important to conduct the time-out before anesthesia for several reasons, including involvement of the patient. An organization may conduct the time-out before anesthesia or may add another time-out at that time. During a time-out, activities are suspended to the extent possible so that team members can focus on active confirmation of the patient, site, and procedure.

A designated member of the team initiates the time-out and it includes active communication among all relevant members of the procedure team. The procedure is not started until all questions or concerns are resolved. The time-out is most effective when it is conducted consistently across the organization.

Elements of Performance for UP.01.03.01

1.   Conduct a time-out immediately before starting the invasive procedure or making the incision. **R**

2.   The time-out has the following characteristics: **R**
     - It is standardized, as defined by the organization.
     - It is initiated by a designated member of the team.
     - It involves the immediate members of the procedure team, including the individual performing the procedure, the anesthesia providers, the circulating nurse, the operating room technician, and other active participants who will be participating in the procedure from the beginning.

     Note: *For organizations providing telehealth surgical services: Based on current UP requirements, telehealth staff who are physically present in the operating room and participating in a surgical procedure are actively involved in the timeout.*

3.   When two or more procedures are being performed on the same patient, and the person performing the procedure changes, perform a time-out before each procedure is initiated. **R**

4.   During the time-out, the team members agree, at a minimum, on the following: **R**
     - Correct patient identity
     - The correct site
     - The procedure to be done

     Note: *For organizations providing telehealth surgical services: Based on current UP requirements, telehealth staff who are physically present in the operating room and participating in a surgical procedure are actively involved in the timeout.*

5.   ⓓ Document the completion of the time-out. **R**

     Note: *The organization determines the amount and type of documentation.*

Provision of Care, Treatment, and Services (PC)

Overview

The standards in the "Provision of Care, Treatment, and Services" (PC) chapter center around the integrated and cyclical process that allows care to be delivered according to patient needs and the organization's scope of services. This care process may occur between multiple organizations or it may be limited to the organization itself. The complexity of providing care, treatment, or services through this process often demands a collaborative, interdisciplinary approach and a mutual effort among those who work in the organization to coordinate care in a manner that is conducive to optimal patient outcomes, quality, and safety.

The provision of care, treatment, or services is composed of the following four core components of the care process:
1. Assessing patient needs
2. Planning care, treatment, or services
3. Providing care, treatment, or services
4. Coordinating care, treatment, or services

Within these core processes, care activities include the following:
- Providing access to levels of care and/or disciplines necessary to meet the patient's needs
- Interventions based on the plan of care, including the education or instruction of patients regarding their care, treatment, or services
- Coordinating care to promote continuity at the end of an episode of care or when patients are referred, discharged, or transferred

The activities are performed by a wide variety of staff and licensed independent practitioners. Therefore, communication, collaboration, and coordination are among the most important work habits that must be adopted so that care, treatment, or services are provided at the highest level.

About This Chapter

The standards in this chapter are placed within a logical framework that demonstrates the continuum of care as a cyclical process that may occur over short or long periods of time and may be continual or episodic in nature. Therefore, the standards are organized to relate to the patient's experience from entry into the organization to the end of an episode of care, or at discharge or transfer.

This chapter addresses the following:

- Accepting the patient for care, treatment, or services
- Assessing and reassessing the patient
- Planning the patient's care
- Providing the patient with care, treatment, or services
- Coordinating the patient's care, treatment, or services
- Providing the patient with education
- Planning the patient's operative or other high-risk procedures, including those that require the administration of moderate or deep sedation
- Caring for the patient who requires the use of restraint for non–behavioral health purposes
- Caring for the patient who requires the use of restraint or seclusion for behavioral health purposes
- Meeting the patient's need for continuing care, treatment, or services at the end of an episode of care or at discharge or transfer

Chapter Outline

Standards, Rationales, and Elements of Performance

Standard PC.01.01.01

The organization accepts the patient for care, treatment, or services based on its ability to meet the patient's needs.

Elements of Performance for PC.01.01.01

7. The organization accepts a patient for care, treatment, or services based on whether its scope of services can meet the patient's needs.

Introduction to Standard PC.01.02.01

The goal of assessment is to determine the care, treatment, or services that will meet the patient's initial and continuing needs. Patient needs must be reassessed throughout the course of care, treatment, or services.

Identifying and delivering the right care, treatment, or services depends on the following three processes:

1. Collecting information about the patient's health history as well as physical, functional, and psychosocial status
2. Analyzing the information in order to understand the patient's needs for care, treatment, or services
3. Making care, treatment, or service decisions based on the analysis of information collected

The depth and frequency of assessment depends on a number of factors, including the patient's needs, program goals, and the care, treatment, or services provided. Assessment activities may vary between settings, as defined by the organization's leaders.

Information gathered at the patient's first contact may indicate the need for more data or a more intensive assessment. At a minimum, the need for further assessment is determined by the care, treatment, or services sought; the patient's presenting condition(s); and whether the patient agrees to the recommended care, treatment, or services.

Standard PC.01.02.01 ▬▬▬▬▬▬▬▬▬▬▬

The organization assesses and reassesses its patients.

Elements of Performance for PC.01.02.01

1. ⒹThe organization defines, in writing, the scope and content of screening, assessment, and reassessment information it collects. Patient information is collected according to these requirements.

    Note 1: *The scope and content are dependent on whether the patient is making an initial or follow-up visit and whether the assessment is focused or comprehensive.*

    Note 2: *In defining the scope and content of the information it collects, the organization may want to consider information that it can obtain, with the patient's consent, from the patient's family and the patient's other care providers, as well as information conveyed on any medical jewelry.*

    (*See also* RC.02.01.01, EP 2)

2. ⒹThe organization defines, in writing, criteria that identify when additional, specialized, or more in-depth assessments are performed.

    Note: *Examples of criteria could include those that identify when a nutritional, functional, or pain assessment should be performed for patients who are at risk.*

Standard PC.01.02.03 ▬▬▬▬▬▬▬▬▬▬▬

The organization assesses and reassesses the patient and the patient's condition according to defined time frames.

Elements of Performance for PC.01.02.03

1. ⒹThe organization conducts the patient's initial assessment in accordance with written time frames it defines and law and regulation.

    (*See also* RC.01.03.01, EP 2)

3. Each patient is reassessed as necessary based on their plan for care or changes in their condition.

    Note: *Reassessments may also be based on the patient's diagnosis; desire for care, treatment, or services; response to previous care, treatment, or services; and/or their setting requirements.*

9. At each patient's visit, the organization documents updates to the patient's condition.

Introduction to Standard PC.01.02.07

The identification and management of pain is an important component of patient-centered care. First, to support individualized pain treatment and management, organizations need to develop systems for pain screening and assessment. The tools required to adequately assess pain may differ depending on a patient's age, condition, ability to understand, and whether pain is acute or chronic. For example, for an episode of acute pain from an identified cause, brief assessment of pain intensity and characteristics may be sufficient. For chronic pain, more extensive patient assessment including various domains of physical and functional impairment is required. Among patients with chronic pain, assessment and reassessment should focus on whether a treatment improves the patient's function and ability to meet treatment goals.

Next, pain management strategies—which may include nonpharmacologic, pharmacologic, or a combination of approaches—should consider the patient's current presentation, type of pain, past medical history, and pain management goals. In many clinical situations, complete elimination of pain is not a reasonable expectation or goal. To arrive at realistic expectations and clear goals, patient involvement in planning pain management is necessary. Finally, patient-centered care can be further supported by discharge education. Whether provided at the end of an episode of care or at discharge or transfer from the organization, it serves as an opportunity for the provider/care team to re-engage the patient in a discussion on the pain management plan and opioid safety.

Standard PC.01.02.07

The organization assesses and manages the patient's pain and minimizes the risks associated with treatment.

Elements of Performance for PC.01.02.07

1. Ⓓ The organization has defined criteria to screen, assess, and reassess pain that are consistent with the patient's age, condition, and ability to understand.

3. The organization treats the patient's pain or refers the patient for treatment.

    Note: *Treatment strategies for pain may include nonpharmacologic, pharmacologic, or a combination of approaches.*

4. Ⓓ The organization develops a pain treatment plan based on evidence-based practices and the patient's clinical condition, past medical history, and pain management goals.

Note: ***For ambulatory surgical centers:*** *A pain treatment plan relates to the procedure and treatment provided by the organization.*

5.   ⒟ The organization involves patients in the pain management treatment planning process through the following:
- Developing realistic expectations and measurable goals that are understood by the patient for the degree, duration, and reduction of pain
- Discussing the objectives used to evaluate treatment progress (for example, relief of pain and improved physical and psychosocial function)
- Providing education on pain management, treatment options, and safe use of opioid and non-opioid medications when prescribed

7.   ⒟ Based on the patient's condition, the organization reassesses and responds to the patient's pain through the following:
- Evaluation and documentation of response(s) to pain intervention(s)
- Progress toward pain management goals including functional ability (for example, improved pain, physical function, quality of life, mental and cognitive symptoms, sleep habits, functioning in life roles)

Note: *This bullet is not applicable to ambulatory surgical centers, episodic care, urgent/immediate care.*
- Side effects of treatment
- Risk factors for adverse events caused by the treatment

8.   ⒟ The organization educates the patient and family on discharge plans related to pain management including the following:
- Pain management plan of care
- Side effects of pain management treatment
- If applicable, activities of daily living, including the home environment, that might exacerbate pain or reduce effectiveness of the pain management plan of care, as well as strategies to address these issues
- Safe use, storage, and disposal of opioids when prescribed

Introduction to Standard PC.01.02.09

People who are victims of abuse or neglect may come to an organization for a variety of reasons. Sometimes the reason a patient seeks health care is not connected to their experience with abuse or neglect; however, by assessing patients who may be possible victims of abuse or neglect, health care organizations fulfill an important role in helping to protect patients.

Standard PC.01.02.09

The organization assesses the patient who may be a victim of possible abuse and neglect.

Elements of Performance for PC.01.02.09

1. The organization uses criteria to identify those patients who may be victims of physical assault, sexual assault, sexual molestation, domestic abuse, or elder or child abuse and neglect.

   Note: *Criteria can be based on age, sex, and circumstance.*

   (*See also* RI.01.06.03, EP 2)

2. Ⓓ To assist with referrals of possible victims of abuse and neglect, the organization maintains a list of private and public community agencies that can provide or arrange for assessment and care.

3. The organization educates staff about how to recognize signs of possible abuse and neglect and about their roles in follow-up.

6. The organization internally reports cases of possible abuse and neglect.

   (*See also* RI.01.06.03, EP 3)

7. The organization reports cases of possible abuse and neglect to external agencies, in accordance with law and regulation.

   (*See also* RI.01.06.03, EP 3)

Standard PC.01.02.15

The organization provides for diagnostic testing.

Elements of Performance for PC.01.02.15

2. Diagnostic testing and procedures are performed as ordered within time frames defined by the organization.

5.   Ⓓ The organization documents the radiation dose index (computed tomography dose index [CTDIvol], dose length product [DLP], or size-specific dose estimate [SSDE]) on every study produced during a diagnostic computed tomography (CT) examination. The radiation dose index must be exam specific, summarized by series or anatomic area, and documented in a retrievable format.

Note 1: *This element of performance is only applicable for systems capable of calculating and displaying radiation dose indices.*

Note 2: *This element of performance does not apply to systems used for therapeutic radiation treatment planning or delivery, or for calculating attenuation coefficients for nuclear medicine studies.*

Note 3: *This element of performance does not apply to dental cone beam CT radiographic imaging studies performed for diagnosis of conditions affecting the maxillofacial region or to obtain guidance for the treatment of such conditions.*

Note 4: *While the CTDIvol, DLP, and SSDE are useful indicators for monitoring radiation dose indices from the CT machine, they do not represent the patient's radiation dose.*

10. **For organizations that provide diagnostic computed tomography (CT), magnetic resonance imaging (MRI), positron emission tomography (PET), or nuclear medicine (NM) services:** Prior to conducting a diagnostic imaging study, the organization verifies the following:
   ■ Correct patient
   ■ Correct imaging site
   ■ Correct patient positioning
   ■ **For CT only:** Correct imaging protocol
   ■ **For CT only:** Correct scanner parameters

Note: *This element of performance does not apply to dental cone beam CT radiographic imaging studies performed for diagnosis of conditions affecting the maxillofacial region or to obtain guidance for the treatment of such conditions.*

12. **For organizations that provide diagnostic computed tomography (CT), magnetic resonance imaging (MRI), positron emission tomography (PET), or nuclear medicine (NM) services:** The organization considers the patient's age and recent imaging exams when deciding on the most appropriate type of imaging exam.

Note 1: *Knowledge of a patient's recent imaging exams can help to prevent unnecessary duplication of these examinations.*

Note 2: *This element of performance does not apply to dental cone beam CT radiographic imaging studies performed for diagnosis of conditions affecting the maxillofacial region or to obtain guidance for the treatment of such conditions.*

13. Ⓓ **For organizations that provide fluoroscopic services:** The, cumulative-air kerma or kerma-area product is documented in a retrievable format. For fluoroscopy equipment that cannot display or provide cumulative-air kerma or kerma-area product, fluoroscopy time and number of images acquired are documented in a retrievable format, such as a picture archiving and communication system.

Note: *This element of performance does not apply to fluoroscopy equipment used for therapeutic radiation treatment planning or delivery or fluoroscopy equipment classified as a mini C-arm.*

Introduction to Standard PC.01.03.01

Planning for care, treatment, or services is individualized to meet the patient's unique needs. The first step in the process includes creating an initial plan for care, treatment, or services that is appropriate to the patient's specific assessed needs. To continue to meet the patient's unique needs, the plan is maintained and revised based on the patient's response. The plan may be modified or terminated based on reassessment; the patient's need for further care, treatment, or services; or the patient's achievement of goals. The modification of the plan for care, treatment, or services may result in planning for the patient's transfer to another setting.

Standard PC.01.03.01

The organization plans the patient's care.

Elements of Performance for PC.01.03.01

1. The organization plans the patient's care, treatment, or services based on needs identified by the patient's assessment, reassessment, and results of diagnostic testing.

25. The organization establishes or adopts diagnostic computed tomography (CT) imaging protocols based on current standards of practice, which address key criteria including the following:
    - Clinical indication
    - Contrast administration
    - Age (to indicate whether the patient is pediatric or an adult)
    - Patient size and body habitus
    - Expected radiation dose index range

    Note: *This element of performance does not apply to dental cone beam CT radiographic imaging studies performed for diagnosis of conditions affecting the maxillofacial region or to obtain guidance for the treatment of such conditions.*

26. Diagnostic computed tomography (CT) imaging protocols are reviewed and kept current with input from an interpreting physician, medical physicist, and lead imaging technologist to make certain that they adhere to current standards of practice and account for changes in CT imaging equipment. These reviews are conducted at time frames identified by the organization.

    Note: *This element of performance does not apply to dental cone beam CT radiographic imaging studies performed for diagnosis of conditions affecting the maxillofacial region or to obtain guidance for the treatment of such conditions.*

44. **For organizations that elect The Joint Commission Primary Care Medical Home option:** Patient self-management goals are developed in partnership with patients, based on criteria established by the organization, and incorporated into the patient's treatment plan.

    Note: *Examples of criteria include the patient's disease process or condition and specific patient populations, such as those with multiple comorbidities or a chronic disease. It is not expected that self-management goals be developed for every patient. (Refer to RI.01.02.01, EP 1)*

45. **For organizations that elect The Joint Commission Primary Care Medical Home option:** The primary care medical home uses clinical decision support tools to guide decision making. (Refer to LD.03.10.01, EPs 1–3)

Standard PC.02.01.01 ▬▬▬▬▬▬▬▬▬▬▬▬▬▬▬▬▬▬

The organization provides care, treatment, or services for each patient.

Elements of Performance for PC.02.01.01

1. The organization provides the patient with care, treatment, or services according to the patient's individualized plan of care.

10. Before initiating a blood or blood component transfusion, the organization follows a process to correctly identify patients that includes the following:
    - Matching the blood or blood component to the order
    - Matching the patient to the blood or blood component
    - Using a two-person verification process or a one-person verification process accompanied by automated identification technology, such as bar coding

    Note: *When using a two-person verification process, one individual conducting the identification verification is the qualified transfusionist who will administer the blood or blood component to the patient. The second individual conducting the identification verification is qualified to participate in the process, as determined by the organization.*

    (*See also* NPSG.01.01.01, EPs 1, 2)

16. **For organizations that elect The Joint Commission Primary Care Medical Home option:** Each patient has a designated primary care clinician.

30. **For organizations that provide fluoroscopic services:** The organization identifies radiation exposure and skin dose threshold levels that, if exceeded, trigger further review and/or patient evaluation to assess for adverse radiation effects.

    Note 1: *Information on radiation exposure thresholds can be found in the National Council on Radiation Protection's (NCRP) report number 168 and on the US Food and Drug Administration's (FDA) Center for Devices for Radiological Health (CDRH) website.*

    Note 2: *Radiation exposure thresholds may be established based on metrics such as reference-air kerma, cumulative-air kerma, kerma-area product, or fluoroscopy time.*

    (*See also* PI.03.01.01, EP 20)

Standard PC.02.01.03 ━━━━━━━━━━

The organization provides care, treatment, and services as ordered or prescribed, and in accordance with law and regulation.

Elements of Performance for PC.02.01.03

1. **For ambulatory surgical centers that elect to use The Joint Commission deemed status option:** Radiologic services are provided based on orders from practitioners with clinical privileges in accordance with professional standards of practice, or from other practitioners authorized by the medical staff and the governing body, consistent with state law.

20. Before taking action on a verbal order or verbal report of a critical test result, staff uses a record and "read back" process to verify the information. **R**

Standard PC.02.01.05 ━━━━━━━━━━

The organization provides interdisciplinary, collaborative care, treatment, or services.

Elements of Performance for PC.02.01.05

1. Care, treatment, or services are provided to the patient in an interdisciplinary, collaborative manner.

Standard PC.02.01.07 ━━━━━━━━━━

The organization safely administers blood and blood component(s).

Elements of Performance for PC.02.01.07

2. Ⓓ The organization's written procedures for acquiring blood or blood component(s) include identifying the following:
   - The source of materials used during acquisition
   - The time frames for acquisition
   - Accountability for acquisition
   - On-site storage

12. **For ambulatory surgical centers that elect to use The Joint Commission deemed status option:** Only physicians or registered nurses administer blood and blood component(s).

Standard PC.02.01.09 ▬▬▬▬▬▬▬▬▬▬▬▬▬▬▬▬▬▬▬▬▬▬▬

The organization plans for and responds to life-threatening emergencies.

Elements of Performance for PC.02.01.09

1. Ⓓ The organization follows written policies and procedures for responding to life-threatening emergencies.

4. **For ambulatory surgical centers that elect to use The Joint Commission deemed status option:** Staff trained in emergency equipment use and cardiopulmonary resuscitation are available whenever a patient is in the ambulatory surgical center. **R**

    (*See also* HR.01.02.05, EP 13)

9. **For ambulatory surgical centers that elect to use The Joint Commission deemed status option:** Emergency equipment is immediately available for use when needed to respond to emergencies. **R**

10. **For ambulatory surgical centers that elect to use The Joint Commission deemed status option:** The types of emergency equipment available are appropriate for the organization's patient population and types of procedures performed. **R**

    (*See also* LD.04.01.11, EP 8)

Standard PC.02.01.21 ▬▬▬▬▬▬▬▬▬▬▬▬▬▬▬▬▬▬▬▬▬▬▬

For organizations that elect The Joint Commission Primary Care Medical Home option: The organization effectively communicates with patients when providing care, treatment, or services.

Elements of Performance for PC.02.01.21

1. **For organizations that elect The Joint Commission Primary Care Medical Home option:** The primary care clinician and the interdisciplinary team identify the patient's oral and written communication needs, including the patient's preferred language for discussing health care.

    Note: *Examples of communication needs include the need for personal devices such as hearing aids or glasses, language interpreters, communication boards, and translated or plain language materials. (Refer to RC.02.01.01, EP 27)*

2. **For organizations that elect The Joint Commission Primary Care Medical Home option:** The primary care clinician and the interdisciplinary team communicate with the patient during the provision of care, treatment, or services in a manner that meets the patient's oral and written communication needs. (Refer to RI.01.01.03, EPs 1, 2, 3)

Introduction to Standard PC.02.02.01

Coordination of care is recognized as a major challenge in the safe delivery of care. The rise of chronic illness means that a patient's care, treatment, or services likely include an array of providers in a variety of health care settings, including the patient's home.

The Institute of Medicine's report "Crossing the Quality Chasm—A New Health System for the 21st Century" notes that "because of the special vulnerability that accompanies illness or injury, coordination of care takes on special importance. Many patients depend on those who provide care to coordinate services—whether tests, consultations, or procedures—to ensure that accurate and timely information reaches those who need it at the appropriate time." Health care providers and organizations need to work together to coordinate their efforts in order to provide safe, quality care.

Standard PC.02.02.01 ━━━━━━━━━━━━━━━━━━━━━━━━━━━━

The organization coordinates the patient's care, treatment, or services based on the patient's needs.

Elements of Performance for PC.02.02.01

1. The organization follows a process to receive or share patient information when the patient is referred to other internal or external providers of care, treatment, or services.

   (*See also* PC.04.02.01, EP 1)

2. The organization's process for hand-off communication provides for the opportunity for discussion between the giver and receiver of patient information.

   Note: *Such information may include the patient's condition, care, treatment, medications, services, and any recent or anticipated changes to any of these.*

3. The organization coordinates the patient's care, treatment, or services within a time frame that meets the patient's needs.

> **Note:** *Coordination involves resolving scheduling conflicts and duplication of care, treatment, or services.*

10. When the organization uses external resources to meet the patient's needs, it participates in coordinating the patient's care, treatment, or services.

15. **For ambulatory surgical centers that elect to use The Joint Commission deemed status option:** Radiologic services may only be provided when they are integral to procedures offered by the ambulatory surgical center.

Standard PC.02.02.03

The organization makes food and nutrition products available to its patients.

Elements of Performance for PC.02.02.03

7. Food and nutrition products are consistent with each patient's care, treatment, or services.

11. Food and nutrition products are managed safely.

> **Note:** *Safe management refers to sanitation, temperature, light, moisture, ventilation, and security.*

Introduction to Standard PC.02.03.01

Chronic disease is on the rise, and patients are becoming increasingly responsible for managing their own health at home. At the end of an episode of care or at discharge, patients are often given instructions for self-care that can range from changing bandages to caring for drains to home infusion. Consequently, patient education continues to take on greater importance in influencing the patient's outcome and in promoting healthy behaviors. To equip the patient to provide for their health care needs, the organization needs to assess the patient's learning needs and use methods of education and instruction that are matched to the patient's level of understanding.

Standard PC.02.03.01

The organization provides patient education and training based on each patient's needs and abilities.

Elements of Performance for PC.02.03.01

1. The organization assesses the patient's learning needs.

4. The organization provides education and training to the patient based on the patient's assessed needs.

5. The organization coordinates the patient education and training provided by all disciplines involved in the patient's care, treatment, or services.

10. Based on the patient's condition and assessed needs, the education and training provided to the patient by the organization include the following:
    ■ An explanation of the plan for care, treatment, or services
    ■ Basic health practices and safety
    ■ Information on the safe and effective use of medications
    ■ Nutrition interventions (for example, supplements) and modified diets
    ■ Discussion of pain, the risk for pain, the importance of effective pain management, the pain assessment process, and methods for pain management
    ■ Information on oral health
    ■ Information on the safe and effective use of medical equipment or supplies provided by the organization
    ■ Habilitation or rehabilitation techniques to help the patient reach maximum independence

    (*See also* MM.06.01.01, EP 9)

25. The organization evaluates the patient's understanding of the education and training it provided.

27. The organization provides the patient education on how to communicate concerns about patient safety issues that occur before, during, and after care is received.

28. **For organizations that elect The Joint Commission Primary Care Medical Home option:** The primary care clinician and the interdisciplinary team educate the patient on self-management tools and techniques based on the patient's individual needs. (Refer to PC.01.03.01, EP 44)

30. **For organizations that elect The Joint Commission Primary Care Medical Home option:** The interdisciplinary team identifies the patient's health literacy needs.

    Note: *Typically this is an interactive process, the goal of which is to ascertain the patient's capacity to process and understand basic health information needed to make appropriate health decisions.*

31. **For organizations that elect The Joint Commission Primary Care Medical Home option:** Patient education is consistent with the patient's health literacy needs.

Standard PC.02.04.01 ▬▬▬▬▬▬▬▬▬▬▬▬▬▬▬▬▬

For organizations that elect The Joint Commission Primary Care Medical Home option: The patient has access to the organization 24 hours a day, 7 days a week.

Note: *Access may be provided through a number of methods, including telephone, e-mail, websites, portals, and flexible hours.*

Elements of Performance for PC.02.04.01

1. **For organizations that elect The Joint Commission Primary Care Medical Home option:** The organization provides patients with the ability to do the following 24 hours a day, 7 days a week:
   - Contact the primary care medical home to obtain a same- or next-day appointment
   - Request prescription renewal
   - Obtain clinical advice for urgent health needs

2. **For organizations that elect The Joint Commission Primary Care Medical Home option:** The organization offers flexible scheduling to accommodate patient care needs.

   Note: *This may include open scheduling, same-day appointments, group visits, expanded hours, and arrangements with other organizations.*

3. **For organizations that elect The Joint Commission Primary Care Medical Home option:** The organization has a process to respond to patient urgent care needs 24 hours a day, 7 days a week.

4. **For organizations that elect The Joint Commission Primary Care Medical Home option:** Primary care medical home patients are provided online access to their health information within four business days after the information is available to the primary care clinician or interdisciplinary team. This information includes diagnostic test results, lab results, summary lists, and medication lists.

5. **For organizations that elect The Joint Commission Primary Care Medical Home option:** The organization uses a certified electronic health record to provide appointment reminders to patients with two or more office visits in the last two years.

Standard PC.02.04.03 ▬▬▬▬▬▬▬

For organizations that elect The Joint Commission Primary Care Medical Home option: The organization is accountable for providing patient care. (Refer to Standard PC.02.04.05)

Elements of Performance for PC.02.04.03

1. **For organizations that elect The Joint Commission Primary Care Medical Home option:** The organization manages transitions in care and provides or facilitates patient access to care, treatment, or services including the following:
    - Acute care
    - Management of chronic care
    - Preventive services that are age- and gender-specific
    - Behavioral health needs
    - Oral health care
    - Optical health
    - Urgent and emergent care
    - Substance abuse treatment
    - Rehabilitative services and equipment (examples include physical, occupational, and speech therapy and equipment such as orthotics, prosthetics, and wheelchairs)

    Note: *Some of these services may be obtained through the use of community resources as available, or in collaboration with other organizations.*

2. **For organizations that elect The Joint Commission Primary Care Medical Home option:** The organization provides care that addresses various phases of a patient's lifespan, including end-of-life care.

3. **For organizations that elect The Joint Commission Primary Care Medical Home option:** The organization provides disease and chronic care management services to its patients.

4. **For organizations that elect The Joint Commission Primary Care Medical Home option:** The organization provides population-based care.

5. **For organizations that elect The Joint Commission Primary Care Medical Home option:** The organization uses a certified electronic health record system to do the following:
    - Support the continuity of care, and the provision of comprehensive and coordinated care, treatment, or services

- Document and track care, treatment, or services
- Support disease management, including providing patient education
- Support preventive care, treatment, or services
- Create reports for internal use
- Create and submit reports to external providers and organizations, including public health agencies, disease-specific registries, immunization registries, and other specialized registries
- Facilitate electronic exchange of information among providers
- Support performance improvement
- Identify and provide patient-specific education resources

Standard PC.02.04.05

For organizations that elect The Joint Commission Primary Care Medical Home option: The primary care clinician and the interdisciplinary team work in partnership with the patient to support the continuity of care and the provision of comprehensive and coordinated care, treatment, or services.

Elements of Performance for PC.02.04.05

1. **For organizations that elect The Joint Commission Primary Care Medical Home option:** The organization identifies the composition of the interdisciplinary team. The team must include a doctor of medicine or doctor of osteopathy.

   Note: *The intent of this requirement is that while a doctor of medicine or doctor of osteopathy is always available to be part of the interdisciplinary team, the doctor's involvement in a patient's care would be determined by the needs of the patient.*

2. **For organizations that elect The Joint Commission Primary Care Medical Home option:** The members of the interdisciplinary team provide comprehensive and coordinated care, treatment, or services and maintain the continuity of care.

   Note: *The provision of care may include making internal and external referrals.*

4. **For organizations that elect The Joint Commission Primary Care Medical Home option:** The primary care clinician and the interdisciplinary team provide care for a panel of patients.

5.   **For organizations that elect The Joint Commission Primary Care Medical Home option:** The primary care clinician is responsible for making certain that the interdisciplinary team provides comprehensive and coordinated care, treatment, or services and maintains the continuity of care as described in EPs 6–12.

      Note: *Coordination of care may include making internal and external referrals, developing and evaluating treatment plans, and resolving conflicts in the provision of care.*

6.   **For organizations that elect The Joint Commission Primary Care Medical Home option:** When a patient is referred internally or externally for care, treatment, or services, the interdisciplinary team reviews and tracks the care provided to the patient and, as needed, acts on recommendations for additional care, treatment, or services.

      Note: *Internal referrals include orders for laboratory tests and imaging.*

8.   **For organizations that elect The Joint Commission Primary Care Medical Home option:** The interdisciplinary team participates in the development of the patient's treatment plan.

9.   **For organizations that elect The Joint Commission Primary Care Medical Home option:** The interdisciplinary team works in partnership with the patient to achieve planned outcomes.

10.   **For organizations that elect The Joint Commission Primary Care Medical Home option:** The interdisciplinary team monitors the patient's progress toward achieving treatment goals.

11.   **For organizations that elect The Joint Commission Primary Care Medical Home option:** The interdisciplinary team involves the patient in the development of the patient's treatment plan.

12.   Ⓓ **For organizations that elect The Joint Commission Primary Care Medical Home option:** The interdisciplinary team assesses patients for health risk behaviors.

Introduction to Standards PC.03.01.01 Through PC.03.01.07

The standards for sedation and anesthesia care apply when patients in any setting receive, for any purpose, by any of the following routes:

- General, spinal, or other major regional anesthesia
- Moderate or deep sedation (with or without analgesia) that, in the manner used, may be expected to result in the loss of protective reflexes

Standard PC.03.01.01

The organization plans operative or other high-risk procedures, including those that require the administration of moderate or deep sedation or anesthesia.

Elements of Performance for PC.03.01.01

2. In addition to the individual performing the procedure, a sufficient number of qualified staff are present to evaluate the patient, to provide the sedation and/or anesthesia, to help with the procedure, and to monitor and recover the patient. **R**

6. For operative or other high-risk procedures, including those that require the administration of moderate or deep sedation or anesthesia, the following is available: **R**
   - Equipment to monitor the patient's physiological status
   - Equipment to administer intravenous fluids and medications and, if needed, blood and blood components

Standard PC.03.01.03

The organization provides the patient with care before initiating operative or other high-risk procedures, including those that require the administration of moderate or deep sedation or anesthesia.

Elements of Performance for PC.03.01.03

1. Before operative or other high-risk procedures are initiated, or before moderate or deep sedation or anesthesia is administered: The organization conducts a presedation or preanesthesia patient assessment.

   (*See also* RC.02.01.01, EP 2)

4. Before operative or other high-risk procedures are initiated, or before moderate or deep sedation or anesthesia is administered: The organization provides the patient with preprocedural education, according to the plan for care.

5. Before operative and other high-risk procedures are initiated or before moderate or deep sedation or anesthesia is administered, the organization does the following: **R**
   - Performs and documents a history and physical examination, as needed
   - Performs and documents diagnostic tests or other data
   - Ascertains and documents the preoperative diagnosis
   - Ascertains and documents the need to administer blood or blood component(s)

8. The organization reevaluates the patient immediately before administering moderate or deep sedation or anesthesia.

   (*See also* RC.02.01.01, EP 2)

9. **For ambulatory surgical centers that elect to use The Joint Commission deemed status option:** A physician or anesthetist (as defined by law and regulation) examines the patient immediately before surgery to evaluate the risks associated with moderate or deep sedation or anesthesia. **R**

10. **For ambulatory surgical centers that elect to use The Joint Commission deemed status option:** The organization records into the patient's clinical record the results of any preoperative diagnostic studies performed to evaluate the patient's risks associated with anesthesia.

12. **For ambulatory surgical centers that elect to use The Joint Commission deemed status option:** Anesthetics must be administered only by one of the following: a qualified anesthesiologist; a physician qualified to administer anesthesia; a certified registered nurse anesthetist or an anesthesiologist's assistant; or a supervised trainee in an approved education program.

13. **For ambulatory surgical centers that elect to use The Joint Commission deemed status option:** In cases in which a non-physician administers the anesthesia, the anesthetist (unless exempt) must be under the supervision of the operating physician and, in the case of an anesthesiologist's assistant, under the supervision of an anesthesiologist.

Note: *An ambulatory surgical center may be exempt from the requirement for physician supervision of certified registered nurse anesthetists (CRNAs) as described in paragraph (b)(2) of 42 CFR 416.42 if the state in which the ambulatory surgical center is located submits a letter to the Centers for Medicare & Medicaid Services (CMS) signed by the governor, following consultation with the state's Boards of Medicine and Nursing, requesting exemption from physician supervision of CRNAs. The letter from the governor must attest that they have consulted with state Boards of Medicine and Nursing about issues related to access to and the quality of anesthesia services in the state and has concluded that it is in the best interests of the state's citizens to opt-out of the current physician supervision requirement, and that the opt-out is consistent with state law. The request for exemption and recognition of state laws as well as the withdrawal of the request may be submitted at any time, and they are effective upon submission.*

15. **For ambulatory surgical centers that elect to use The Joint Commission deemed status option:** Each patient has a presurgical assessment completed upon admission by a physician or other qualified practitioner, in accordance with applicable state health and safety laws, standards of practice, and organization policy. This assessment includes documentation of any allergies to drugs and biologicals.

16. **For ambulatory surgical centers that elect to use The Joint Commission deemed status option:** A physician examines the patient immediately before surgery to evaluate patient risk for the procedure to be performed.

17. **For ambulatory surgical centers that elect to use The Joint Commission deemed status option:** The ambulatory surgical center completes the appropriate presurgical assessments for each patient, including all elements required for discharge.

19. Ⓓ The organization develops and maintains a policy that identifies those patients who require a medical history and physical examination prior to surgery. The policy is based on nationally recognized guidelines and standards of practice and applicable state and local health and safety laws, and the policy addresses the following:
    - The time frame for medical history and physical examination to be completed prior to surgery

- Patient-specific factors that include the patient's age, diagnosis, the type and number of procedures scheduled to be performed on the same surgery date, known comorbidities, and the planned anesthesia level

Standard PC.03.01.05

The organization monitors the patient during operative or other high-risk procedures and/or during the administration of moderate or deep sedation or anesthesia.

Elements of Performance for PC.03.01.05

1. During operative or other high-risk procedures, including those that require the administration of moderate or deep sedation or anesthesia, the patient's oxygenation, ventilation, and circulation are monitored continuously. **R**

   (*See also* RC.02.01.03, EP 8)

Standard PC.03.01.07

The organization provides care to the patient after operative or other high-risk procedures and/or the administration of moderate or deep sedation or anesthesia.

Elements of Performance for PC.03.01.07

1. The organization assesses the patient's physiological status immediately after the operative or other high-risk procedure and/or as the patient recovers from moderate or deep sedation or anesthesia. **R**

   (*See also* RC.02.01.03, EP 8)

2. The organization monitors the patient's physiological status, mental status, and pain level at a frequency and intensity consistent with the potential effect of the operative or other high-risk procedure and/or the sedation or anesthesia administered. **R**

4. A qualified licensed independent practitioner discharges the patient from the recovery area or from the organization. In the absence of a qualified licensed independent practitioner, patients are discharged according to criteria approved by clinical leaders.

   (*See also* RC.02.01.03, EPs 9, 10)

5. **For ambulatory surgical centers that elect to use The Joint Commission deemed status option:** Each patient is evaluated by a physician (as defined in section 1861(r) of the Social Security Act), or an anesthetist (as defined by law and regulation) for proper recovery before discharge from the ambulatory surgical center.

6. Patients who have received sedation or anesthesia are discharged in the company of an individual who accepts responsibility for the patient.

9. **For ambulatory surgical centers that elect to use The Joint Commission deemed status option:** The ambulatory surgical center completes the appropriate postsurgical assessments for each patient, including all elements required for discharge.

Standard PC.03.02.03

Written policies and procedures guide the organization's safe use of restraint.

Elements of Performance for PC.03.02.03

1. ⒟ The organization's written policies and procedures on the use of restraint specify the frequency, format, and content of entries in the patient's clinical record for each episode of restraint.

    (*See also* RC.02.01.05, EP 1)

Standard PC.03.02.07

The organization monitors patients who are restrained.

Rationale for PC.03.02.07

Monitoring a patient who is restrained is important because it provides an opportunity to do the following:

- Determine whether the restraint has been correctly applied.
- Evaluate whether less restrictive methods are possible.
- Assess the patient for changes in behavior or clinical condition that might warrant the removal of restraints.
- Assess the patient's physical and emotional well-being.
- Make sure the patient's rights, dignity, and safety are maintained.

Elements of Performance for PC.03.02.07

1. The frequency and extent of monitoring patients who are restrained are determined by the following:

- Organization policies and procedures
- Protocols
- Individual orders
- The care setting
- Individual patient needs
- Applicable law and regulation

(*See also* RC.02.01.05, EP 1)

2. A patient in restraint is monitored either every two hours or more frequently if required by their needs and organization policy.

    (*See also* RC.02.01.05, EP 1)

3. Qualified staff monitor a patient in restraint.

    Note: *Monitoring may occur using observation, interaction with the patient, or direct examination.*

Standard PC.04.01.01

The organization follows a process that addresses the patient's need for continuing care, treatment, or services after discharge or transfer.

Elements of Performance for PC.04.01.01

1. The organization describes the following:
    - The reason(s) for and conditions under which the patient is discharged or transferred
    - The method for shifting responsibility for a patient's care from one clinician, organization, program, or service to another

11. **For ambulatory surgical centers that elect to use The Joint Commission deemed status option:** The ambulatory surgical center has procedures for immediately transferring a patient who requires emergency care that is beyond its capability.

12. **For ambulatory surgical centers that elect to use The Joint Commission deemed status option:** Patients are transferred to local hospitals that meet requirements for payment of emergency services.

    Note: *CMS requires patients to be transferred to hospitals that are either participating in Medicare, or meet the requirements at 42 CFR 482.2 "Provision of emergency services by nonparticipating hospitals."*

13. **Ⓓ For ambulatory surgical centers that elect to use The Joint Commission deemed status option:** The ambulatory surgical center periodically provides the local hospital with written notice of its operations and patient population served.

Standard PC.04.01.03 ▬▬▬▬▬▬▬▬▬▬▬▬▬▬▬▬

The organization discharges or transfers the patient based on the patient's assessed needs and the organization's ability to meet those needs.

Elements of Performance for PC.04.01.03

2. The organization identifies any needs the patient may have for continuing psychosocial or physical care.

3. The patient, the patient's family, licensed independent practitioners, physicians, and staff involved in the patient's care, treatment, or services participate in planning the patient's discharge or transfer.

4. Prior to discharge, the organization arranges or assists in arranging the services required by the patient after discharge in order to meet the patient's ongoing needs for care and services.

Standard PC.04.01.05 ▬▬▬▬▬▬▬▬▬▬▬▬▬▬▬▬

Before the organization discharges or transfers a patient, it informs and educates the patient about their follow-up care, treatment, or services.

Elements of Performance for PC.04.01.05

1. When the organization determines the patient's needs at the end of an episode of care, or at discharge or transfer, it promptly shares this information with the patient.

7. The organization educates the patient about how to obtain any continuing care, treatment, or services the patient will need.

9. **For ambulatory surgical centers that elect to use The Joint Commission deemed status option:** The ambulatory surgical center informs all patients of their prescriptions, postoperative instructions, and physician contact information for follow-up care either in advance of their surgical procedure or prior to leaving the ambulatory surgical center. **R**

10. **For ambulatory surgical centers that elect to use The Joint Commission deemed status option:** The patient's postsurgical needs are addressed and included in the discharge notes.

11. **For ambulatory surgical centers that elect to use The Joint Commission deemed status option:** The ambulatory surgical center provides each patient with written discharge instructions and overnight supplies.

12. **For ambulatory surgical centers that elect to use The Joint Commission deemed status option:** The ambulatory surgical center provides each patient with a follow-up appointment with a physician, as necessary.

13. **For ambulatory surgical centers that elect to use The Joint Commission deemed status option:** Each patient has a discharge order signed by the physician who performed the surgery or procedure, in accordance with applicable state health and safety laws, standards of practice, and organization policy. **R**

14. **For ambulatory surgical centers that elect to use The Joint Commission deemed status option:** Patients are discharged from the ambulatory surgical center in the company of a responsible adult, unless the patient is exempted from this requirement by the attending physician. **R**

Standard PC.04.02.01

When a patient is discharged or transferred, the organization gives information about the care, treatment, or services provided to the patient to other service providers who will provide the patient with care, treatment, or services.

Elements of Performance for PC.04.02.01

1. At the end of an episode of care, or at the time of the patient's discharge or transfer, the organization informs other service providers who will provide care, treatment, or services to the patient about the following:
   - The reason for the patient's discharge or transfer
   - The patient's physical and psychosocial status
   - A summary of care, treatment, or services it provided to the patient
   - The patient's progress toward goals

   Note: *This bullet is not applicable to settings that do not provide continuing care, such as urgent care and convenient care clinics.*
   - A list of community resources or referrals made or provided to the patient
   - A list of the patient's current medications, including any allergies to medications

   (*See also* PC.02.02.01, EP 1)

Performance Improvement (PI)

Overview

All organizations want better patient outcomes and, therefore, are concerned about improving the safety and quality of the care, treatment, or services they provide. The best way to achieve better care is by first measuring the performance of processes that support care and then using that data to make improvements. The standards in this chapter stress the importance of using data to inform positive change.

About This Chapter

The standards in this chapter address the fundamental principles of performance improvement: collecting data, analyzing data, and taking action to improve and monitor performance. Leaders have ultimate responsibility for performance improvement. They set performance improvement priorities and provide the resources needed to achieve improvement. They make sure that all individuals who work in the organization participate in performance improvement activities. The leaders' responsibilities are more fully described in the "Leadership" (LD) chapter. (Standards LD.03.01.01 through LD.03.06.01 describe the management of important organizationwide systems that support safety and quality. Standard LD.03.07.01 addresses the need for leaders to establish performance improvement priorities.)

Collecting data is the foundation of performance improvement (*see* Standard IM.01.01.01, addressing the planning of managing information, and Standard IM.02.02.03, regarding retrieving, disseminating, and transmitting health information in usable formats). Based on its setting, scope, and services, the organization selects measures that are meaningful to the organization and that address the needs of the patients it serves. In addition, The Joint Commission has identified important processes (*see* Standard PI.01.01.01) that should always be measured because they involve risk and can harm patients.

Regardless of how much data the organization collects, data are not useful if not analyzed. Analysis identifies trends, patterns, and performance levels that suggest opportunities for improvement. The organization can then make improvements based on the analysis. Of course, there is always the chance that analysis may reveal that more opportunities for improvement exist than an organization can manage at one time. In this case, leaders need to set priorities for improvement.

After a change has been made, the organization monitors that change by collecting and analyzing data to make sure the desired improvement is achieved and sustained. Organizations should identify the results that will signify sustained improvement. If the improvement does not meet expectations, the organization makes additional changes, and the cycle starts again. These principles of performance improvement also apply whenever the organization wants to design new processes, such as a new service or an information management system (*see* Standard LD.03.08.01).

Chapter Outline

Standards, Rationales, and Elements of Performance

Introduction to Standard PI.01.01.01

Data provide organizations with important information that can be used in a variety of ways. Collecting and analyzing data on performance, outcomes, and other activities can help the organization improve its ability to provide quality care, treatment, or services. The organization can collect data from many areas, including internal data obtained from staff, patients, records, and observations. Data are also available from quality control, risk management activities, and research studies. Other valuable data can be obtained from external sources, such as regulators, insurers, and the community. The Joint Commission has identified important areas that should be measured regularly. In addition, the organization should establish data priorities particular to its needs.

Note: *The organization also collects data on evaluation and improvement of conditions in the environment, infection control, and the medication management system. Standards addressing this data collection are located in the "Environment of Care" (EC), "Infection Prevention and Control" (IC), and "Medication Management" (MM) chapters.*

Standard PI.01.01.01 ━━━━━━━━━━━━━━━━━

The organization collects data to monitor its performance.

Elements of Performance for PI.01.01.01

The organization collects data on the following:

2. Performance improvement priorities identified by leaders.

(*See also* LD.03.07.01, EP 2)

3. Ⓓ Operative or other procedures that place patients at risk of disability or death.

(*See also* LD.03.07.01, EP 2)

4. Ⓓ All significant discrepancies between preoperative and postoperative diagnoses, including pathologic diagnoses.

5. Ⓓ Adverse events related to using moderate or deep sedation or

anesthesia.

(*See also* LD.03.07.01, EP 2)

  6. ⓓ The use of blood and blood components.

(*See also* LD.03.07.01, EP 2)

  7. ⓓ All confirmed transfusion reactions.

(*See also* LD.03.07.01, EP 2)

  12. ⓓ Significant medication errors.

(*See also* LD.03.07.01, EP 2; MM.08.01.01, EP 1)

  13. ⓓ Significant adverse drug reactions.

(*See also* LD.03.07.01, EP 2; MM.08.01.01, EP 1)

  14. ⓓ Patient perception of the safety and quality of care, treatment, or services.

26. ⓓ **For ambulatory surgical centers that elect to use The Joint Commission deemed status option:** The ambulatory surgical center documents the improvement projects it is conducting. The documentation includes, at a minimum, the reason(s) for implementing the project and a description of the project's results.

For organizations that elect The Joint Commission Primary Care Medical Home option: The organization collects data on the following:

  28. ⓓ Disease management outcomes.

  29. ⓓ Patient access to care within time frames established by the organization.

30. ⓓ **For organizations that elect The Joint Commission Primary Care Medical Home option:** The organization collects data on the following:
- Patient experience and satisfaction related to access to care, treatment, or services and communication
- Patient perception of the comprehensiveness of care, treatment, or services
- Patient perception of the coordination of care, treatment, or services
- Patient perception of the continuity of care, treatment, or services

34. ⓓ The organization collects data on patient thermal injuries that occur during magnetic resonance imaging exams.

35. Ⓓ The organization collects data on the following:
    - Incidents where ferromagnetic objects unintentionally entered the magnetic resonance imaging (MRI) scanner room
    - Injuries resulting from the presence of ferromagnetic objects in the MRI scanner room

Standard PI.02.01.01

The organization has a performance improvement plan.

Rationale for PI.02.01.01

Planning is essential to achieving and sustaining improved performance. Leaders who monitor data related to organizational processes and outcomes have a better awareness of how well they are performing and where opportunities for improvement exist. When leaders identify the processes and outcomes that will be the focus for improvement, a detailed plan will communicate to staff the goals, expectations, data to collect, and timelines for activity. This detailed plan provides structure and focus for both leaders and staff that will lead to meaningful and sustainable change.

The regularity and visibility of leadership review and updates to the plan affirm the commitment being made to quality and improvement throughout the organization. Leaders can use this opportunity to recognize staff achievement of successful changes and identify new priorities to include in the next round of planning. The message this sends is one that ongoing attention and vigilance at all levels of the organization are critical in the quest for health care high reliability.

Elements of Performance for PI.02.01.01

1. Ⓓ Performance improvement priorities established by organization leaders are described in a written plan that includes the following:
    - The defined process(es) needing improvement, along with any stakeholder (for example, patient, staff, regulatory) requirements, project goals, and improvement activities
    - Method(s) for measuring performance of the process(es) identified for improvement
    - Analysis method(s) for identifying causes of variation and poor performance in the process(es)
    - Methods implemented to address process deficiencies and improve performance
    - Methods for monitoring and sustaining the improved process(es)

(*See also* LD.03.07.01, EP 2)

2. ⓄⒹ Leadership reviews the plan for addressing performance improvement priorities at least annually and updates it to reflect any changes in strategic priorities and in response to changes in the internal or external environment.

Introduction to Standard PI.03.01.01

When data are collected, they are analyzed using statistical tools and techniques. When the organization analyzes data over time, it transforms raw data into useful information. Analysis of data from internal sources allows the organization to identify patterns and trends and monitor its performance. The organization may also have access to external databases that allow it to compare its performance with other organizations on a specific topic, such as a procedure or outcome.

A data display helps with analysis. There are many different ways to display data, including simple bar or pie charts or more sophisticated run or control charts. The display should match the question being studied. For example, something being studied over time might be displayed in a run chart or histogram. The display can be hand-written, created in a simple spreadsheet, or generated by more complex statistical software.

Standard PI.03.01.01

The organization compiles and analyzes data.

Elements of Performance for PI.03.01.01

4. The organization analyzes and compares internal data over time to identify levels of performance, patterns, trends, and variations.

6. The organization reviews and analyzes incidents where the radiation dose index (computed tomography dose index [CTDIvol], dose length product [DLP], or size-specific dose estimate [SSDE]) from diagnostic CT examinations exceeded expected dose index ranges identified in imaging protocols. These incidents are then compared to external benchmarks.

   Note 1: *While the CTDIvol, DLP, and SSDE are useful indicators for monitoring radiation dose indices from the CT machine, they do not represent the patient's radiation dose.*

Note 2: *This element of performance does not apply to dental cone beam CT radiographic imaging studies performed for diagnosis of conditions affecting the maxillofacial region or to obtain guidance for the treatment of such conditions.*

8.   The organization uses the results of data analysis to identify improvement opportunities.

11.   **For ambulatory surgical centers that elect to use The Joint Commission deemed status option:** The number and scope of distinct improvement projects conducted annually reflects the scope and complexity of the ambulatory surgical center's services and operations.

19.   The organization monitors the use of opioids to determine if they are being prescribed safely.

(*See also* LD.04.03.13, EP 1)

20.   **For organizations that provide fluoroscopic services:** The organization reviews and analyzes instances where the radiation exposure and skin dose threshold levels identified by the organization are exceeded.

Note: *Radiation exposure thresholds may be established based on metrics such as reference-air kerma, cumulative-air kerma, kerma-area product, or fluoroscopy time.*

(*See also* PC.02.01.01, EP 30)

21.   The organization provides incidence data to key stakeholders, including leaders, licensed independent practitioners, nursing staff, and other clinicians on surgical site infections.

Standard PI.04.01.01

The organization improves performance.

Rationale for PI.04.01.01

Data have been collected, monitoring is underway, and data analysis has revealed an opportunity for improvement. Some opportunities are resolved with minimal work and immediate acceptance, but many are more complex, involve and impact more people, and require more careful efforts to achieve improvement and make it last. Tested and proven improvement tools and methodologies can make the difference between an actual improvement with lasting change versus a quick fix that is just as quickly forgotten. Knowing that highly reliable processes provide for a zero-harm environment for patients, organizations must explore available tools and methodologies and determine what will best facilitate and sustain their improvement successes.

Elements of Performance for PI.04.01.01

2. The organization acts on improvement priorities.

   (*See also* MM.08.01.01, EP 6)

3. The organization uses improvement tools or methodologies to improve its performance.

5. The organization acts when it does not achieve or sustain planned improvements.

   (*See also* MM.09.01.03, EP 5)

10. **For ambulatory surgical centers that elect to use The Joint Commission deemed status option:** The ambulatory surgical center implements preventive strategies throughout the facility targeting adverse patient events and makes certain that all staff are familiar with these strategies.

    (*See also* LD.03.09.01, EPs 2, 3, 4, 9)

11. **For organizations that elect The Joint Commission Primary Care Medical Home option:** The organization uses the data it collects on the patient's perception of the safety and quality of care, treatment, or services to improve its performance. This data includes the following:
    - Patient experience and satisfaction related to access to care, treatment, or services and communication
    - Patient perception of the comprehensiveness of care, treatment, or services
    - Patient perception of the coordination of care, treatment, or services
    - Patient perception of the continuity of care, treatment, or services

12. **For ambulatory surgical centers that elect to use The Joint Commission deemed status option:** The organization's quality assurance and performance improvement activities demonstrate the following:
    - Measurable improvement in patient health outcomes
    - Improvements in patient safety by using quality indicators or performance measures associated with improved health outcomes
    - Improvements in patient safety through efforts to identify and reduce medical errors

Record of Care, Treatment, and Services (RC)

Overview

The "Record of Care, Treatment, and Services" (RC) chapter contains a wealth of information about the components of a complete clinical record. A highly detailed document when seen in its entirety, the clinical record comprises all data and information gathered about a patient from the moment they enter the organization to the moment of discharge or transfer. As such, the clinical record functions not only as a historical record of a patient's episode(s) of care, but also as a method of communication between practitioners and staff that can facilitate the continuity of care and aid in clinical decision making.

In many organizations, patient care is episodic. The organization may only see the patient once or twice, depending on the patient's need and the organization's scope of services. For example, a diagnostic imaging center may only see the patient for magnetic resonance imaging (MRI). However, other organizations, such as college-based student health centers, may see a patient for a limited number of visits over a few years. In either case, the patient's episode(s) of care must be carefully documented.

Whether the organization keeps paper records, electronic records, or both, the contents of the record remain the same. Special care should be taken, however, by organizations that are transitioning from paper to electronic systems, as the period of transition can present increased opportunity for errors in recordkeeping that can affect the delivery of safe, quality care.

About This Chapter

Within this chapter is a comprehensive set of requirements for compiling and maintaining the clinical record. The separate components of a complete clinical record are listed and arranged within common groups (demographic, clinical, and additional information). This chapter also contains documentation requirements for screenings, assessments, and reassessments; pre- and postoperative procedures; the administration of moderate or deep sedation or anesthesia; restraint and seclusion; the clinical procedures themselves; and discharge. Standards provide policies and procedures that guide the compilation, completion, authentication, retention, and release of records.

Chapter Outline

I. Plan
    A. Clinical Record Components (RC.01.01.01)
    B. Authentication (RC.01.02.01)
    C. Timeliness (RC.01.03.01)
    D. Audit (RC.01.04.01)
    E. Retention (RC.01.05.01)

II. Implement
    A. Care, Treatment, or Services (RC.02.01.01, RC.02.01.03, RC.02.01.05)
    B. Orders (RC.02.03.07)

Standards, Rationales, and Elements of Performance

Standard RC.01.01.01 ▬▬▬▬▬▬▬▬▬▬▬▬▬▬▬

The organization maintains complete and accurate clinical records.

Elements of Performance for RC.01.01.01

1. The organization defines the components of a complete clinical record.

5. The clinical record includes the following:
    - Information needed to support the patient's diagnosis and condition
    - Information needed to justify the patient's care, treatment, or services
    - Information that documents the course and result of the patient's care, treatment, or services
    - Information about the patient's care, treatment, or services that promotes continuity of care among providers

    Note: *For organizations that elect The Joint Commission Primary Care Medical Home option:* *This requirement refers to care provided by both internal and external providers.*

7. All entries in the clinical record are dated.

9. When needed to provide care, summaries of care, treatment, or services are forwarded to other care providers.

Standard RC.01.02.01 ▬▬▬▬▬▬▬▬▬▬▬▬▬▬▬

Entries in the clinical record are authenticated.

Elements of Performance for RC.01.02.01

1. Only authorized individuals make entries in the clinical record.

2. The organization defines the types of entries in the clinical record made by nonindependent practitioners that require countersigning, in accordance with law and regulation.

3. The author of each clinical record entry is identified in the clinical record.

4. Entries in the clinical record are authenticated by the author. Information introduced into the clinical record through transcription or dictation is authenticated by the author.

Note 1: *Authentication can be verified through electronic signatures, written signatures or initials, rubber-stamp signatures, or computer key.*

Note 2: *For paper-based records, signatures entered for purposes of authentication after transcription or for verbal orders are dated when required by law or regulation or organization policy. For electronic records, electronic signatures will be date-stamped.*

5. The individual identified by the signature stamp or method of electronic authentication is the only individual who uses it.

Standard RC.01.03.01

Documentation in the clinical record is entered in a timely manner.

Elements of Performance for RC.01.03.01

1. The organization defines the time frame for completion of the clinical record.

2. Ⓓ The organization follows its written policy requiring timely entry of information into the patient's clinical record.

   (*See also* PC.01.02.03, EP 1)

Standard RC.01.04.01

The organization audits its clinical records.

Elements of Performance for RC.01.04.01

1. According to a time frame it defines, the organization reviews its clinical records to confirm that the required information is present, accurate, legible, authenticated, and completed on time.

Standard RC.01.05.01

The organization retains its clinical records.

Elements of Performance for RC.01.05.01

1. Ⓓ The retention time of the clinical record is determined by its use and organization policy, in accordance with law and regulation.

   Note: *For ambulatory surgical centers that elect to use The Joint Commission deemed status option:* *The Centers for Medicare & Medicaid Services requires the ambulatory surgical center to retain the original or legally reproduced medical record for at least five years, including applicable films, scans, and other images.*

8. Original clinical records are not released unless the organization is responding to law and regulation.

Standard RC.02.01.01 ▬▬▬▬▬▬▬▬▬▬▬▬▬▬▬▬▬▬▬▬▬▬▬▬▬

The clinical record contains information that reflects the patient's care, treatment, or services.

Elements of Performance for RC.02.01.01

1. The clinical record contains the following demographic information:
    - The patient's name, address, phone number, and date of birth and the name of any legally authorized representative
    - The patient's sex, height, and weight
    - The legal status of any patient receiving behavioral health care services
    - The patient's language and communication needs

    Note: *If the patient is a minor, is incapacitated, or has a designated advocate, the communication needs of the parent or legal guardian, surrogate decision-maker, or legally authorized representative are documented in the clinical record.*

2. The clinical record contains the following clinical information:
    - The patient's initial diagnosis, diagnostic impression(s), or condition(s)
    - Any findings of assessments and reassessments
    - Any allergies to food
    - Any allergies to medications
    - Any conclusions or impressions drawn from the patient's medical history and physical examination
    - Any diagnoses or conditions established during the patient's course of care, treatment, or services
    - Any consultation reports
    - Any progress notes
    - Any medications ordered or prescribed
    - Any medications administered, including the strength, dose, route, date and time of administration

    Note 1: *When rapid titration of a medication is necessary, the organization defines in policy the urgent/emergent situations in which block charting would be an acceptable form of documentation.*

    Note 2: *For the definition and a further explanation of block charting, refer to the Glossary.*

- Any access site for medication, administration devices used, and rate of administration
- The patient's response to any medication administered
- Any adverse drug reactions
- Plans for care and any revisions to the plan for care
- Orders for diagnostic and therapeutic tests and procedures and their results

(*See also* PC.01.02.01, EP 1; PC.03.01.03, EPs 1, 8)

4. As needed to provide care, treatment, or services, the clinical record contains the following additional information:
   - Any advance directives

   Note: *For ambulatory surgical centers that elect to use The Joint Commission deemed status option:* The organization documents in a prominent place in the clinical record whether or not the patient has advance directives in place.
   - *Any informed consent*
   - *Any documentation of clinical research interventions distinct from entries related to regular patient care, treatment, or services*
   - *Any records of communication with the patient, such as telephone calls or e-mail*
   - *Any referrals or communications made to internal or external care providers and community agencies*
   - *Any patient-generated information*

   (*See also* RI.01.03.05, EP 4)

18. The clinical record of a patient who receives urgent or immediate care, treatment, or services contains the following:
    - The time and means of arrival
    - Indication that the patient left against medical advice, when applicable
    - Conclusions reached at the termination of care, treatment, or services, including the patient's final disposition, condition, and instructions given for follow-up care, treatment, or services
    - A copy of any information made available to the practitioner or medical organization providing follow-up care, treatment, or services

25. **For organizations that elect The Joint Commission Primary Care Medical Home option:** The clinical record contains the patient's:
    - Gender, race, and ethnicity
    - Family history

- Work history (including any occupational risk factors or exposures)

26. **For organizations that elect The Joint Commission Primary Care Medical Home option:** The clinical record includes the patient's self-management goals and the patient's progress toward achieving those goals. (Refer to PC.01.03.01, EP 44)

27. **For organizations that elect The Joint Commission Primary Care Medical Home option:** The clinical record contains the patient's preferred language for discussing health care.

30. **For ambulatory surgical centers that elect to use The Joint Commission deemed status option:** The clinical record contains any significant medical history and results of physical examination, as applicable.

Standard RC.02.01.03 ▬▬▬▬▬▬▬

The patient's clinical record contains documentation on any operative or other high-risk procedures and the use of moderate or deep sedation or anesthesia.

Elements of Performance for RC.02.01.03

1. The organization documents in the patient's clinical record any operative or other high-risk procedure and/or the administration of moderate or deep sedation or anesthesia. **R**

2. A licensed independent practitioner involved in the patient's care documents the provisional diagnosis in the clinical record before an operative or other high-risk procedure is performed.

4. **For ambulatory surgical centers that elect to use The Joint Commission deemed status option:** The patient's clinical record contains the results of preoperative diagnostic studies. The results are included in the patient's clinical record prior to the start of the surgical procedure.

5. An operative or other high-risk procedure report is written or dictated upon completion of the operative or other high-risk procedure and before the patient is transferred to the next level of care.

   Note 1: *The exception to this requirement occurs when an operative or other high-risk procedure progress note is written immediately after the procedure, in which case the full report can be written or dictated within a time frame defined by the organization.*

> **Note 2:** *If the practitioner performing the operation or high-risk procedure accompanies the patient from the operating room to the next unit or area of care, the report can be written or dictated in the new unit or area of care.*

6.   The operative or other high-risk procedure report includes the following information:
- The name(s) of the licensed independent practitioner(s) who performed the procedure and their assistant(s)
- The name of the procedure performed
- A description of the procedure
- Findings of the procedure
- Any estimated blood loss
- Any specimen(s) removed
- The postoperative diagnosis

7.   When a full operative or other high-risk procedure report cannot be entered immediately into the patient's clinical record, a note is entered immediately. This note includes the name(s) of the primary surgeon(s) and their assistant(s), procedure performed and a description of each procedure finding, estimated blood loss, specimens removed, and postoperative diagnosis. **R**

8.   The clinical record contains the following postoperative information:
- The patient's vital signs and level of consciousness
- Any medications, including intravenous fluids and any administered blood, blood products, and blood components
- Any unanticipated events or complications (including blood transfusion reactions) and the management of those events

(*See also* PC.03.01.05, EP 1; PC.03.01.07, EP 1)

9.   The clinical record contains documentation that the patient was discharged from the recovery phase of the operation or procedure either by the licensed independent practitioner responsible for the patient's care or according to discharge criteria.

(*See also* PC.03.01.07, EP 4)

10.   The clinical record contains documentation of the use of approved discharge criteria that determine the patient's readiness for discharge.

(*See also* PC.03.01.07, EP 4)

11. The postoperative documentation contains the name of the licensed independent practitioner responsible for discharge.

12. **For ambulatory surgical centers that elect to use The Joint Commission deemed status option:** The clinical record contains the discharge diagnosis.

13. **For ambulatory surgical centers that elect to use The Joint Commission deemed status option:** The patient's medical history and physical assessment (if any) is placed in the patient's medical record prior to the surgical procedure. **R**

14. **For ambulatory surgical centers that elect to use The Joint Commission deemed status option:** The patient's postsurgical condition is assessed and documented in the medical record by a physician, other qualified practitioner, or registered nurse with, at a minimum, postoperative care experience, in accordance with applicable state health and safety laws, standards of practice, and organizational policy. **R**

Standard RC.02.01.05

The clinical record contains documentation of the use of restraint.

Elements of Performance for RC.02.01.05

1. The organization documents the use of restraint in the clinical record, including the following:
   - Orders for use
   - Results of patient monitoring
   - Reassessment
   - Unanticipated changes in the patient's condition

   (*See also* PC.03.02.03, EP 1; PC.03.02.07, EPs 1, 2)

Standard RC.02.03.07

Qualified staff receive and record verbal orders.

Elements of Performance for RC.02.03.07

1. ⒹThe organization identifies, in writing, the staff who are authorized to receive and record verbal orders, in accordance with law and regulation.

2. Only authorized staff receive and record verbal orders.

3. Documentation of verbal orders includes the date and the names of individuals who gave, received, recorded, and implemented the orders.

4. Verbal orders are authenticated within the time frame specified by law and regulation.

Rights and Responsibilities of the Individual (RI)

Overview
When the organization recognizes and respects patient rights, it is providing an important aspect of care that has been shown to encourage patients to become more informed and involved in their care. These empowered patients ask questions and develop better relationships with their caregivers. This acknowledgement of patient rights also helps patients feel supported by the organization and those people directly involved in their care, treatment, or services. In a climate of respect and trust, communication is enhanced, and issues that could lead to problems in safety or quality may be prevented or addressed.

Recognizing and respecting patient rights are, however, only part of the story. Patients also have the obligation to take on certain responsibilities. The organization defines these responsibilities and then relays them to the patient. When patients understand and accept their responsibilities, the concept of the patient as a partner in care becomes a dynamic component of the patient's episode of care.

In summary, the standards in this chapter address the following processes and activities as they relate to patient rights:
- Informing patients of their rights
- Helping patients understand and exercise their rights
- Respecting patients' values, beliefs, and preferences
- Informing patients of their responsibilities regarding their care, treatment, or services

About This Chapter
This chapter presents a series of requirements that help organizations to recognize and respect patient rights. These requirements address the following:
- Identification of fundamental, overarching patient rights
- The right to effective communication
- The right to participate in care decisions
- The right to informed consent
- The right to know care providers

- The right to participate in end-of-life decisions
- Individual rights of patients
- Patient responsibilities

Note: *This chapter talks about the role of a surrogate decision-maker who may participate in circumstances in which the patient cannot or chooses not to make decisions. Instead of stating "patient or surrogate decision-maker" in each occurrence where the surrogate decision-maker may need to play a role, "patient" is used with the understanding that if the patient is unable to make decisions, the surrogate decision-maker will do so.*

Chapter Outline

I. Patient Rights
    A. Developing and Communicating Patient Rights
        1. Charge to Organizations (RI.01.01.01)
        2. Effective Communication (RI.01.01.03)
    B. Participation in Care Decisions (RI.01.02.01)
    C. Informed Consent (RI.01.03.01, RI.01.03.05)
    D. Right to Know (RI.01.04.01, RI.01.04.03)
    E. End-of-Life Issues (RI.01.05.01)
    F. Personal Rights (RI.01.06.03)
    G. Services Provided by Organizations to Respect Patient Rights (RI.01.07.01)

II. Patient Responsibilities (RI.02.01.01)

Standards, Rationales, and Elements of Performance

Introduction to Standard RI.01.01.01

This standard focuses on how the organization respects the rights of the patient during their encounter with the organization. Rights such as treating the patient in a dignified and respectful manner, providing effective communication, and respecting the patient's cultural and personal values are covered in this standard. An organization puts its respect for the patient's rights into action by showing its support of these rights through the ways that staff and caregivers interact with the patient and involve the patient in care, treatment, or services.

Standard RI.01.01.01

The organization respects patient rights.

Elements of Performance for RI.01.01.01

1. Ⓓ The organization has written policies on patient rights.

2. Information about patient rights is available to the patient.

    (*See also* RI.01.01.03, EPs 1, 2, 3)

4. The organization treats the patient in a dignified and respectful manner that supports the patient's dignity.

5. The organization respects the patient's right to and need for effective communication.

    (*See also* RI.01.01.03, EPs 1, 2, 3)

6. The organization respects the patient's cultural and personal values, beliefs, and preferences.

7. The organization respects the patient's right to privacy.

    Note: *This element of performance (EP) addresses a patient's personal privacy. For EPs addressing the privacy of a patient's health information, please refer to Standard IM.02.01.01.*

(*See also* IM.02.01.01, EPs 1, 3, 4)

10. The organization allows the patient to access, request amendment to, and obtain information on disclosures of the patient's health information, in accordance with law and regulation.

13. **For ambulatory surgical centers that elect to use The Joint Commission deemed status option:** The organization respects the patient's right to receive care in a safe setting.

Introduction to Standard RI.01.01.03

Because communication is a cornerstone of patient safety and quality care, every patient has the right to receive information in a manner they understand. Effective communication allows patients to participate more fully in their care. When a patient understands what is being said about their care, treatment, or services, that patient is more likely to fulfill critical health care responsibilities. Communicating effectively with patients is also critical to the informed consent process and helps practitioners and organizations give the best possible care. For communication to be effective, the information provided must be complete, accurate, timely, unambiguous, and under-stood by the patient.

Many patients of varying circumstances require alternative communication methods: patients who speak and/or read languages other than English; patients who have limited literacy in any language; patients who have visual or hearing impairments; patients on ventilators; patients with cognitive impairments; and children. The organization has many options available to assist in communication with these individuals, such as interpreters, translated written materials, pen and paper, communication boards, and speech therapy. It is up to the organization to determine which method is the best for each patient.

There are laws, regulations, and a body of literature that are relevant to the use of interpreters. These include Title VI of the Civil Rights Act, 1964; Executive Order 13166; policy guidance from the Office of Civil Rights regarding compliance with Title VI, 2004; Title III of the Americans with Disabilities Act, 1990; state laws (many states have laws and regulations that require the provision of language assistance); and the American Medical Association Office Guide to Limited English Proficiency (LEP) Patient Care. Organizations may wish to reference these sources for additional information on providing interpreting and translation services to their patients.

Standard RI.01.01.03

The organization respects the patient's right to receive information in a manner the patient understands.

Elements of Performance for RI.01.01.03

1. The organization provides information in a manner tailored to the patient's age, language, and ability to understand.

    (*See also* RI.01.01.01, EPs 2, 5)

2. The organization provides interpreting and translation services, as necessary.

    Note: *For organizations that elect The Joint Commission Primary Care Medical Home option:* *Language interpreting options may include trained bilingual staff, contract interpreting services, or employed language interpreters. These options may be provided in person or via telephone or video. The documents translated, and the languages into which they are translated, are dependent on the organization's patient population.*

    (*See also* RI.01.01.01, EPs 2, 5)

3. The organization communicates with the patient who has vision, speech, hearing, or cognitive impairments in a manner that meets the patient's needs.

    (*See also* RI.01.01.01, EPs 2, 5)

4. Ⓓ **For ambulatory surgical centers that elect to use The Joint Commission deemed status option:** The ambulatory surgical center provides the patient or the patient's surrogate decision-maker with verbal and written notice of the patient's rights prior to the start of the surgical procedure in a language and manner that the patient or their surrogate decision-maker understands.

5.   ⑩ **For ambulatory surgical centers that elect to use The Joint Commission deemed status option:** The ambulatory surgical center posts a copy of its notice of patient rights in a location where it is likely to be noticed by patients. The notice of rights includes contact information for reporting complaints to the state agency and the website for the Office of the Medicare Beneficiary Ombudsman.

Standard RI.01.02.01 ▬▬▬▬▬▬▬▬▬▬▬▬▬▬▬▬▬▬▬▬▬▬▬▬

The organization respects the patient's right to participate in decisions about their care, treatment, or services.

Elements of Performance for RI.01.02.01

1.   The organization involves the patient in making decisions about their care, treatment, or services.

2.   When a patient is unable to make decisions about their care, treatment, or services, the organization involves a surrogate decision-maker in making these decisions.

     (*See also* RI.01.03.01, EP 1)

4.   The organization respects the right of the patient or surrogate decision-maker to refuse care, treatment, or services in accordance with law and regulation.

8.   The organization involves the patient's family in care, treatment, or services decisions to the extent permitted by the patient or surrogate decision-maker, in accordance with law and regulation.

20. The organization provides the patient or surrogate decision-maker with the information about the following:
     ■ Outcomes of care, treatment, or services that the patient needs in order to participate in current and future health care decisions
     ■ Unanticipated outcomes of the patient's care, treatment, or services that are sentinel events as defined by The Joint Commission (Refer to the Glossary for a definition of sentinel event.)

31. **For organizations that elect The Joint Commission Primary Care Medical Home option:** The organization respects the patient's right to make decisions about the management of the patient's care.

32. **For organizations that elect The Joint Commission Primary Care Medical Home option:** The organization respects the patient's right and provides the patient the opportunity to do the following:
    - Obtain care from other clinicians of the patient's choosing within the primary care medical home
    - Seek a second opinion from a clinician of the patient's choosing
    - Seek specialty care

    Note: *This element of performance does not imply financial responsibility for any activities associated with these rights.*

Standard RI.01.03.01 ▬▬▬▬▬▬▬▬▬▬▬▬▬▬▬▬▬▬▬

The organization honors the patient's right to give or withhold informed consent.

Rationale for RI.01.03.01

Obtaining informed consent presents an opportunity to establish a mutual understanding between the patient and the licensed independent practitioner or other licensed practitioners with privileges about the care, treatment, or services that the patient will receive. Informed consent is not merely a signed document. It is a process that considers patient needs and preferences, complies with law and regulation, and includes patient education. Utilizing the informed consent process helps the patient to participate fully in decisions about their care, treatment, or services.

Elements of Performance for RI.01.03.01

1. Ⓓ The organization follows a written policy on informed consent that describes the following:
   - The specific care, treatment, or services that require informed consent
   - Circumstances that would allow for exceptions to obtaining informed consent
   - When a surrogate decision-maker may give informed consent

   (*See also* RI.01.02.01, EP 2)

2. The informed consent process includes a discussion about the following:
   - The patient's proposed care, treatment, or services.
   - Potential benefits, risks, and side effects of the patient's proposed care, treatment, or services; the likelihood of the patient achieving their goals; and any potential problems that might occur during recuperation.

- Reasonable alternatives to the patient's proposed care, treatment, or services. The discussion encompasses risks, benefits, and side effects related to the alternatives and the risks related to not receiving the proposed care, treatment, or services.

3. Ⓓ The organization obtains and documents informed consent in advance when it makes and uses recordings, films, or other images of patients for internal use other than the identification, diagnosis, or treatment of the patient (for example, performance improvement and education).

    Note 1: *The term "recordings, films, or other images" refers to photographic, video, digital, electronic, or audio media.*

    Note 2: *This element of performance does not apply to the use of security cameras.*

15. **For ambulatory surgical centers that elect to use The Joint Commission deemed status option:** Informed consent is obtained before a treatment or procedure is performed.

Standard RI.01.03.05

The organization protects the patient and respects the patient's rights during research, investigation, and clinical trials.

Elements of Performance for RI.01.03.05

2. To help the patient determine whether or not to participate in research, investigation, or clinical trials, the organization provides the patient with all of the following information:
    - An explanation of the purpose of the research
    - The expected duration of the patient's participation
    - A clear description of the procedures to be followed
    - A statement of the potential benefits, risks, discomforts, and side effects
    - Alternative care, treatment, or services available to the patient that might prove advantageous to the patient

3. The organization informs the patient that refusing to participate in research, investigation, or clinical trials or discontinuing participation at any time will not jeopardize the patient's access to care, treatment, or services unrelated to the research.

4. Ⓓ The organization documents the following in the research consent form:

- That the patient received information to help determine whether or not to participate in the research, investigation, or clinical trials
- That the patient was informed that refusing to participate in research, investigation, or clinical trials or discontinuing participation at any time will not jeopardize their access to care, treatment, or services unrelated to the research
- The name of the person who provided the information and the date the form was signed
- The patient's right to privacy, confidentiality, and safety

(*See also* RC.02.01.01, EP 4)

Standard RI.01.04.01 ━━━━━━━━━━━━━━

The organization respects the patient's right to receive information about the individual(s) responsible for the patient's care, treatment, or services.

Elements of Performance for RI.01.04.01

1. The organization informs the patient of the following:
   - The name of the physician or other practitioner who has primary responsibility for the patient's care, treatment, or services
   - The name of the physician(s) or other practitioner(s) who will provide the patient's care, treatment, or services

7. **For organizations that elect The Joint Commission Primary Care Medical Home option:** The organization allows the patient to select their primary care clinician.

Standard RI.01.04.03 ━━━━━━━━━━━━━━

For organizations that elect The Joint Commission Primary Care Medical Home option: The organization provides patients with information about the functions and services of the primary care medical home.

Elements of Performance for RI.01.04.03

1. **For organizations that elect The Joint Commission Primary Care Medical Home option:** The organization provides information to the patient about the mission, vision, and goals of the primary care medical home. (Refer to LD.02.01.01, EP 3)

Note: *This may include how it provides for patient-centered and team-based comprehensive care, a systems-based approach to quality and safety, and enhanced patient access.*

2. **For organizations that elect The Joint Commission Primary Care Medical Home option:** The organization provides information to the patient about how the primary care medical home functions, its scope of care, and its types of services. (For more information, refer to Standards PC.01.01.01 and LD.01.03.01)

3. **For organizations that elect The Joint Commission Primary Care Medical Home option:** The organization provides information to the patient about the following:
   - Selection of a primary care clinician
   - Involvement in the patient's own treatment plan
   - Management of referrals
   - Coordination of care
   - Collaboration with patient-selected clinicians who provide specialty care or second opinions
   - Communication with the primary care medical home about health care concerns or other information

5. **For organizations that elect The Joint Commission Primary Care Medical Home option:** The organization provides information to the patient about patient responsibilities, including providing health history and current medications, and participating in self-management activities. (Refer to RI.02.01.01, EP 2)

6. **For organizations that elect The Joint Commission Primary Care Medical Home option:** The organization provides information to the patient about the patient's right to obtain care from other clinicians within the primary care medical home, to seek a second opinion, and to seek specialty care. (Refer to PC.02.03.01, EP 4; RI.01.01.03, EPs 1 and 3)

7. **For organizations that elect The Joint Commission Primary Care Medical Home option:** The primary care medical home provides patients with information regarding the credentials and educational background of individuals serving in the role of primary care clinician.

Standard RI.01.05.01 ━━━━━━━━━━━━━━━

The organization addresses patient decisions about care, treatment, or services received at the end of life.

Elements of Performance for RI.01.05.01

1. Ⓓ The organization follows written policies on advance directives that specify whether the organization will honor advance directives. The organization communicates its policies on advance directives to patients upon request.

7. Ⓓ **For ambulatory surgical centers that elect to use The Joint Commission deemed status option:** Prior to the start of the surgical procedure the ambulatory surgical center provides the patient or the patient's surrogate decision-maker with written information concerning its policies on advance directives, including a description of applicable state health and safety laws and, if requested, official state advance directive forms.

10. Upon request, the organization shares with the patient possible sources of help in formulating advance directives.

Standard RI.01.06.03 ━━━━━━━━━━━━━━━

The patient has the right to be free from neglect; exploitation; and verbal, mental, physical, and sexual abuse.

Elements of Performance for RI.01.06.03

1. The organization determines how it will protect the patient from neglect, exploitation, and abuse that could occur while the patient is receiving care, treatment, or services.

2. The organization evaluates all allegations, observations, and suspected cases of neglect, exploitation, and abuse that occur within the organization.

    (*See also* PC.01.02.09, EP 1)

3. The organization reports allegations, observations, and suspected cases of neglect, exploitation, and abuse to appropriate authorities based on its evaluation of the suspected events.

    (*See also* PC.01.02.09, EPs 6, 7)

6. **For ambulatory surgical centers that elect to use The Joint Commission deemed status option:** The organization respects the patient's right to be free from all forms of abuse or harassment. **R**

Standard RI.01.07.01

The patient and their family have the right to have complaints reviewed by the organization.

Elements of Performance for RI.01.07.01

1. The organization establishes a complaint resolution process and informs the patient and the patient's family about it.

4. The organization reviews and, when possible, resolves complaints from the patient and the patient's family.

10. **For ambulatory surgical centers that elect to use The Joint Commission deemed status option:** The patient has the right to exercise their rights without being subject to coercion, discrimination, reprisal, or interruption of care that could adversely affect the patient.

11. **For ambulatory surgical centers that elect to use The Joint Commission deemed status option:** The patient has the right to voice grievances regarding treatment or care that are (or fail to be) furnished.

21. Ⓓ **For ambulatory surgical centers that elect to use The Joint Commission deemed status option:** The ambulatory surgical center establishes a written procedure for documenting the existence, submission, investigation, and disposition of a patient's written or verbal grievance(s).

22. **For ambulatory surgical centers that elect to use The Joint Commission deemed status option:** All allegations, violations, or grievances related to, but not limited to, mistreatment, neglect or verbal, mental, sexual or physical abuse, are immediately reported to a person in authority in the ambulatory surgical center.

23. Ⓓ **For ambulatory surgical centers that elect to use The Joint Commission deemed status option:** All alleged violations or grievances related to, but not limited to, mistreatment, neglect or verbal, mental, sexual or physical abuse, are fully documented.

24. **For ambulatory surgical centers that elect to use The Joint Commission deemed status option:** Substantiated allegations related to, but not limited to, mistreatment, neglect or verbal, mental, sexual or physical abuse, are reported to the state authority or the local authority, or both.

25. **For ambulatory surgical centers that elect to use The Joint Commission deemed status option:** The grievance process specifies time frames for review of the grievance and the provision of a response.

26. **For ambulatory surgical centers that elect to use The Joint Commission deemed status option:** The ambulatory surgical center, in responding to the grievance, investigates all grievances made by a patient or the patient's representative regarding treatment or care that is (or fails to be) furnished.

27. ⓓ **For ambulatory surgical centers that elect to use The Joint Commission deemed status option:** The ambulatory surgical center documents how the grievance was addressed and provides the patient with written notice of its decision. The decision contains the name of an ambulatory surgical center contact person, the steps taken to investigate the grievance, the results of the grievance process, and the date the grievance process was completed.

Introduction to Standard RI.02.01.01

The safety of patients is enhanced when patients are partners in the health care process. In addition, organizations are entitled to reasonable and responsible behavior on the part of patients and their families. When organizations inform patients and their families about their responsibilities, some of the topics that are discussed could include the following:

- Providing information. Patients should provide, to the best of their knowledge, accurate information about present complaints, past illnesses, hospitalizations, medications, and other matters related to their health.
- Sharing expectations. Patients should provide the organization with information about their expectations of and satisfaction with the organization.
- Asking questions. Patients should ask questions when they do not understand their care, treatment, or services or what they are expected to do.

- Following instructions. Patients should follow their plan of care, treatment, or services. They should also express any concerns about their ability to follow the proposed plan of care, treatment, or services.

- Accepting consequences. Patients should accept their share of responsibility for the outcomes of care, treatment, or services if they do not follow the care, treatment, or services plan.

- Following policies and procedures. Patients should follow the organization's policies and procedures.

- Showing respect and consideration. Patients should be considerate of the organization's staff and property, as well as other patients and their property.

- Meeting financial commitments. Patients should meet any financial obligation agreed to with the organization.

Standard RI.02.01.01

The organization informs the patient about the patient's responsibilities related to their care, treatment, or services.

Elements of Performance for RI.02.01.01

2.   The organization informs the patient about the patient's responsibilities.

   Note: *Information about patient responsibilities can be shared verbally, in writing, or both.*

Transplant Safety (TS)

Overview

Transplantation of tissues is sometimes the only option for treatment of a wide range of diseases. In the past 10 years, advances in transplantation have led to a greater success rate for transplanted tissues. More and more people receive transplants every year. Tissue transplants are used most often to enhance the lives of recipients; they are also used at times to save lives. Tissues that are transplanted include bones, tendons, corneas, heart valves, veins, and skin. A single donor can save many lives, as well as improve the quality of life for many more.

Transplantation is not free from risk. Transmission of infections from the donor to the recipient is a significant safety concern. With the increased number of tissue transplants, the number of opportunities for transmission of infectious pathogens has also increased. Instances of tissue-borne infection in recipients of donor tissues are well documented. Diseases with documented transmission from infected donors subsequent to transplant include, to name a few, human immunodeficiency virus (HIV), hepatitis B and C, and Creutzfeldt-Jakob disease (CJD). Recipients may also contract bacterial or fungal infections through contamination during transportation, storage, or handling. The opportunity for transmission of infectious disease will continue to increase as the number of transplants continues to rise.

Effective communication of an adverse event directly related to tissue use is critical to patient safety. The organization may become aware of an adverse event directly related to tissue use through external notification or internal detection. Prompt investigation of each adverse event provides response and treatment to recipients affected by the infected tissue and could prevent further transplantation from an infected donor.

About This Chapter

The standards in this chapter focus on the development and implementation of policies and procedures for safe tissue transplantation.

Chapter Outline

Standards, Rationales, and Elements of Performance

Introduction to Standards TS.03.01.01, TS.03.02.01, and TS.03.03.01

The following standards apply to organizations that store or issue tissue. This includes any areas outside of the clinical laboratory that store or issue tissue; for example, surgery and outpatient centers or tissue banks. They apply to human and nonhuman cellular-based transplantable and implantable products whether classified by the US Food and Drug Administration (FDA) as a tissue or a medical device. Collagen and tissue products derived from plastics and polymers are not considered cellular-based products and are not evaluated under these standards.

Specific tissue transplant requirements apply to autologous tissue. This includes policies and procedures for identifying, tracking, storing, and handling autologous tissue, in addition to investigating tissue adverse events. Also, if the state in which an organization resides classifies something as tissue that falls outside the scope of The Joint Commission definition, the standards would apply.

Examples of Tissue and Cell Products

- Amnion/Amniotic Membrane
- Arteries
- Autologous Cells
- Autologous Tissue
- Bone
- Bone Marrow
- Bone Paste
- Bone Powder
- Bone Putty
- Cancellous Chips
- Cardiac (Heart) Valves (Aortic, Pulmonary)
- Cartilage
- Chondrocytes
- Cornea
- Demineralized Bone Matrix

- Dendritic Cells
- Dermal Matrix
- Dermis
- Dura Mater
- Embryo
- Fascia/Fascia Lata
- Hematopoietic Stem Cell
- Leukocytes
- Ligaments
- Limbal Graft
- Limbal Stem Cells
- Lymphocytes
- Marrow
- Membrane
- Meniscus
- Nerves
- Non-valved Conduits
- Oocyte/Ovarian Cells
- Ovarian Tissue
- Pancreatic Islet Cells
- Parathyroid
- Pericardium
- Peripheral Blood Stem Cells
- Progenitor Cells
- Sclera
- Semen, Sperm
- Skin
- Somatic Cells
- Tendons
- Testicular Tissue
- Therapeutic Cells (T-Cell Pheresis)/T-Cells
- Tissue (also Synthetic Tissue)
- Trachea
- Umbilical Cord Blood Stem Cells
- Vascular Graft
- Veins (Saphenous, Femoral, Iliac)
- Other cellular- and tissue-based transplant or implant products whether classified by

the FDA as a tissue or a medical device

■ Other tissues that are classified as tissues by state law and regulation

Standard TS.03.01.01

The organization uses standardized procedures for managing tissues.

Elements of Performance for TS.03.01.01

1. The organization assigns responsibility to one or more individuals for overseeing the acquisition, receipt, storage, and issuance of tissues throughout the organization.

    Note: *Responsibility for this oversight involves coordinating efforts to provide standardized practices throughout the organization. An organization may have a centralized process (one department responsible for the ordering, receipt, storage, and issuance of tissue throughout the organization) or a decentralized process (multiple departments responsible for the ordering, receipt, storage, and issuance of tissue throughout the organization).*

2. ⒹThe organization develops and maintains standardized written procedures for the acquisition, receipt, storage, and issuance of tissues.

    (See also TS.03.02.01, EP 5)

3. The organization confirms that tissue suppliers are registered with the US Food and Drug Administration (FDA) as a tissue establishment and maintain a state license when required.*

    Note: *This element of performance does not apply to autologous tissue- or cellular-based products considered tissue for the purposes of these standards but classified as medical devices by the FDA.*

5. The organization follows the tissue suppliers' or manufacturers' written directions for transporting, handling, storing, and using tissue. **R**

6. ⒹThe organization documents the receipt of all tissues.

    (See also TS.03.02.01, EPs 3, 6)

7. ⒹThe organization verifies at the time of receipt that package integrity is met

---

* For US Food and Drug Administration (FDA) registration, the supplier registration status may also be checked annually by using the FDA's online database: https://www.fda.gov/vaccines-blood-biologics/biologics-establishment-registration/find-tissue-establishment.

and transport temperature range was controlled and acceptable for tissues requiring a controlled environment. This verification is documented.

Note 1: *If the distributor uses validated shipping containers, then the receiver may document that the shipping container was received undamaged and within the stated time frame.*

Note 2: *Tissues requiring no greater control than "ambient temperature" (generally defined as the temperature of the immediate environment) for transport and storage would not need to have the temperature verified on receipt.*

(*See also* TS.03.02.01, EP 5)

8. Ⓓ The organization maintains daily records to demonstrate that tissues requiring a controlled environment are stored at the required temperatures.

Note 1: *Types of tissue storage include room temperature, refrigerated, frozen (for example, deep freezing colder than -40°C), and liquid nitrogen storage.*

Note 2: *Tissues requiring no greater control than "ambient temperature" (defined as the temperature of the immediate environment) for storage would not require temperature monitoring.*

(*See also* TS.03.02.01, EP 5)

9. The organization continuously monitors the temperature of refrigerators, freezers, nitrogen tanks, and other storage equipment used to store tissues.

Note 1: *Continuous temperature recording is not required but may be available with some continuous temperature monitoring systems.*

Note 2: *For tissue stored at room temperature, continuous temperature monitoring is not required.*

10. Refrigerators, freezers, nitrogen tanks, and other storage equipment used to store tissues at a controlled temperature have functional alarms and an emergency backup plan. **R**

Note: *For tissue stored at room temperature, alarm systems are not required.*

Standard TS.03.02.01 ▬▬▬▬▬▬▬▬▬▬▬▬▬
The organization traces all tissues bi-directionally.

Elements of Performance for TS.03.02.01

1.   ⓓ The organization's records allow any tissue to be traced from the donor or tissue supplier to the recipient(s) or other final disposition, including discard, and from the recipient(s) or other final disposition back to the donor or tissue supplier. **R**

2.   ⓓ The organization identifies, in writing, the materials and related instructions used to prepare or process tissues.

3.   ⓓ The organization documents the dates, times, and staff involved when tissue is accepted, prepared, and issued.

     (*See also* TS.03.01.01, EP 6)

4.   The organization documents in the recipient's clinical record the tissue type and its unique identifier.

5.   The organization retains tissue records on storage temperatures, outdated procedures, manuals, and publications for a minimum of 10 years. If required by state and/or federal laws, organizations may have to retain tissue records longer than 10 years.

     (*See also* TS.03.01.01, EPs 2, 7, 8)

6.   The organization retains tissue records for a minimum of 10 years beyond the date of distribution, transplantation, disposition, or expiration of tissue (whichever is latest). If required by state and/or federal laws, organizations may have to retain tissue records longer than 10 years. Records are kept on all of the following:
     ■ The tissue supplier

     Note: *For medical devices, the manufacturer may be the tissue supplier.*
     ■ The original numeric or alphanumeric donor and lot identification
     ■ The name(s) of the recipient(s) or the final disposition of each tissue
     ■ The expiration dates of all tissues

     (*See also* TS.03.01.01, EP 6)

7.   The organization completes and returns tissue usage information cards requested

by the tissue supplier.[†]

Standard TS.03.03.01

The organization investigates adverse events related to tissue use or donor infections.

Elements of Performance for TS.03.03.01

1. Ⓓ The organization has a written procedure to investigate tissue adverse events, including disease transmission or other complications that are suspected of being directly related to the use of tissue.

2. The organization investigates tissue adverse events, including disease transmission or other complications that are suspected of being directly related to the use of tissue.

3. As soon as the organization becomes aware of a post-transplant infection or other adverse event related to the use of tissue, it reports the infection or adverse event to the tissue supplier. **R**

4. The organization sequesters tissue whose integrity may have been compromised or that is reported by the tissue supplier as a suspected cause of infection. **R**

5. The organization identifies and informs tissue recipients of infection risk when donors are subsequently found to have human immunodeficiency virus (HIV), human T-lymphotropic virus-I/II (HTLV-I/II), viral hepatitis, or other infectious agents known to be transmitted through tissue. **R**

[†] According to the Health Insurance Portability and Accountability Act (HIPAA) regulations regarding protected health information, "A covered entity may disclose protected health information for public health activities or other purposes to a person subject to the jurisdiction of the Food and Drug Administration (FDA) for the following purposes:

■ To track products if the disclosure is made to a person required or directed by the FDA to track the product

■ To enable product recalls, repairs or replacement (including locating and notifying individuals who have received products of product recalls, withdrawals, or other problems" (Refer to 45 CFR 164.512(b)(1)(iii)(B) and (C))

Waived Testing (WT)

Overview

A laboratory test is an activity that evaluates a substance(s) removed from a human body and translates the evaluation into a result. A result can be stated as a number, presence or absence of a cell or reaction, or an interpretation. Tests that produce a result measured as a discrete number are termed "quantitative." Tests that produce a negative or positive result, such as occult bloods and urine pregnancy screens, are termed "qualitative." A test that is more precise than a qualitative test (pos/neg), but less precise than a quantitative test (numerical), is usually scored on a graded scale (1+, 2+, 3+) and is termed "semiquantitative." Tests with analysis steps that rely on the use of an instrument to produce a result are instrument-based tests. These can be qualitative, semiquantitative, or quantitative.

Test results that are used to assess a patient condition or make a clinical decision about a patient are governed by the federal regulations known as the Clinical Laboratory Improvement Amendments of 1988 (CLIA '88). CLIA '88 classifies testing into four complexity levels: high complexity, moderate complexity, provider performed microscopy (PPM) procedures (a subset of moderate complexity), and waived testing. The high, moderate, and PPM levels, otherwise called nonwaived testing, have specific and detailed requirements regarding personnel qualifications, quality assurance, quality control, and other systems. Waived testing, on the other hand, has few requirements and is less stringent than the requirements for nonwaived testing.

The waived testing requirements are supported by the *Morbidity and Mortality Weekly Report*, November 11, 2005, on "Good Laboratory Practices for Waived Testing Sites." This report indicates quality and safety concerns related to waived testing. Although by law waived tests should have insignificant risk of erroneous results, these tests are not completely error proof; some waived tests have potential for serious health impacts if performed incorrectly. This report draws attention to these pertinent risks:

- Lack of current manufacturers' instructions, including manufacturers' updates
- Failure to follow manufacturers' instructions, including performing quality control
- Reporting of incorrect results
- Lack of adherence to expiration dates
- Inappropriate storage requirements
- Not performing test system function checks or calibration checks

- Lack of documentation, including quality control and tests performed
- Inadequate training
- Lack of understanding about good laboratory practices

These errors could cause inaccurate results that could lead to inaccurate diagnoses, inappropriate or unnecessary medical treatment, and poor patient outcomes.

Waived testing is the most common complexity level performed by caregivers at the patient bedside or point of care. The list of methods that are approved as waived is under constant revision, so it is advisable to check the US Food and Drug Administration (FDA), Centers for Disease Control and Prevention, or Centers for Medicare & Medicaid Services (CMS) websites for the most up-to-date information regarding test categorization and complete CLIA '88 requirements such as the following:

- http://www.accessdata.fda.gov/scripts/cdrh/cfdocs/cfClia/testswaived.cfm
- https://www.cdc.gov/labquality/waived-tests.html?CDC_AA_refVal
  =https%3A%2F%2Fwww.cdc.gov%2Fclia%2Fwaived-tests.html
- https://www.cms.gov/Regulations-and-Guidance/Legislation/CLIA/index.html

About This Chapter

When a patient performs their own test (for example, whole blood glucose testing by a patient on their own meter cleared by the FDA for home use), the action is not regulated. Only testing performed by staff on patients is an activity regulated by CLIA '88. The Joint Commission standards apply to staff using instruments owned by staff, owned by the organization, or owned by the patient in performing waived laboratory tests. If staff are providing only instruction or cueing the patient, then these standards do not apply. This distinction is important when caring for patients who monitor their own health care (for example, testing of glucose or prothrombin times with home devices).

Currently, The Joint Commission allows for an organization to use the patient's results for treatment decisions. When using a patient's results from self-testing, health care providers do not have the same type of assurance about quality as they would if they conducted the testing themselves. The following processes are not specific Joint Commission requirements and are provided only as examples of how organizations have dealt with these concerns in practice:

- Verification of competency by either confirming the patient has been previously trained or observing the patient perform their first test

- Requiring the patient to perform quality control, if available for the meter, each day results are used
- Correlation of the patient's first glucose result with testing by a main laboratory
- Confirmation of all critical and nonlinear instrument values with testing by the main laboratory
- Demonstration of proper equipment maintenance

Note: *The Joint Commission requirements for laboratories or sites that perform nonwaived testing are located in the "Quality System Assessment for Nonwaived Testing" (QSA) chapter of the* Comprehensive Accreditation Manual for Laboratory and Point-of-Care Testing.

Chapter Outline

I.   Policies and Procedures (WT.01.01.01)

II.   Identification of Staff Performing and Supervising Waived Testing (WT.02.01.01)

III. Competency of Staff Performing Waived Testing (WT.03.01.01)

IV. Performance of Quality Control Checks (WT.04.01.01)

V.   Recordkeeping (WT.05.01.01)

Standards, Rationales, and Elements of Performance

Standard WT.01.01.01 ▬▬▬▬▬▬▬▬▬▬▬▬▬▬▬▬

Policies and procedures for waived tests are established, current, approved, and readily available.

Elements of Performance for WT.01.01.01

1. The director named on the Clinical Laboratory Improvement Amendments of 1988 (CLIA '88) certificate approves a consistent approach for when waived test results can be used for diagnosis and treatment and when follow-up testing is required.

    (*See also* LD.04.01.01, EP 1)

2. Ⓓ The person from the organization whose name appears on the Clinical Laboratory Improvement Amendments of 1988 (CLIA '88) certificate, or a qualified designee, establishes written policies and procedures for waived testing that address the following:
    - Clinical usage and limitations of the test methodology
    - Need for confirmatory testing (for example, recommendations made by the manufacturer for rapid tests) and result follow-up recommendations (for example, a recommendation to repeat the test when results are higher or lower than the reportable range of the test)
    - Specimen type, collection, and identification, and required labeling
    - Specimen preservation, if applicable
    - Instrument maintenance and function checks, such as calibration
    - Storage conditions for test components
    - Reagent use, including not using a reagent after its expiration date
    - Quality control (including frequency and type) and corrective action when quality control is unacceptable
    - Test performance
    - Result reporting, including not reporting individual patient results unless quality control is acceptable
    - Equipment performance evaluation

    Note 1: *Policies and procedures for waived testing are made available to testing personnel.*

Note 2: *The designee should be knowledgeable by virtue of training, experience, and competence about the waived testing performed.*

3. Ⓓ If manufacturers' manuals or package inserts are used as the policies or procedures for each waived test, they are enhanced to include specific operational policies (that is, detailed quality control protocols and any other institution-specific procedures regarding the test or instrument).

4. Ⓓ The person from the organization whose name appears on the Clinical Laboratory Improvement Amendments of 1988 (CLIA '88) certificate, or a qualified designee, approves in writing policies and procedures for waived testing at the following times:
    - Before initial use of the test for patient testing
    - Periodically thereafter, as defined by the person whose name appears on the CLIA certificate but at least once every three years
    - When changes in procedures occur (for example, when manufacturers' updates to package inserts include procedural changes or when a different manufacturer is used)

Standard WT.02.01.01

The person from the organization whose name appears on the Clinical Laboratory Improvement Amendments of 1988 (CLIA '88) certificate identifies the staff responsible for performing and supervising waived testing.

Note 1: *Responsible staff may be employees of the organization, contracted staff, or employees of a contracted service.*

Note 2: *Responsible staff may be identified within job descriptions or by listing job titles or individual names.*

Elements of Performance for WT.02.01.01

1. Ⓓ The person from the organization whose name appears on the Clinical Laboratory Improvement Amendments of 1988 (CLIA '88) certificate, or a qualified designee, identifies, in writing, the staff responsible for performing waived testing.

2. Ⓓ The person from the organization whose name appears on the Clinical Laboratory Improvement Amendments of 1988 (CLIA '88) certificate, or a qualified designee, identifies in writing the staff responsible for supervising waived testing.

Standard WT.03.01.01 ━━━━━━━

Staff and licensed independent practitioners performing waived tests are competent.

Elements of Performance for WT.03.01.01

1. The person from the organization whose name appears on the Clinical Laboratory Improvement Amendments of 1988 (CLIA '88) certificate, or a qualified designee, provides orientation and training to and assesses the competency of, staff and licensed independent practitioners who perform waived testing.

2. ⓓ Staff and licensed independent practitioners who perform waived testing have received orientation in accordance with the organization's specific services. The orientation for waived testing is documented.

3. ⓓ Staff and licensed independent practitioners who perform waived testing have been trained for each test that they are authorized to perform. The training for each waived test is documented.

4. ⓓ Staff and licensed independent practitioners who perform waived testing that requires the use of an instrument have been trained on its use and maintenance. The training on the use and maintenance of an instrument for waived testing is documented.

5. Competency for waived testing is assessed using at least two of the following methods per person per test: **R**
    - Performance of a test on a blind specimen
    - Periodic observation of routine work by the supervisor or qualified designee
    - Monitoring of each user's quality control performance
    - Use of a written test specific to the test assessed

6. ⓓ Competence for waived testing is assessed according to organization policy at defined intervals, but at least at the time of orientation and annually thereafter. This competency is documented.

Note 1: *When a licensed independent practitioner performs waived testing that does not involve an instrument and the test falls within their specialty, the organization may use the credentialing and privileging process to document evidence of training and competency in lieu of annual competency assessment. In this circumstance, individual practitioner privileges include the specific waived tests appropriate to their scope of practice that they are authorized to perform. At the discretion of the person from the organization whose name appears on the Clinical Laboratory Improvement Amendments of 1988 (CLIA '88) certificate or according to organization policy, more stringent competency requirements may be implemented.*

Note 2: *Provider-performed microscopy (PPM) procedures are not waived tests.*

Standard WT.04.01.01

The organization performs quality control checks for waived testing on each procedure.

Note: *Internal quality controls may include electronic, liquid, or control zone. External quality controls may include electronic or liquid.*

Elements of Performance for WT.04.01.01

1. Ⓓ The person from the organization whose name appears on the Clinical Laboratory Improvement Amendments of 1988 (CLIA '88) certificate establishes a written quality control plan for waived testing that specifies the method(s) for controlling procedures for quality, establishes timetables, and explains the rationale for choice of procedures and timetables.

   (*See also* LD.04.01.01, EP 1)

2. The documented quality control rationale for waived testing is based on the following:
   - How the test is used
   - Reagent stability
   - Manufacturers' recommendations
   - The organization's experience with the test
   - Currently accepted guidelines

3. For non-instrument-based waived testing, quality control checks are performed at the frequency and number of levels recommended by the manufacturer and as defined by the organization's policies. **R**

   Note: *If these elements are not defined by the manufacturer, the organization defines the frequency and number of levels for quality control.*

4. For instrument-based waived testing, quality control checks are performed on each instrument used for patient testing per manufacturers' instructions. **R**

5. For instrument-based waived testing, quality control checks require two levels of control, if commercially available.

Standard WT.05.01.01

The organization maintains records for waived testing.

Elements of Performance for WT.05.01.01

1. Ⓓ Quality control results, including internal and external controls for waived testing, are documented.

    Note 1: *Internal quality controls may include electronic, liquid, or control zone. External quality controls may include electronic or liquid.*

    Note 2: *Quality control results may be located in the clinical record.*

2. Test results for waived testing are documented in the patient's clinical record.

3. Quantitative test result reports in the clinical record for waived testing are accompanied by reference intervals (normal values) specific to the test method used and the population served.

    Note 1: *Semiquantitative results, such as urine macroscopic and urine dipsticks, are not required to comply with this element of performance.*

    Note 2: *If the reference intervals (normal values) are not documented on the same page as and adjacent to the waived test result, they must be located elsewhere within the permanent clinical record. The result must have a notation directing the reader to the location of the reference intervals (normal values) in the clinical record.*

4. Individual test results for waived testing are associated with quality control results and instrument records.

    Note: *A formal log is not required, but a functional audit trail is maintained that allows retrieval of individual test results and their association with quality control and instrument records.*

5. Quality control result records, test result records, and instrument records for waived testing are retained for at least two years.

Standards Applicability Process (SAP)

Ambulatory care organizations provide a wide range of care, treatment, or services in a variety of settings, and they even may deliver services on a mobile platform. (*See* the "Glossary" (GL) chapter for a definition of *mobile delivery of health care services*.) Not all of the standards/requirements in the *CAMAC* apply to all types of ambulatory care organizations. Based on the particular care, treatment, or services provided by your ambulatory care organization, you should use this grid to identify which standards/requirements are applicable. It allows you to quickly identify the services, as you identified them in your E-App, and find related standards that apply to your ambulatory care organization.

In contrast, the E-dition® on your *Joint Commission Connect®* extranet site provides a customized manual based on the settings and services checked on your E-App. The selection of the specific settings and services in the E-App drives the standards displayed in your organization-specific E-dition (against which you will be surveyed). To view your organization's services in E-dition, click "Service Profile" on the top navigation bar. Check with your Joint Commission account executive if you have questions or to help ensure your E-App is complete and accurate.

Services are listed horizontally along the top of this grid. The standard/requirement and element of performance (EP) numbers are listed vertically. Applicability is indicated with an "**X**".

The following services are listed in the Ambulatory Care Services applicability grid (starting on page SAP-3):
- Ambulatory Surgery Centers
- Endoscopy
- Medical Centers
- Dental Centers
- Diagnostic/Therapeutic
- Diagnostic Imaging Services
- Diagnostic Sleep Centers

- Kidney Care/Dialysis
- Telehealth/Nonsurgical
- Telehealth/Surgical
- Episodic Care
- Occupational/Worksite Health
- Urgent/Immediate Care
- Convenient Care

Ambulatory Care Services Applicability

Standard/Requirement Number	EP #	Ambulatory Surgery Centers	Endoscopy	Medical Centers	Dental Centers	Diagnostic/Therapeutic	Diagnostic Imaging Services	Diagnostic Sleep Centers	Kidney Care/Dialysis	Telehealth/Nonsurgical	Telehealth/Surgical	Episodic Care	Occupational/Worksite Health	Urgent/Immediate Care	Convenient Care
APR.01.01.01	1	X	X	X	X	X	X	X	X	X	X	X	X	X	X
APR.01.02.01	1	X	X	X	X	X	X	X	X	X	X	X	X	X	X
APR.01.03.01	1	X	X	X	X	X	X	X	X	X	X	X	X	X	X
	2	X													
APR.02.01.01	1	X	X	X	X	X	X	X	X	X	X	X	X	X	X
APR.05.01.01	1	X	X	X	X	X	X	X	X	X	X	X	X	X	X
APR.06.01.01	1	X	X	X	X	X	X	X	X	X	X	X	X	X	X
APR.07.01.01	1	X	X	X	X	X	X	X	X	X	X	X	X	X	X
APR.08.01.01	1	X	X	X	X	X	X	X	X	X	X	X	X	X	X
	2	X	X	X	X	X	X	X	X	X	X	X	X	X	X
APR.09.01.01	1	X	X	X	X	X	X	X	X			X	X	X	X
	2	X	X	X	X	X	X	X	X			X	X	X	X
APR.09.02.01	1	X	X	X	X	X	X	X	X	X	X	X	X	X	X
	2	X	X	X	X	X	X	X	X	X	X	X	X	X	X
	3	X	X	X	X	X	X	X	X	X	X	X	X	X	X
APR.09.03.01	1	X	X	X	X	X	X	X	X	X	X	X	X	X	X
APR.09.04.01	1	X	X	X	X	X	X	X	X	X	X	X	X	X	X
EC.01.01.01	1	X	X	X	X	X	X	X	X			X	X	X	X
	3	X	X	X	X	X	X	X	X			X	X	X	X
	4	X	X	X	X	X	X	X	X			X	X	X	X
	5	X	X	X	X	X	X	X	X			X	X	X	X
	6	X	X	X	X	X	X	X	X			X	X	X	X
	7	X	X	X	X	X	X	X	X			X	X	X	X
	8	X	X	X	X	X	X	X	X		X	X	X	X	X
	9	X	X	X	X	X	X	X	X	X	X	X	X	X	X
EC.02.01.01	1	X	X	X	X	X	X	X	X			X	X	X	X
	3	X	X	X	X	X	X	X	X			X	X	X	X
	5	X	X												

Standard/Requirement Number	EP #	Ambulatory Surgery Centers	Endoscopy	Medical Centers	Dental Centers	Diagnostic/Therapeutic	Diagnostic Imaging Services	Diagnostic Sleep Centers	Kidney Care/Dialysis	Telehealth/Nonsurgical	Telehealth/Surgical	Episodic Care	Occupational/Worksite Health	Urgent/Immediate Care	Convenient Care
	6	X	X	X	X	X	X	X	X			X	X	X	X
	8	X	X	X	X	X	X	X	X			X	X	X	X
	11	X	X	X	X	X	X	X	X			X	X	X	X
	14						X								
	16	X	X	X		X	X					X		X	
EC.02.01.03	1	X	X	X	X	X	X	X	X			X	X	X	X
EC.02.02.01	1	X	X	X	X	X	X	X	X			X	X	X	X
	3	X	X	X	X	X	X	X	X			X	X	X	X
	4	X	X	X	X	X	X	X	X			X	X	X	X
	5	X	X	X	X	X	X	X	X			X	X	X	X
	6	X	X	X		X	X					X			
	7	X	X	X	X	X	X					X	X	X	X
	8	X	X	X		X	X		X			X		X	
	9	X	X	X	X	X	X					X		X	
	10	X	X	X	X	X	X					X		X	
	11	X	X	X	X	X	X	X	X			X	X	X	X
	12	X	X	X	X	X	X	X	X			X	X	X	X
	14	X	X												
	15	X	X												
	17	X	X	X		X	X					X		X	
EC.02.03.01	1	X	X	X	X	X	X	X	X			X	X	X	X
	4	X	X	X	X	X	X	X	X			X	X	X	X
	9	X	X	X	X	X	X	X	X			X	X	X	X
	11	X	X	X	X							X		X	
	12	X	X	X	X							X		X	
	13	X	X	X	X	X	X	X	X			X	X	X	X
EC.02.03.03	1	X	X	X	X							X			
	2	X	X	X	X	X	X	X	X			X	X	X	X
	3	X	X	X	X	X	X	X	X			X	X	X	X
	5	X	X	X	X	X	X	X	X			X	X	X	X

Standard/ Requirement Number	EP #	Ambulatory Surgery Centers	Endoscopy	Medical Centers	Dental Centers	Diagnostic/Therapeutic	Diagnostic Imaging Services	Diagnostic Sleep Centers	Kidney Care/Dialysis	Telehealth/Nonsurgical	Telehealth/Surgical	Episodic Care	Occupational/Worksite Health	Urgent/Immediate Care	Convenient Care
EC.02.03.05	1	X	X	X	X	X	X	X	X			X	X	X	X
	2	X	X	X	X	X	X	X	X			X	X	X	X
	3	X	X	X	X	X	X	X	X			X	X	X	X
	4	X	X	X	X	X	X	X	X			X	X	X	X
	5	X	X	X	X	X	X	X	X			X	X	X	X
	6	X	X	X	X	X	X	X	X			X	X	X	X
	7	X	X	X	X	X	X	X	X			X	X	X	X
	8	X	X	X	X	X	X	X	X			X	X	X	X
	9	X	X	X	X	X	X	X	X			X	X	X	X
	10	X	X	X	X	X	X	X	X			X	X	X	X
	11	X	X	X	X	X	X	X	X			X	X	X	X
	12	X	X	X	X	X	X	X	X			X	X	X	X
	14	X	X	X	X	X	X	X	X			X	X	X	X
	15	X	X	X	X	X	X	X	X			X	X	X	X
	16	X	X	X	X	X	X	X	X			X	X	X	X
	17	X	X	X	X	X	X	X	X			X	X	X	X
	18	X	X	X	X	X	X	X	X			X	X	X	X
	19	X	X	X	X	X	X	X	X			X	X	X	X
	20	X	X	X	X	X	X	X	X			X	X	X	X
	25	X	X	X	X	X	X	X	X			X	X	X	X
	27	X	X	X	X	X	X	X	X			X	X	X	X
	28	X	X	X	X	X	X	X	X			X	X	X	X
EC.02.04.01	2	X	X	X	X	X	X	X	X			X	X	X	X
	3	X	X	X	X	X	X	X	X			X	X	X	X
	5	X	X	X	X	X	X	X	X			X	X	X	X
	6	X	X	X	X	X	X		X			X	X	X	X
	10	X	X	X		X	X					X		X	
EC.02.04.03	1	X	X	X	X	X	X	X	X			X	X	X	X
	2	X	X	X	X	X	X	X	X			X	X		
	3	X	X	X	X	X	X	X	X			X	X	X	X

Standard/Requirement Number	EP #	Ambulatory Surgery Centers	Endoscopy	Medical Centers	Dental Centers	Diagnostic/Therapeutic	Diagnostic Imaging Services	Diagnostic Sleep Centers	Kidney Care/Dialysis	Telehealth/Nonsurgical	Telehealth/Surgical	Episodic Care	Occupational/Worksite Health	Urgent/Immediate Care	Convenient Care
	4	X	X	X	X							X		X	
	5					X			X						
	8	X	X	X	X	X	X	X	X			X	X	X	X
	10	X	X												
	18						X								
	19	X	X												
	20	X		X		X	X					X			
	21	X	X	X		X	X					X		X	
	22	X		X		X	X					X		X	
	23	X	X	X		X	X					X		X	
	24	X	X	X		X	X					X		X	
	25	X	X	X		X	X					X		X	
	26	X	X	X	X							X		X	
	27	X	X	X	X	X	X	X	X			X	X	X	X
	34	X	X	X	X	X	X					X		X	
EC.02.05.01	2	X	X	X	X	X	X	X	X			X	X	X	X
	4	X	X	X	X	X	X	X	X			X	X	X	X
	5	X	X												
	7	X	X	X	X							X		X	X
	8	X	X	X	X	X			X			X	X	X	X
	9	X	X	X	X	X			X			X	X	X	X
	10	X	X	X	X	X	X	X	X	X	X	X	X	X	X
	11	X	X	X	X	X	X	X	X			X	X	X	X
	12	X	X	X	X	X			X			X	X	X	X
	13	X	X	X	X	X	X	X	X	X	X	X	X	X	X
	16	X	X	X	X	X	X	X	X			X	X	X	X
	18	X	X	X	X	X	X	X	X			X	X	X	X
	19	X	X	X	X	X	X	X	X			X	X	X	X
	20	X	X	X	X							X		X	
	21	X	X	X	X	X	X	X	X			X	X	X	X

Standard/Requirement Number	EP #	Ambulatory Surgery Centers	Endoscopy	Medical Centers	Dental Centers	Diagnostic/Therapeutic	Diagnostic Imaging Services	Diagnostic Sleep Centers	Kidney Care/Dialysis	Telehealth/Nonsurgical	Telehealth/Surgical	Episodic Care	Occupational/Worksite Health	Urgent/Immediate Care	Convenient Care
	22	X	X												
	23	X	X	X	X	X	X	X	X			X	X	X	X
	24	X	X	X	X	X	X	X	X			X	X	X	X
	25	X	X									X			
	26	X	X									X			
	27	X	X	X	X	X	X	X	X			X	X	X	X
EC.02.05.03	1	X	X												
	2	X	X												
	3	X	X												
	4	X	X												
	5	X	X												
	6	X	X	X	X	X						X		X	
	7	X	X	X	X	X			X			X		X	
	11	X	X	X	X	X	X	X	X			X		X	
	12	X	X	X	X	X	X	X	X			X	X	X	X
	14	X	X	X	X	X			X			X		X	
	15	X	X	X	X	X			X			X	X	X	X
EC.02.05.05	1	X	X	X	X	X	X	X	X			X	X	X	X
	2	X	X	X	X	X	X	X	X			X	X	X	X
	3	X	X	X	X	X	X	X	X			X	X	X	X
	7	X	X	X	X	X	X	X	X			X	X	X	X
	8	X	X	X	X	X	X	X	X			X	X	X	X
EC.02.05.07	1	X	X	X	X	X	X	X				X	X	X	X
	2	X	X	X	X	X	X	X				X	X	X	X
	3	X	X	X	X	X	X	X				X	X	X	X
	4	X	X	X	X	X	X	X				X	X	X	X
	5	X	X	X	X	X	X	X				X	X	X	X
	6	X	X	X	X	X	X	X				X	X	X	X
	7	X	X	X	X	X	X	X				X	X	X	X
	8	X	X	X	X	X	X	X				X	X	X	X

Standard/Requirement Number	EP #	Ambulatory Surgery Centers	Endoscopy	Medical Centers	Dental Centers	Diagnostic/Therapeutic	Diagnostic Imaging Services	Diagnostic Sleep Centers	Kidney Care/Dialysis	Telehealth/Nonsurgical	Telehealth/Surgical	Episodic Care	Occupational/Worksite Health	Urgent/Immediate Care	Convenient Care
	9	X	X	X	X	X	X	X				X	X	X	X
	10	X	X	X	X	X	X	X				X	X	X	X
EC.02.05.09	1	X	X	X	X	X	X	X	X			X	X	X	X
	2	X	X	X	X	X						X		X	
	3	X	X	X	X	X	X	X	X			X	X	X	X
	4	X	X	X	X	X	X	X	X			X	X	X	X
	5	X	X	X	X	X	X	X	X			X	X	X	X
	6	X	X	X	X	X	X	X	X			X	X	X	X
	7	X	X	X	X	X						X		X	
	8	X	X	X	X	X						X		X	
	9	X	X	X	X	X						X		X	
	10	X	X	X	X	X						X		X	
	11	X	X	X	X	X						X		X	
	12	X	X	X	X	X	X	X	X			X	X	X	X
	13	X	X	X	X	X	X	X	X			X	X	X	X
	14	X	X	X	X	X			X			X		X	
EC.02.06.01	1	X	X	X	X	X	X	X	X			X	X	X	X
	7	X	X												
	11	X	X	X	X	X	X	X	X			X	X	X	X
	20	X	X	X	X	X	X	X	X			X	X	X	X
EC.02.06.05	1	X	X	X	X	X	X	X	X			X	X	X	X
	2	X	X	X	X	X	X	X	X			X	X	X	X
	3	X	X	X	X	X	X	X	X			X	X	X	X
	4	X	X	X		X	X					X		X	
	6	X	X	X		X	X					X		X	
EC.03.01.01	1	X	X	X	X	X	X	X	X			X	X	X	X
	2	X	X	X	X	X	X	X	X			X	X	X	X
EC.04.01.01	1	X	X	X	X	X	X	X	X			X	X	X	X
	2	X	X	X	X	X	X	X	X			X	X	X	X
	3	X	X	X	X	X	X	X	X			X	X	X	X

Standard/ Requirement Number	EP #	Ambulatory Surgery Centers	Endoscopy	Medical Centers	Dental Centers	Diagnostic/Therapeutic	Diagnostic Imaging Services	Diagnostic Sleep Centers	Kidney Care/Dialysis	Telehealth/Nonsurgical	Telehealth/Surgical	Episodic Care	Occupational/Worksite Health	Urgent/Immediate Care	Convenient Care
	4	X	X	X	X	X	X	X	X			X	X	X	X
	5	X	X	X	X	X	X	X	X			X	X	X	X
	15	X	X	X	X	X	X	X	X			X	X	X	X
EC.04.01.03	2	X	X	X	X	X	X	X	X			X	X	X	X
EC.04.01.05	1	X	X	X	X	X	X	X	X			X	X	X	X
EM.01.01.01	1	X	X	X	X	X	X	X	X	X	X	X	X	X	X
	2	X	X	X	X	X	X	X	X	X	X	X	X	X	X
	3	X	X	X	X	X	X	X	X	X	X	X	X	X	X
	4	X	X	X	X	X	X	X	X			X	X	X	X
	5	X	X	X	X	X	X	X	X	X	X	X	X	X	X
	6	X	X	X	X	X	X	X	X	X	X	X	X	X	X
	9	X	X	X											
	10	X	X	X											
EM.02.01.01	1	X	X	X	X	X	X	X	X	X	X	X	X	X	X
	2	X	X	X	X	X	X	X	X	X	X	X	X	X	X
	4	X	X	X	X	X	X	X	X	X	X	X	X	X	X
	5	X	X	X	X	X	X	X	X	X	X	X	X	X	X
	6	X	X	X	X	X	X	X	X	X	X	X	X	X	X
	7	X	X	X											
	8	X	X	X	X	X	X	X	X	X	X	X	X	X	X
	10	X	X	X											
	11	X	X	X											
	12	X	X	X											
	14	X	X	X											
	15	X	X												
	20	X	X	X											
	21	X	X	X											
	22	X	X	X											
EM.02.02.01	1	X	X	X	X	X	X	X	X	X	X	X	X	X	X
	3	X	X	X	X	X	X	X	X			X	X	X	X

Standard/Requirement Number	EP #	Ambulatory Surgery Centers	Endoscopy	Medical Centers	Dental Centers	Diagnostic/Therapeutic	Diagnostic Imaging Services	Diagnostic Sleep Centers	Kidney Care/Dialysis	Telehealth/Nonsurgical	Telehealth/Surgical	Episodic Care	Occupational/Worksite Health	Urgent/Immediate Care	Convenient Care
	4	X	X	X											
	7	X	X	X											
	12	X	X	X											
	14	X	X	X	X	X	X	X	X	X	X	X	X	X	X
	17	X	X	X	X	X	X	X	X	X	X	X	X	X	X
	20	X	X	X											
	21	X	X	X											
	22	X	X	X											
	23	X	X	X											
	30	X	X	X											
	31	X	X	X											
	32	X	X	X											
	33	X	X	X											
	34	X	X	X											
EM.02.02.03	1	X	X	X		X	X		X			X	X	X	X
	2	X	X	X		X	X	X	X			X	X	X	X
	3	X	X	X		X	X	X	X			X	X	X	X
	9	X	X	X											
	12	X	X	X		X	X	X	X	X	X	X	X	X	X
EM.02.02.05	1	X	X	X		X	X	X	X	X	X	X	X	X	X
	5	X	X	X		X	X	X	X			X	X	X	X
	10	X	X	X		X	X	X	X	X	X	X	X	X	X
EM.02.02.07	1	X	X	X		X	X	X	X	X	X	X	X	X	X
	2	X	X	X		X	X	X	X			X	X	X	X
	3	X	X	X		X	X	X	X			X	X	X	X
	4	X	X	X		X	X	X	X	X	X	X	X	X	X
	7	X	X	X											
	9	X	X	X		X	X	X	X			X	X	X	X
	10	X	X	X		X	X	X	X	X	X	X	X	X	X
	11	X	X	X											

Standard/ Requirement Number	EP #	Ambulatory Surgery Centers	Endoscopy	Medical Centers	Dental Centers	Diagnostic/Therapeutic	Diagnostic Imaging Services	Diagnostic Sleep Centers	Kidney Care/Dialysis	Telehealth/Nonsurgical	Telehealth/Surgical	Episodic Care	Occupational/Worksite Health	Urgent/Immediate Care	Convenient Care
	12			X											
	13	X	X	X											
	14	X	X												
	18	X	X	X											
	19	X	X	X											
	20	X	X	X											
	21	X	X												
EM.02.02.09	1	X	X	X		X	X	X	X			X	X	X	X
	8	X	X	X		X	X	X	X	X	X	X	X	X	X
EM.02.02.11	1	X	X	X	X	X	X	X	X			X	X	X	X
	3	X	X	X	X	X	X	X	X			X	X	X	X
	11	X	X	X	X	X	X	X	X			X	X	X	X
	12	X	X	X											
	13	X	X	X											
	15	X	X	X											
	16	X	X	X											
EM.02.02.13	1	X	X	X		X	X					X		X	
	2	X	X	X		X	X					X		X	
	3	X	X	X		X	X					X		X	
	4	X	X	X		X	X					X		X	
	5	X	X	X		X	X					X		X	
	6	X	X	X		X	X					X		X	
	7	X	X	X		X	X					X		X	
	8	X	X	X		X	X					X		X	
	9	X	X	X		X	X					X		X	
EM.02.02.15	1	X	X	X		X	X					X		X	
	2	X	X	X		X	X					X		X	
	3	X	X	X		X	X					X		X	
	4	X	X	X		X	X					X		X	
	5	X	X	X		X	X					X		X	

Standard/Requirement Number	EP #	Ambulatory Surgery Centers	Endoscopy	Medical Centers	Dental Centers	Diagnostic/Therapeutic	Diagnostic Imaging Services	Diagnostic Sleep Centers	Kidney Care/Dialysis	Telehealth/Nonsurgical	Telehealth/Surgical	Episodic Care	Occupational/Worksite Health	Urgent/Immediate Care	Convenient Care
	6	X	X	X		X	X					X		X	
	7	X	X	X		X	X					X		X	
	8	X	X	X		X	X					X		X	
	9	X	X	X		X	X					X		X	
EM.03.01.03	3	X	X	X	X	X	X	X	X	X	X	X	X	X	X
	5	X	X	X	X	X	X	X	X	X	X	X	X	X	X
	10	X	X	X											
	13	X	X	X	X	X	X	X	X	X	X	X	X	X	X
	14	X	X	X	X	X	X	X	X	X	X	X	X	X	X
	16	X	X	X	X	X	X	X	X	X	X	X	X	X	X
	17	X	X	X	X	X	X	X	X	X	X	X	X	X	X
	22	X	X	X											
EM.04.01.01	1	X	X	X											
	2	X	X	X											
	3	X	X	X											
	5	X	X	X											
	6	X	X	X											
	7	X	X	X											
HR.01.01.01	1	X	X	X	X	X	X	X	X	X	X	X	X	X	X
	2	X	X	X	X	X	X	X	X	X	X	X	X	X	X
	3	X	X	X	X	X	X	X	X	X	X	X	X	X	X
	4	X	X	X	X	X	X	X	X	X	X	X	X	X	X
	5	X	X	X	X	X	X	X	X	X	X	X	X	X	X
	7	X	X	X	X	X	X	X	X	X	X	X	X	X	X
	32	X	X	X		X	X					X		X	
	33	X	X	X		X	X					X		X	
HR.01.02.05	10	X	X												
	11	X	X												
	12	X	X												
	13	X	X												

Standard/Requirement Number	EP #	Ambulatory Surgery Centers	Endoscopy	Medical Centers	Dental Centers	Diagnostic/Therapeutic	Diagnostic Imaging Services	Diagnostic Sleep Centers	Kidney Care/Dialysis	Telehealth/Nonsurgical	Telehealth/Surgical	Episodic Care	Occupational/Worksite Health	Urgent/Immediate Care	Convenient Care
HR.01.02.07	1	X	X	X	X	X	X	X	X	X	X	X	X	X	X
	2	X	X	X	X	X	X	X	X	X	X	X	X	X	X
	3			X											
	5	X	X	X	X	X	X	X	X	X	X	X	X	X	X
HR.01.04.01	1	X	X	X	X	X	X	X	X	X	X	X	X	X	X
	3	X	X	X	X	X	X	X	X	X	X	X	X	X	X
HR.01.05.03	1	X	X	X	X	X	X	X	X	X	X	X	X	X	X
	14	X	X	X		X	X					X		X	
	25	X	X	X		X	X					X		X	
HR.01.06.01	1	X	X	X	X	X	X	X	X	X	X	X	X	X	X
	3	X	X	X	X	X	X	X	X	X	X	X	X	X	X
	5	X	X	X	X	X	X	X	X	X	X	X	X	X	X
	6	X	X	X	X	X	X	X	X	X	X	X	X	X	X
HR.01.07.01	1	X	X	X	X	X	X	X	X	X	X	X	X	X	X
	2	X	X	X	X	X	X	X	X	X	X	X	X	X	X
	5	X	X	X	X	X	X	X	X	X	X	X	X	X	
HR.02.01.03	1	X	X	X	X	X	X	X	X	X	X	X	X	X	X
	2	X	X	X	X	X	X	X	X	X	X	X	X	X	X
	3	X	X	X	X	X	X	X	X	X	X	X	X	X	X
	4	X	X	X	X	X	X	X	X	X	X	X	X	X	X
	5	X	X	X	X	X	X	X	X	X	X	X	X	X	X
	6	X	X	X	X	X	X	X	X	X	X	X	X	X	X
	7	X	X	X	X	X	X	X	X	X	X	X	X	X	X
	10	X	X	X	X	X	X	X	X	X	X	X	X	X	X
	11	X	X	X	X	X	X	X	X	X	X	X	X	X	X
	19	X	X	X	X	X	X	X	X	X	X	X	X	X	X
	20	X	X	X	X	X	X	X	X	X	X	X	X	X	X
	21	X	X	X	X	X	X	X	X	X	X	X	X	X	X
	24	X	X	X	X	X	X	X	X	X	X	X	X	X	X
	25	X	X	X	X	X	X	X	X	X	X	X	X	X	X

Standard/Requirement Number	EP #	Ambulatory Surgery Centers	Endoscopy	Medical Centers	Dental Centers	Diagnostic/Therapeutic	Diagnostic Imaging Services	Diagnostic Sleep Centers	Kidney Care/Dialysis	Telehealth/Nonsurgical	Telehealth/Surgical	Episodic Care	Occupational/Worksite Health	Urgent/Immediate Care	Convenient Care
	27									X	X				
	29									X	X				
	30									X	X				
	31	X	X												
	32	X	X												
	33	X	X												
	34	X	X												
	35							X							
HR.02.01.05	1	X	X	X	X	X	X	X	X	X	X	X	X	X	X
	2	X	X	X	X	X	X	X	X	X	X	X	X	X	X
	9	X	X	X	X	X	X	X	X	X	X	X	X	X	X
	10	X	X	X	X	X	X	X	X	X	X	X	X	X	X
HR.02.02.01	1	X	X	X	X	X	X	X	X	X	X	X	X	X	X
	3	X	X	X	X	X	X	X	X	X	X	X	X	X	X
HR.02.03.01	1	X	X	X	X	X	X	X	X	X	X	X	X	X	X
	6	X	X	X	X	X	X	X	X	X	X	X	X	X	X
HR.02.04.01	1									X	X				
	2									X	X				
	3									X	X				
	4									X	X				
	5									X	X				
	6									X	X				
	7									X	X				
	8									X	X				
	9									X	X				
HR.02.04.03	1									X	X				
	2									X	X				
	3									X	X				
	4									X	X				
	5									X	X				

Standard/Requirement Number	EP #	Ambulatory Surgery Centers	Endoscopy	Medical Centers	Dental Centers	Diagnostic/Therapeutic	Diagnostic Imaging Services	Diagnostic Sleep Centers	Kidney Care/Dialysis	Telehealth/Nonsurgical	Telehealth/Surgical	Episodic Care	Occupational/Worksite Health	Urgent/Immediate Care	Convenient Care
	6									X	X				
	7									X	X				
	8									X	X				
	9									X	X				
HR.03.01.01	1			X											
IC.01.01.01	3	X	X	X	X	X	X	X	X			X	X	X	X
	5	X	X												
IC.01.02.01	1	X	X	X	X	X	X	X	X			X	X	X	X
	2	X	X	X	X	X			X			X	X	X	X
	3	X	X	X	X	X	X	X	X			X	X	X	X
IC.01.03.01	1	X	X	X	X	X	X	X	X			X	X	X	X
	3	X	X	X	X	X	X	X	X			X	X	X	X
IC.01.04.01	1	X	X	X	X	X	X	X	X			X	X	X	X
IC.01.05.01	1	X	X	X	X	X	X	X	X			X	X	X	X
	2	X	X	X	X	X	X	X	X			X	X	X	X
	5	X	X	X		X	X	X	X			X	X	X	X
	6	X	X	X	X	X	X	X	X			X	X	X	X
	9	X	X												
	11	X	X												
IC.01.06.01	2	X	X	X					X			X		X	
	3	X	X	X					X			X		X	
	4	X	X	X					X			X		X	
IC.02.01.01	1	X	X	X	X	X	X	X	X			X	X	X	X
	2	X	X	X	X	X	X	X	X			X	X	X	X
	3	X	X	X	X	X	X	X	X			X	X	X	X
	5	X	X	X	X	X	X	X	X			X	X	X	X
	6	X	X	X	X	X	X	X	X			X	X	X	X
	7	X	X	X	X	X	X	X	X			X	X	X	X
	8	X	X	X	X	X	X	X	X			X	X	X	X
	9	X	X	X	X	X	X	X	X			X	X	X	X

Standard/Requirement Number	EP #	Ambulatory Surgery Centers	Endoscopy	Medical Centers	Dental Centers	Diagnostic/Therapeutic	Diagnostic Imaging Services	Diagnostic Sleep Centers	Kidney Care/Dialysis	Telehealth/Nonsurgical	Telehealth/Surgical	Episodic Care	Occupational/Worksite Health	Urgent/Immediate Care	Convenient Care
	10	X	X	X		X			X			X	X	X	X
	11	X	X	X	X	X			X			X		X	
IC.02.02.01	1	X	X	X	X	X	X	X	X			X	X	X	X
	2	X	X	X	X	X	X	X	X			X		X	
	3	X	X	X	X	X	X	X	X			X	X	X	X
	4	X	X	X	X	X	X	X	X			X	X	X	X
	5	X	X	X	X	X						X			
IC.02.03.01	1	X	X	X	X	X	X	X	X			X	X	X	X
	2	X	X	X	X	X	X	X	X			X	X	X	X
	4	X	X	X	X	X	X	X	X			X	X	X	X
IC.02.04.01	1	X	X	X	X	X	X	X	X			X	X	X	X
	2	X	X	X	X	X	X	X	X			X	X	X	X
	3	X	X	X	X	X	X	X	X			X	X	X	X
	4	X	X	X	X	X	X	X	X			X	X	X	X
	6	X	X	X	X	X	X	X	X			X	X	X	X
	7	X	X	X	X	X	X	X	X			X	X	X	X
	8	X	X	X	X	X	X	X	X			X	X	X	X
	9	X	X	X	X	X	X	X	X			X	X	X	X
IC.02.05.01	1	X		X	X							X		X	X
	2	X		X	X							X			
	3	X		X	X							X			
IC.03.01.01	1	X	X	X	X	X	X	X	X			X	X	X	X
	6	X	X	X	X	X	X	X	X			X	X	X	X
	7	X	X	X	X	X	X	X	X			X	X	X	X
IM.01.01.01	2	X	X	X	X	X	X	X	X	X	X	X	X	X	X
IM.01.01.03	1	X	X	X	X	X	X	X	X	X	X	X	X	X	X
	2	X	X	X	X	X	X	X	X	X	X	X	X	X	X
	5	X	X	X											
	6	X	X	X											
IM.02.01.01	1	X	X	X	X	X	X	X	X	X	X	X	X	X	X

Standard/ Requirement Number	EP #	Ambulatory Surgery Centers	Endoscopy	Medical Centers	Dental Centers	Diagnostic/Therapeutic	Diagnostic Imaging Services	Diagnostic Sleep Centers	Kidney Care/Dialysis	Telehealth/Nonsurgical	Telehealth/Surgical	Episodic Care	Occupational/Worksite Health	Urgent/Immediate Care	Convenient Care
	3	X	X	X	X	X	X	X	X	X	X	X	X	X	X
	4	X	X	X	X	X	X	X	X	X	X	X	X	X	X
IM.02.01.03	1	X	X	X	X	X	X	X	X	X	X	X	X	X	X
	2	X	X	X	X	X	X	X	X	X	X	X	X	X	X
	5	X	X	X	X	X	X	X	X	X	X	X	X	X	X
	6	X	X	X	X	X	X	X	X	X	X	X	X	X	X
	7	X	X	X	X	X	X	X	X	X	X	X	X	X	X
IM.02.02.01	2	X	X	X	X	X	X	X	X	X	X	X	X	X	X
	3	X	X	X	X	X	X	X	X	X	X	X	X	X	X
IM.02.02.03	2	X	X	X	X	X	X	X	X	X	X	X	X	X	X
	3	X	X	X	X	X	X	X	X	X	X	X	X	X	X
	13	X		X	X	X	X					X			
IM.03.01.01	1	X	X	X	X	X	X	X	X	X	X	X	X	X	X
LD.01.01.01	1	X	X	X	X	X	X	X	X	X	X	X	X	X	X
	2	X	X	X	X	X	X	X	X	X	X	X	X	X	X
	3	X	X	X	X	X	X	X	X	X	X	X	X	X	X
LD.01.03.01	1	X	X	X	X	X	X	X	X	X	X	X	X	X	X
	2	X	X	X	X	X	X	X	X	X	X	X	X	X	X
	3	X	X	X	X	X	X	X	X	X	X	X	X	X	X
	4	X	X	X	X	X	X	X	X	X	X	X	X	X	X
	5	X	X	X	X	X	X	X	X	X	X	X	X	X	X
	6	X	X	X	X	X	X	X	X	X	X	X	X	X	X
	12	X	X												
	22	X	X												
LD.01.04.01	1	X	X	X	X	X	X	X	X	X	X	X	X	X	X
LD.01.07.01	2	X	X	X	X	X	X	X	X	X	X	X	X	X	X
	3	X	X	X	X	X	X	X	X	X	X	X	X	X	X
LD.02.01.01	1	X	X	X	X	X	X	X	X	X	X	X	X	X	X
	2	X	X	X	X	X	X	X	X	X	X	X	X	X	X
	3	X	X	X	X	X	X	X	X	X	X	X	X	X	X

Standard/Requirement Number	EP #	Ambulatory Surgery Centers	Endoscopy	Medical Centers	Dental Centers	Diagnostic/Therapeutic	Diagnostic Imaging Services	Diagnostic Sleep Centers	Kidney Care/Dialysis	Telehealth/Nonsurgical	Telehealth/Surgical	Episodic Care	Occupational/Worksite Health	Urgent/Immediate Care	Convenient Care
LD.02.03.01	1	X	X	X	X	X	X	X	X	X	X	X	X	X	X
	2	X	X	X	X	X	X	X	X	X	X	X	X	X	X
LD.03.01.01	1	X	X	X	X	X	X	X	X	X	X	X	X	X	X
	2	X	X	X	X	X	X	X	X	X	X	X	X	X	X
	4	X	X	X	X	X	X	X	X	X	X	X	X	X	X
	5	X	X	X	X	X	X	X	X	X	X	X	X	X	X
LD.03.02.01	1	X	X	X	X	X	X	X	X	X	X	X	X	X	X
	2	X	X	X	X	X	X	X	X	X	X	X	X	X	X
LD.03.03.01	1	X	X	X	X	X	X	X	X	X	X	X	X	X	X
	2	X	X	X	X	X	X	X	X	X	X	X	X	X	X
	3	X	X	X	X	X	X	X	X	X	X	X	X	X	X
LD.03.04.01	1	X	X	X	X	X	X	X	X	X	X	X	X	X	X
	2	X	X	X	X	X	X	X	X	X	X	X	X	X	X
LD.03.05.01	1	X	X	X	X	X	X	X	X	X	X	X	X	X	X
	2	X	X	X	X	X	X	X	X	X	X	X	X	X	X
	3	X	X	X	X	X	X	X	X	X	X	X	X	X	X
LD.03.06.01	1	X	X	X	X	X	X	X	X	X	X	X	X	X	X
	2	X	X	X	X	X	X	X	X	X	X	X	X	X	X
	3	X	X	X	X	X	X	X	X	X	X	X	X	X	X
	4	X	X	X	X	X	X	X	X	X	X	X	X	X	X
	5	X	X	X	X	X	X	X	X	X	X	X	X	X	X
LD.03.07.01	1	X	X	X	X	X	X	X	X	X	X	X	X	X	X
	2	X	X	X	X	X	X	X	X	X	X	X	X	X	X
	4			X											
	13	X	X												
	14	X	X												
	15	X	X												
	16	X	X												
	17	X	X												
	18	X	X												

Standard/Requirement Number	EP #	Ambulatory Surgery Centers	Endoscopy	Medical Centers	Dental Centers	Diagnostic/Therapeutic	Diagnostic Imaging Services	Diagnostic Sleep Centers	Kidney Care/Dialysis	Telehealth/Nonsurgical	Telehealth/Surgical	Episodic Care	Occupational/Worksite Health	Urgent/Immediate Care	Convenient Care
	19	X	X												
	20	X	X												
	21		X												
	23	X	X												
LD.03.08.01	1	X	X	X	X	X	X	X	X	X	X	X	X	X	X
	2	X	X	X	X	X	X	X	X	X	X	X	X	X	X
LD.03.09.01	1	X	X	X	X	X	X	X	X	X	X	X	X	X	X
	2	X	X	X	X	X	X	X	X	X	X	X	X	X	X
	3	X	X	X	X	X	X	X	X	X	X	X	X	X	X
	4	X	X	X	X	X	X	X	X	X	X	X	X	X	X
	5	X	X	X	X	X	X	X	X	X	X	X	X	X	X
	6	X	X	X	X	X	X	X	X	X	X	X	X	X	X
	8	X	X	X	X	X	X	X	X	X	X	X	X	X	X
	9	X	X	X	X	X	X	X	X	X	X	X	X	X	X
	10	X	X	X	X	X	X	X	X	X	X	X	X	X	X
	11	X	X	X	X	X	X	X	X	X	X	X	X	X	X
	13	X	X												
LD.03.10.01	1	X	X	X	X	X	X	X	X	X	X	X	X	X	X
	2	X	X	X	X	X	X	X	X	X	X	X	X	X	X
	3	X	X	X	X	X	X	X	X	X	X	X	X	X	X
LD.04.01.01	1	X	X	X	X	X	X	X	X	X	X	X	X	X	X
	2	X	X	X	X	X	X	X	X	X	X	X	X	X	X
	3	X	X	X	X	X	X	X	X	X	X	X	X	X	X
	15	X	X												
	19	X	X												
	21	X	X												
LD.04.01.03	1	X	X	X	X	X	X	X	X	X	X	X	X	X	X
	3	X	X	X	X	X	X	X	X	X	X	X	X	X	X
	4	X	X	X	X	X	X	X	X	X	X	X	X	X	X
LD.04.01.05	2	X	X	X	X	X	X	X	X	X	X	X	X	X	X

Standard/Requirement Number	EP #	Ambulatory Surgery Centers	Endoscopy	Medical Centers	Dental Centers	Diagnostic/Therapeutic	Diagnostic Imaging Services	Diagnostic Sleep Centers	Kidney Care/Dialysis	Telehealth/Nonsurgical	Telehealth/Surgical	Episodic Care	Occupational/Worksite Health	Urgent/Immediate Care	Convenient Care
	3	X	X	X	X	X	X	X	X	X	X	X	X	X	X
	4	X	X	X	X	X	X	X	X	X	X	X	X	X	X
	5	X	X	X	X	X	X	X	X	X	X	X	X	X	X
	11			X		X	X					X		X	
	13	X	X												
	25	X	X	X	X	X	X					X		X	
LD.04.01.07	1	X	X	X	X	X	X	X	X	X	X	X	X	X	X
	10	X	X												
LD.04.01.11	3	X	X	X	X	X	X	X	X	X	X	X	X	X	X
	4	X	X	X	X	X	X	X	X	X	X	X	X	X	X
	5	X	X	X	X	X	X	X	X	X	X	X	X	X	X
	8	X	X												
LD.04.02.01	2	X	X	X	X	X	X	X	X	X	X	X	X	X	X
	3	X	X	X	X	X	X	X	X	X	X	X	X	X	X
	4	X	X	X	X	X	X	X	X	X	X	X	X	X	X
	5	X	X	X	X	X	X	X	X	X	X	X	X	X	X
	6	X	X												
LD.04.02.03	1	X	X	X	X	X	X	X	X	X	X	X	X	X	X
	5	X	X	X	X	X	X	X	X	X	X	X	X	X	X
	7	X	X	X	X	X	X	X	X	X	X	X	X	X	X
	10	X	X	X	X	X	X	X		X	X	X	X	X	X
LD.04.03.01	1	X	X	X	X	X	X	X	X	X	X	X	X	X	X
	25	X	X												
LD.04.03.07	1	X	X	X	X	X	X	X	X	X	X	X	X	X	X
LD.04.03.09	1	X	X	X	X	X	X	X	X	X	X	X	X	X	X
	2	X	X	X	X	X	X	X	X	X	X	X	X	X	X
	3	X	X	X	X	X	X	X	X	X	X	X	X	X	X
	4	X	X	X	X	X	X	X	X	X	X	X	X	X	X
	5	X	X	X	X	X	X	X	X	X	X	X	X	X	X
	6	X	X	X	X	X	X	X	X	X	X	X	X	X	X

Standard/ Requirement Number	EP #	Ambulatory Surgery Centers	Endoscopy	Medical Centers	Dental Centers	Diagnostic/Therapeutic	Diagnostic Imaging Services	Diagnostic Sleep Centers	Kidney Care/Dialysis	Telehealth/Nonsurgical	Telehealth/Surgical	Episodic Care	Occupational/Worksite Health	Urgent/Immediate Care	Convenient Care
	7	X	X	X	X	X	X	X	X	X	X	X	X	X	X
	8	X	X	X	X	X	X	X	X	X	X	X	X	X	X
	10	X	X	X	X	X	X	X	X	X	X	X	X	X	X
LD.04.03.13	1	X		X	X				X			X		X	
	3	X		X	X				X			X		X	
	4	X		X	X				X			X		X	
	6			X	X				X			X		X	
LS.01.01.01	1	X	X		X										
	2	X	X												
	3	X	X												
	4	X	X												
	6	X	X												
	7	X	X												
LS.01.02.01	2	X	X												
	3	X	X												
	4	X	X												
	5	X	X												
	6	X	X												
	7	X	X												
	8	X	X												
	9	X	X												
	10	X	X												
	11	X	X												
	12	X	X												
	13	X	X												
	14	X	X												
	15	X	X												
LS.03.01.10	1	X	X												
	2	X	X												
	3	X	X												

Standard/Requirement Number	EP #	Ambulatory Surgery Centers	Endoscopy	Medical Centers	Dental Centers	Diagnostic/Therapeutic	Diagnostic Imaging Services	Diagnostic Sleep Centers	Kidney Care/Dialysis	Telehealth/Nonsurgical	Telehealth/Surgical	Episodic Care	Occupational/Worksite Health	Urgent/Immediate Care	Convenient Care
	4	X	X												
	5	X	X												
	6	X	X												
	7	X	X												
	8	X	X												
	9	X	X												
	10	X	X												
	11	X	X												
LS.03.01.20	1	X	X												
	2	X	X												
	3	X	X												
	4	X	X												
	5	X	X												
	6	X	X												
	7	X	X												
	8	X	X												
	9	X	X												
	10	X	X												
	11	X	X												
	12	X	X												
	13	X	X												
	14	X	X												
	15	X	X												
	16	X	X												
	17	X	X												
LS.03.01.30	1	X	X												
	2	X	X												
	3	X	X												
	4	X	X												
	5	X	X						X						

Standard/ Requirement Number	EP #	Ambulatory Surgery Centers	Endoscopy	Medical Centers	Dental Centers	Diagnostic/Therapeutic	Diagnostic Imaging Services	Diagnostic Sleep Centers	Kidney Care/Dialysis	Telehealth/Nonsurgical	Telehealth/Surgical	Episodic Care	Occupational/Worksite Health	Urgent/Immediate Care	Convenient Care
	6	X	X												
	7	X	X												
	8	X	X												
	9	X	X												
	10	X	X												
	11	X	X												
	12	X	X												
	13	X	X												
	14	X	X												
	15	X	X												
	16	X	X												
	17	X	X												
LS.03.01.34	1	X	X												
	2	X	X												
	3	X	X												
	4	X	X												
	5	X	X												
	6	X	X												
	7	X	X												
	8	X	X												
	9	X	X												
	10	X	X												
LS.03.01.35	1	X	X												
	2	X	X												
	3	X	X												
	4	X	X												
	5	X	X												
	6	X	X												
	7	X	X												
	10	X	X												

Standard/Requirement Number	EP #	Ambulatory Surgery Centers	Endoscopy	Medical Centers	Dental Centers	Diagnostic/Therapeutic	Diagnostic Imaging Services	Diagnostic Sleep Centers	Kidney Care/Dialysis	Telehealth/Nonsurgical	Telehealth/Surgical	Episodic Care	Occupational/Worksite Health	Urgent/Immediate Care	Convenient Care
	11	X	X												
LS.03.01.40	1	X	X												
	2	X	X												
	3	X	X												
LS.03.01.50	1	X	X												
	2	X	X												
	3	X	X												
	4	X	X												
	5	X	X												
	6	X	X												
	7	X	X												
	8	X	X												
	9	X	X												
	10	X	X												
LS.03.01.70	1	X	X												
	2	X	X												
	3	X	X												
	4	X	X												
	5	X	X												
	6	X	X												
	7	X	X												
	8	X	X												
	9	X	X												
MM.01.01.01	1	X	X	X	X	X	X	X	X			X	X	X	X
	3	X	X												
	4	X	X												
MM.01.01.03	1	X	X	X	X	X	X		X			X	X	X	
	2	X	X	X	X	X	X		X			X	X	X	
MM.01.02.01	1	X	X	X	X	X	X		X			X	X	X	X
	2	X	X	X	X	X	X		X			X	X	X	X

Standard/Requirement Number	EP #	Ambulatory Surgery Centers	Endoscopy	Medical Centers	Dental Centers	Diagnostic/Therapeutic	Diagnostic Imaging Services	Diagnostic Sleep Centers	Kidney Care/Dialysis	Telehealth/Nonsurgical	Telehealth/Surgical	Episodic Care	Occupational/Worksite Health	Urgent/Immediate Care	Convenient Care
	3	X	X	X	X	X	X		X			X	X	X	X
MM.02.01.01	1	X	X	X	X	X	X		X			X	X	X	X
	2	X	X	X	X	X	X		X			X	X	X	X
	3	X	X	X		X	X		X			X	X	X	X
	4	X	X	X	X	X	X		X			X	X	X	X
	6	X	X	X	X	X	X		X			X	X	X	X
	7	X	X	X		X	X		X			X	X	X	X
	9	X	X	X	X	X	X		X			X	X	X	X
	10	X	X	X		X	X		X			X	X	X	X
	12	X	X	X		X	X		X			X	X	X	X
	14	X	X	X		X	X		X			X	X	X	X
MM.03.01.01	2	X	X	X	X	X	X		X			X	X	X	X
	3	X	X	X	X	X	X		X			X	X	X	X
	4	X	X	X	X	X	X		X			X	X	X	X
	6	X	X	X	X	X	X		X			X	X	X	X
	7	X	X	X	X	X	X		X			X	X	X	X
	8	X	X	X	X	X	X		X			X	X	X	X
	9	X	X	X		X	X		X			X			
	18	X	X	X	X	X	X		X			X	X	X	X
MM.03.01.03	1	X	X	X	X	X	X	X	X			X	X	X	
	6	X	X	X	X	X	X	X	X			X	X	X	
MM.03.01.05	1	X	X	X		X	X	X	X			X	X		
	2	X	X	X		X	X	X	X			X	X		
MM.04.01.01	1	X	X	X		X	X	X	X			X	X	X	X
	2	X	X	X	X	X	X		X			X	X	X	X
	7	X	X	X	X	X	X		X			X	X	X	X
	8	X	X	X	X	X	X		X			X			
	12	X	X												
	14			X								X	X	X	X
	21			X											

Standard/Requirement Number	EP #	Ambulatory Surgery Centers	Endoscopy	Medical Centers	Dental Centers	Diagnostic/Therapeutic	Diagnostic Imaging Services	Diagnostic Sleep Centers	Kidney Care/Dialysis	Telehealth/Nonsurgical	Telehealth/Surgical	Episodic Care	Occupational/Worksite Health	Urgent/Immediate Care	Convenient Care
MM.05.01.01	1	X	X	X	X	X			X			X	X	X	X
	4	X	X	X	X	X			X			X	X	X	X
	11	X	X	X	X	X			X			X	X		
MM.05.01.07	1	X	X	X		X	X					X			
	2	X	X	X	X	X	X		X			X	X	X	X
	3	X	X	X	X	X	X		X			X	X	X	X
	4			X		X						X			
MM.05.01.09	1	X	X	X	X	X	X		X			X	X	X	X
	2	X	X	X	X	X	X		X			X	X	X	X
	3	X	X	X	X	X	X		X			X	X	X	X
	7	X	X	X	X	X	X		X			X	X	X	
	10	X	X	X	X	X	X					X	X	X	X
MM.05.01.11	2	X	X	X	X	X						X	X	X	X
MM.05.01.15	1	X	X	X	X	X	X		X			X	X	X	X
MM.05.01.17	1	X	X	X	X	X	X		X			X	X	X	X
	3	X	X	X	X	X	X		X			X	X	X	X
	4	X	X	X	X	X	X		X			X	X	X	X
MM.05.01.19	1	X	X	X		X	X					X	X	X	X
	2	X	X	X		X	X					X	X	X	X
	3	X	X	X		X	X					X	X	X	X
MM.06.01.01	1	X	X	X	X	X	X		X			X	X	X	X
	3	X	X	X	X	X	X		X			X	X	X	X
	9	X	X	X		X	X		X			X	X	X	X
	13	X		X		X	X					X		X	
MM.06.01.05	1	X	X	X		X	X					X		X	
	2	X	X	X		X						X		X	
	3	X	X	X		X						X		X	
MM.07.01.01	1	X	X	X	X	X	X		X			X	X	X	X
	2	X	X	X	X	X	X		X			X	X	X	X
MM.07.01.03	1	X	X	X	X	X	X		X			X	X	X	X

Standard/ Requirement Number	EP #	Ambulatory Surgery Centers	Endoscopy	Medical Centers	Dental Centers	Diagnostic/Therapeutic	Diagnostic Imaging Services	Diagnostic Sleep Centers	Kidney Care/Dialysis	Telehealth/Nonsurgical	Telehealth/Surgical	Episodic Care	Occupational/Worksite Health	Urgent/Immediate Care	Convenient Care
	2	X	X	X	X	X	X		X			X	X	X	X
	3	X	X	X	X	X	X		X			X	X	X	X
	4	X	X												
MM.08.01.01	1	X	X	X	X	X	X		X			X	X	X	X
	5	X	X	X	X	X	X		X			X	X	X	X
	6	X	X	X	X	X	X		X			X	X	X	X
	8	X	X	X	X	X	X		X			X	X	X	X
	16	X	X	X	X	X						X		X	
MM.09.01.03	1			X	X							X	X	X	X
	2			X	X							X	X	X	X
	3			X	X							X	X	X	X
	4			X	X							X	X	X	X
	5			X	X							X	X	X	X
NPSG.01.01.01	1	X	X	X	X	X	X	X	X			X	X	X	X
	2	X	X	X	X	X	X		X			X	X	X	X
NPSG.03.04.01	1	X	X	X	X	X	X		X			X	X	X	X
	2	X	X	X	X	X	X		X			X	X	X	X
	3	X	X	X	X	X	X		X			X	X	X	X
	4	X	X	X	X	X	X		X			X	X	X	X
	5	X	X	X	X	X	X		X			X	X	X	X
	6	X	X	X	X	X	X		X			X	X	X	X
	7	X	X	X	X	X	X		X			X	X	X	X
	8	X	X	X	X	X	X		X			X	X	X	X
NPSG.03.05.01	1			X											
	2			X											
	4			X											
	5			X											
	6			X											
NPSG.03.06.01	1	X	X	X	X	X	X	X	X			X	X	X	X
	2	X	X	X	X	X	X	X	X			X	X	X	X

Standard/Requirement Number	EP #	Ambulatory Surgery Centers	Endoscopy	Medical Centers	Dental Centers	Diagnostic/Therapeutic	Diagnostic Imaging Services	Diagnostic Sleep Centers	Kidney Care/Dialysis	Telehealth/Nonsurgical	Telehealth/Surgical	Episodic Care	Occupational/Worksite Health	Urgent/Immediate Care	Convenient Care
	3	X	X	X	X	X	X					X	X	X	X
	4	X	X	X	X	X	X					X	X	X	X
	5	X	X	X	X	X	X					X	X	X	X
NPSG.07.01.01	1	X	X	X	X	X	X	X	X			X	X	X	X
	2	X	X	X	X	X	X	X	X			X	X	X	X
	3	X	X	X	X	X	X	X	X			X	X	X	X
UP.01.01.01	1	X	X	X	X	X			X			X			
	2	X	X	X	X	X			X			X			
	3	X	X	X	X	X			X			X			
UP.01.02.01	1	X		X	X	X						X			
	2	X		X	X	X						X			
	3	X		X	X	X						X			
	4	X		X	X	X						X			
	5	X		X	X	X						X			
UP.01.03.01	1	X	X	X	X	X			X			X			
	2	X	X	X	X	X			X		X	X			
	3	X	X	X	X	X			X			X			
	4	X	X	X	X	X			X		X	X			
	5	X	X	X	X	X			X			X			
PC.01.01.01	7	X	X	X	X	X	X	X	X	X	X	X	X	X	X
PC.01.02.01	1	X	X	X	X	X	X	X	X	X	X	X	X	X	X
	2	X	X	X		X	X	X	X	X	X	X	X	X	X
PC.01.02.03	1	X	X	X	X	X	X	X	X	X	X	X	X	X	X
	3	X	X	X	X	X	X	X	X	X	X	X	X	X	X
	9	X	X	X	X	X	X	X	X	X	X	X	X		
PC.01.02.07	1	X		X	X				X			X		X	X
	3	X		X	X				X			X		X	X
	4	X		X					X						
	5	X		X					X						
	7	X		X					X			X		X	

Standard/Requirement Number	EP #	Ambulatory Surgery Centers	Endoscopy	Medical Centers	Dental Centers	Diagnostic/Therapeutic	Diagnostic Imaging Services	Diagnostic Sleep Centers	Kidney Care/Dialysis	Telehealth/Nonsurgical	Telehealth/Surgical	Episodic Care	Occupational/Worksite Health	Urgent/Immediate Care	Convenient Care
	8	X		X	X				X			X		X	
PC.01.02.09	1	X	X	X	X	X	X	X	X			X	X	X	X
	2	X	X	X	X	X	X	X	X			X	X	X	X
	3	X	X	X	X	X	X	X	X			X	X	X	X
	6	X	X	X	X	X	X	X	X			X	X	X	X
	7	X	X	X		X	X	X	X			X	X	X	X
PC.01.02.15	2	X	X	X	X	X	X	X		X	X	X	X	X	X
	5	X		X	X	X	X					X			
	10	X	X	X		X	X					X		X	
	12	X	X	X		X	X					X		X	
	13	X	X	X	X	X	X					X		X	
PC.01.03.01	1	X	X	X	X	X	X	X	X	X	X	X	X	X	X
	25	X	X	X		X	X					X		X	
	26	X	X	X		X	X					X		X	
	44			X											
	45			X											
PC.02.01.01	1	X	X	X	X	X	X	X	X	X	X	X	X	X	X
	10	X		X					X			X			
	16			X											
	30	X	X	X	X	X	X					X		X	
PC.02.01.03	1	X	X												
	20	X	X	X		X	X	X	X			X	X	X	X
PC.02.01.05	1	X	X	X	X	X	X	X	X	X	X	X	X	X	X
PC.02.01.07	2	X	X	X								X			
	12	X	X												
PC.02.01.09	1	X	X	X	X	X	X	X	X			X	X	X	X
	4	X	X												
	9	X	X												
	10	X	X												
PC.02.01.21	1			X											

Standard/Requirement Number	EP #	Ambulatory Surgery Centers	Endoscopy	Medical Centers	Dental Centers	Diagnostic/Therapeutic	Diagnostic Imaging Services	Diagnostic Sleep Centers	Kidney Care/Dialysis	Telehealth/Nonsurgical	Telehealth/Surgical	Episodic Care	Occupational/Worksite Health	Urgent/Immediate Care	Convenient Care
	2			X											
PC.02.02.01	1	X	X	X	X	X	X	X	X	X	X	X	X	X	X
	2	X	X	X	X	X	X		X			X	X		
	3	X	X	X	X	X	X	X	X			X	X	X	X
	10	X	X	X	X	X	X	X	X			X	X	X	X
	15	X	X												
PC.02.02.03	7	X	X	X		X	X	X	X			X	X	X	
	11	X	X	X		X	X	X	X			X	X		
PC.02.03.01	1	X	X	X	X	X	X	X	X			X	X	X	X
	4	X	X	X	X	X	X	X	X			X	X	X	X
	5	X	X	X	X	X			X			X	X	X	
	10	X	X	X		X	X	X	X			X	X	X	X
	25	X	X	X	X	X	X	X	X			X	X	X	X
	27	X	X	X	X	X	X	X	X			X	X	X	X
	28			X											
	30			X											
	31			X											
PC.02.04.01	1			X											
	2			X											
	3			X											
	4			X		X	X					X		X	
	5			X		X	X					X		X	
PC.02.04.03	1			X											
	2			X											
	3			X											
	4			X											
	5			X											
PC.02.04.05	1			X											
	2			X											
	4			X											

Standard/Requirement Number	EP #	Ambulatory Surgery Centers	Endoscopy	Medical Centers	Dental Centers	Diagnostic/Therapeutic	Diagnostic Imaging Services	Diagnostic Sleep Centers	Kidney Care/Dialysis	Telehealth/Nonsurgical	Telehealth/Surgical	Episodic Care	Occupational/Worksite Health	Urgent/Immediate Care	Convenient Care
	5			X											
	6			X											
	8			X											
	9			X											
	10			X											
	11			X											
	12			X											
PC.03.01.01	2	X	X	X	X	X						X			
	6	X	X	X	X	X						X			
PC.03.01.03	1	X	X	X	X	X						X		X	
	4	X	X	X	X	X						X		X	
	5	X	X	X	X	X						X		X	
	8	X	X	X	X	X						X		X	
	9	X	X												
	10	X	X												
	12	X	X												
	13	X	X												
	15	X	X												
	16	X	X												
	17	X	X												
	19	X	X		X										
PC.03.01.05	1	X	X	X	X	X						X		X	
PC.03.01.07	1	X	X	X	X	X						X		X	
	2	X	X	X	X	X						X		X	
	4	X	X	X	X	X						X		X	
	5	X	X												
	6	X	X	X	X	X						X		X	
	9	X	X												
PC.03.02.03	1	X	X	X	X				X			X		X	X
PC.03.02.07	1	X	X	X	X				X			X		X	

Standard/Requirement Number	EP #	Ambulatory Surgery Centers	Endoscopy	Medical Centers	Dental Centers	Diagnostic/Therapeutic	Diagnostic Imaging Services	Diagnostic Sleep Centers	Kidney Care/Dialysis	Telehealth/Nonsurgical	Telehealth/Surgical	Episodic Care	Occupational/Worksite Health	Urgent/Immediate Care	Convenient Care
	2	X	X	X					X			X		X	
	3	X	X	X	X				X			X		X	X
PC.04.01.01	1	X	X	X		X	X	X				X	X	X	X
	11	X	X												
	12	X	X												
	13	X	X												
PC.04.01.03	2	X	X	X		X	X	X				X	X	X	X
	3	X	X	X		X	X	X				X	X	X	
	4	X	X	X		X	X	X				X	X	X	X
PC.04.01.05	1	X	X	X	X	X	X	X				X	X	X	X
	7	X	X	X	X	X	X	X				X	X	X	X
	9	X	X												
	10	X	X												
	11	X	X												
	12	X	X												
	13	X	X												
	14	X	X												
PC.04.02.01	1	X	X	X	X	X	X	X				X	X	X	
PI.01.01.01	2	X	X	X	X	X	X	X	X	X	X	X	X	X	X
	3	X	X	X	X	X	X		X		X	X			
	4	X	X	X	X							X	X		
	5	X	X			X									
	6	X	X			X									
	7	X	X			X									
	12	X	X	X	X	X	X		X			X	X	X	X
	13	X	X	X	X	X	X		X			X	X	X	X
	14	X	X	X	X	X	X	X	X			X	X	X	X
	26	X	X												
	28			X											
	29			X											

Standard/Requirement Number	EP #	Ambulatory Surgery Centers	Endoscopy	Medical Centers	Dental Centers	Diagnostic/Therapeutic	Diagnostic Imaging Services	Diagnostic Sleep Centers	Kidney Care/Dialysis	Telehealth/Nonsurgical	Telehealth/Surgical	Episodic Care	Occupational/Worksite Health	Urgent/Immediate Care	Convenient Care
	30			X	X										
	34	X	X	X		X	X					X		X	
	35	X	X	X		X	X					X		X	
PI.02.01.01	1	X	X	X	X	X	X	X	X	X	X	X	X	X	X
	2	X	X	X	X	X	X	X	X	X	X	X	X	X	X
PI.03.01.01	4	X	X	X	X	X	X	X	X	X	X	X	X	X	X
	6	X	X	X		X	X					X		X	
	8	X	X	X	X	X	X	X	X	X	X	X	X	X	X
	11	X	X												
	19	X		X	X				X			X		X	
	20	X	X	X	X	X	X					X		X	
	21	X		X	X							X			
PI.04.01.01	2	X	X	X	X	X	X	X	X	X	X	X	X	X	X
	3	X	X	X	X	X	X	X	X	X	X	X	X	X	X
	5	X	X	X	X	X	X	X	X	X	X	X	X	X	X
	10	X	X												
	11			X											
	12	X	X												
RC.01.01.01	1	X	X	X	X	X	X	X	X	X	X	X	X	X	X
	5	X	X	X	X	X	X	X	X	X	X	X	X	X	X
	7	X	X	X	X	X	X	X	X	X	X	X	X	X	X
	9	X	X	X	X	X	X	X	X	X	X	X	X	X	X
RC.01.02.01	1	X	X	X	X	X	X	X	X	X	X	X	X	X	X
	2	X	X	X	X	X	X	X	X	X	X	X	X	X	X
	3	X	X	X	X	X	X	X	X	X	X	X	X	X	X
	4	X	X	X	X	X	X	X	X	X	X	X	X	X	X
	5	X	X	X	X	X	X	X	X	X	X	X	X	X	X
RC.01.03.01	1	X	X	X	X	X	X	X	X	X	X	X	X	X	X
	2	X	X	X	X	X	X	X	X	X	X	X	X	X	X
RC.01.04.01	1	X	X	X	X	X	X	X	X	X	X	X	X	X	X

Standard/ Requirement Number	EP #	Ambulatory Surgery Centers	Endoscopy	Medical Centers	Dental Centers	Diagnostic/Therapeutic	Diagnostic Imaging Services	Diagnostic Sleep Centers	Kidney Care/Dialysis	Telehealth/Nonsurgical	Telehealth/Surgical	Episodic Care	Occupational/Worksite Health	Urgent/Immediate Care	Convenient Care
RC.01.05.01	1	X	X	X	X	X	X	X	X	X	X	X	X	X	X
	8	X	X	X	X	X	X	X	X	X	X	X	X	X	X
RC.02.01.01	1	X	X	X		X	X	X	X	X	X	X	X	X	X
	2	X	X	X	X	X	X	X	X	X	X	X	X	X	X
	4	X	X	X	X	X	X	X	X	X	X	X	X	X	X
	18			X									X	X	X
	25			X											
	26			X											
	27			X	X										
	30	X	X												
RC.02.01.03	1	X	X	X	X	X			X		X	X		X	
	2	X	X	X	X	X					X	X		X	
	4	X	X												
	5	X	X	X	X	X					X	X		X	
	6	X	X	X	X	X					X	X		X	
	7	X	X	X	X	X					X	X		X	
	8	X	X	X	X	X					X	X		X	
	9	X	X	X	X	X					X	X		X	
	10	X	X	X	X	X					X	X		X	
	11	X	X	X	X	X					X	X		X	
	12	X	X												
	13	X	X												
	14	X	X												
RC.02.01.05	1	X	X	X			X	X	X			X		X	
RC.02.03.07	1	X	X	X	X	X	X	X	X			X	X	X	X
	2	X	X	X	X	X	X	X	X			X	X	X	X
	3	X	X	X	X	X	X	X	X			X	X	X	X
	4	X	X	X	X	X	X	X	X			X	X	X	X
RI.01.01.01	1	X	X	X	X	X	X	X	X	X	X	X	X	X	X
	2	X	X												

Standard/Requirement Number	EP #	Ambulatory Surgery Centers	Endoscopy	Medical Centers	Dental Centers	Diagnostic/Therapeutic	Diagnostic Imaging Services	Diagnostic Sleep Centers	Kidney Care/Dialysis	Telehealth/Nonsurgical	Telehealth/Surgical	Episodic Care	Occupational/Worksite Health	Urgent/Immediate Care	Convenient Care
	4	X	X	X	X	X	X	X	X			X	X	X	X
	5	X	X	X	X	X	X	X	X			X	X	X	X
	6	X	X	X	X	X	X	X	X			X	X	X	X
	7	X	X	X	X	X	X	X	X	X	X	X	X	X	X
	10	X	X	X	X	X	X	X	X			X	X	X	X
	13	X	X												
RI.01.01.03	1	X	X	X	X	X	X	X	X			X	X	X	X
	2	X	X	X	X	X	X	X	X			X	X	X	X
	3	X	X	X	X	X	X	X	X			X	X	X	X
	4	X	X												
	5	X	X												
RI.01.02.01	1	X	X	X	X	X	X	X	X		X	X	X	X	X
	2	X	X	X	X	X	X	X	X		X	X	X	X	X
	4	X	X	X	X	X	X	X	X		X	X	X	X	X
	8	X	X	X	X	X	X	X	X		X	X	X	X	X
	20	X	X	X	X	X	X	X	X		X	X	X	X	X
	31			X											
	32			X											
RI.01.03.01	1	X	X	X	X	X	X	X	X		X	X	X	X	X
	2	X	X	X	X	X	X	X	X		X	X	X	X	X
	3	X	X	X	X	X	X	X	X		X	X	X	X	X
	15	X	X												
RI.01.03.05	2	X	X	X	X	X	X	X	X		X	X		X	
	3	X	X	X	X	X	X	X	X		X	X		X	
	4	X	X	X	X	X	X	X	X		X	X		X	
RI.01.04.01	1	X	X	X	X	X	X	X	X			X	X	X	X
	7			X											
RI.01.04.03	1			X											
	2			X											
	3			X											

Standard/Requirement Number	EP #	Ambulatory Surgery Centers	Endoscopy	Medical Centers	Dental Centers	Diagnostic/Therapeutic	Diagnostic Imaging Services	Diagnostic Sleep Centers	Kidney Care/Dialysis	Telehealth/Nonsurgical	Telehealth/Surgical	Episodic Care	Occupational/Worksite Health	Urgent/Immediate Care	Convenient Care
	5			X											
	6			X											
	7			X		X	X					X		X	
RI.01.05.01	1	X	X	X		X	X	X	X			X	X	X	X
	7	X	X												
	10	X	X	X		X	X	X	X			X		X	
RI.01.06.03	1	X	X	X	X	X	X	X	X			X	X	X	X
	2	X	X	X	X	X	X	X	X			X	X	X	X
	3	X	X	X	X	X	X	X	X			X	X	X	X
	6	X	X												
RI.01.07.01	1	X	X	X	X	X	X	X	X			X	X	X	X
	4	X	X	X	X	X	X	X	X			X	X	X	X
	10	X	X												
	11	X	X												
	21	X	X												
	22	X	X												
	23	X	X												
	24	X	X												
	25	X	X												
	26	X	X												
	27	X	X												
RI.02.01.01	2	X	X	X	X	X	X	X	X			X	X	X	X
TS.03.01.01	1	X		X	X							X			
	2	X		X	X							X			
	3	X		X	X							X			
	5	X		X	X							X			
	6	X		X	X							X			
	7	X		X	X							X			
	8	X		X	X							X			
	9	X		X	X							X			

Standard/ Requirement Number	EP #	Ambulatory Surgery Centers	Endoscopy	Medical Centers	Dental Centers	Diagnostic/Therapeutic	Diagnostic Imaging Services	Diagnostic Sleep Centers	Kidney Care/Dialysis	Telehealth/Nonsurgical	Telehealth/Surgical	Episodic Care	Occupational/Worksite Health	Urgent/Immediate Care	Convenient Care
	10	X		X	X							X			
TS.03.02.01	1	X		X	X							X			
	2	X		X	X							X			
	3	X		X	X							X			
	4	X		X	X							X			
	5	X		X	X							X			
	6	X		X	X							X			
	7	X		X	X							X			
TS.03.03.01	1	X		X	X							X			
	2	X		X	X							X			
	3	X		X	X							X			
	4	X		X	X							X			
	5	X		X	X							X			
WT.01.01.01	1	X	X	X	X	X	X		X			X	X	X	X
	2	X	X	X	X	X	X		X			X	X	X	X
	3	X	X	X	X	X	X		X			X	X	X	X
	4	X	X	X	X	X	X		X			X	X	X	X
WT.02.01.01	1	X	X	X	X	X	X		X			X	X	X	X
	2	X	X	X	X	X	X		X			X	X	X	X
WT.03.01.01	1	X	X	X	X	X	X		X			X	X	X	X
	2	X	X	X	X	X	X		X			X	X	X	X
	3	X	X	X	X	X	X		X			X	X	X	X
	4	X	X	X	X	X	X		X			X	X	X	X
	5	X	X	X	X	X	X		X			X	X	X	X
	6	X	X	X	X	X	X		X			X	X	X	X
WT.04.01.01	1	X	X	X	X	X	X		X			X	X	X	X
	2	X	X	X	X	X	X		X			X	X	X	X
	3	X	X	X	X	X	X		X			X	X	X	X
	4	X	X	X	X	X	X		X			X	X	X	X
	5	X	X	X	X	X	X		X			X	X	X	X

Standard/Requirement Number	EP #	Ambulatory Surgery Centers	Endoscopy	Medical Centers	Dental Centers	Diagnostic/Therapeutic	Diagnostic Imaging Services	Diagnostic Sleep Centers	Kidney Care/Dialysis	Telehealth/Nonsurgical	Telehealth/Surgical	Episodic Care	Occupational/Worksite Health	Urgent/Immediate Care	Convenient Care
WT.05.01.01	1	X	X	X	X	X	X		X			X	X	X	X
	2	X	X	X	X	X	X		X			X	X	X	X
	3	X	X	X	X	X	X		X			X	X	X	X
	4	X	X	X	X	X	X		X			X	X	X	X
	5	X	X	X	X	X	X		X			X	X	X	X

Glossary (GL)

abuse Intentional mistreatment that may cause either physical or psychological injury. *See also* mental abuse, neglect, physical abuse, sexual abuse.

accreditation Determination by The Joint Commission that an eligible organization complies with applicable Joint Commission accreditation requirements.

accreditation contract The primary document that establishes the terms of the relationship between the organization and The Joint Commission.

accreditation decisions Categories of accreditation that an organization can achieve based on a Joint Commission survey. These decision categories are as follows:

- **Limited, Temporary Accreditation** The organization demonstrates compliance with selected standards in surveys conducted under the Early Survey Policy.
- **Accredited** The organization is in compliance with all applicable standards at the time of the on-site survey or has successfully addressed all Requirements for Improvement (RFIs) in an Evidence of Standards Compliance (ESC) within 60 days following the posting of the Final Accreditation Report and does not meet any other rules for other accreditation decisions.

- **Accreditation with Follow-up Survey** The organization is in compliance with all standards, as determined by an acceptable ESC submission. A follow-up survey is required within 6 months to assess sustained compliance.
- **Preliminary Denial of Accreditation** There is justification to deny accreditation to the organization as evidenced by
  - An Immediate Threat to Health or Safety to patients or the public, and/or
  - Submission of falsified documents or misrepresented information, and/or
  - Lack of a required license or similar issue at the time of survey, and/or
  - Significant noncompliance with Joint Commission standards, and/or
  - Patients having been placed at risk for serious adverse outcomes due to significant and pervasive patterns/trends/repeat findings

  The decision is subject to review and appeal by the organization prior to the determi-nation to deny accreditation.
- **Denial of Accreditation** The organization has been denied accreditation. All review and appeal opportunities have been exhausted.

accreditation manual A Joint Commission publication, either in print or online, consisting of policies, procedures, and accreditation requirements relating to ambulatory care, assisted living communities, behavioral health care and human services, critical access hospital, home care, hospital, nursing care centers, office-based surgery, and clinical laboratory and point-of-care testing. Organizations should use the manual that contains the set of accreditation requirements that is most appropriate to the primary focus or mission of the organization.

accreditation process A continuous process whereby organizations are required to demonstrate to The Joint Commission that they are providing safe, high-quality care, as determined by compliance with Joint Commission standards, National Patient Safety Goals, and performance measurement requirements (as applicable). Key components of this process are an evaluation of the organization by a Joint Commission surveyor(s) and, where applicable, quarterly submission of performance measurement data to The Joint Commission.

Accreditation Quality Report *See* Quality Report.

accreditation survey An evaluation of an organization to assess its level of compliance with applicable Joint Commission accreditation requirements and to make determinations regarding its accreditation status. The survey includes evaluation of documentation of compliance provided by organization staff; verbal information concerning the implementation of standards or examples of their implementation that en-

able a determination of compliance to be made; observations by the surveyor(s); and an opportunity for education and consultation regarding standards compliance and performance improvement.

accreditation survey findings Findings from an evaluation conducted by Joint Commission surveyors that result in an organization's accreditation decision.

admitting privileges Authority issued to admit individuals to a health care organization. Individuals with admitting privileges may practice only within the scope of the clinical privileges granted by the organization's governing body.

advance directive A document or documentation allowing a person to give directions about future health care or to designate another person(s) to make health care decisions if the individual loses decision-making capacity. Advance directives may include living wills, durable powers of attorney, do-not-resuscitate (DNR) orders, right-to-die documents, or similar documents listed in the Patient Self-Determination Act that express the person's preferences.

adverse drug event (ADE) An injury resulting from a medical intervention related to a medication, including harm from an adverse drug reaction or a medication error. *See also* medication error.

adverse drug reaction (ADR) A response to a medicinal product that is noxious and unintended and that occurs at doses normally used in humans for the prophylaxis, diagnosis, or treatment of disease or for the restoration, correction, or modification of physiological or psychological function. *See also* significant adverse drug reaction.

adverse event   A patient safety event that resulted in harm to a patient.

adverse medication event   *See* adverse drug event (ADE).

adverse medication reaction   *See* adverse drug reaction (ADR).

ALARA   An acronym for "as low as reasonably achievable," which means making every reasonable effort to maintain exposures to ionizing radiation as far below NRC dose limits as practical.

ambulatory health care   Health services provided to individuals who are not confined to institutional beds as inpatients during the time services are rendered. Ambulatory care services are provided in many settings ranging from freestanding ambulatory surgery facilities, to primary care settings, to diagnostic radiology; outpatient behavioral health services are not included.

ambulatory surgical center (ASC)   Any distinct entity that operates exclusively for the purpose of providing surgical services to patients not requiring hospitalization and in which the expected duration of services would not exceed 24 hours following an admission. The entity must have an agreement with Centers for Medicare & Medicaid Services (CMS) to participate in Medicare as an ASC, and must meet other specific conditions as designated by CMS.

anesthesia and sedation   The administration to an individual, in any setting, for any purpose, by any route, of medication to induce a partial or total loss of sensation for the purpose of conducting an operative or other procedure. Definitions of four levels of sedation and anesthesia include the following:

1. Minimal sedation (anxiolysis): A drug-induced state during which patients respond normally to verbal commands. Although cognitive function and coordination may be impaired, ventilatory and cardiovascular functions are unaffected.

2. Moderate sedation/analgesia ("conscious sedation"): A drug-induced depression of consciousness during which patients respond purposefully to verbal commands, either alone or accompanied by light tactile stimulation. Reflex withdrawal from a painful stimulus is not considered a purposeful response. No interventions are required to maintain a patent airway, and spontaneous ventilation is adequate. Cardiovascular function is usually maintained.

3. Deep sedation/analgesia: A drug-induced depression of consciousness during which patients cannot be easily aroused, but respond purposefully following repeated or painful stimulation. The ability to independently maintain ventilatory function may be impaired. Patients may require assistance in maintaining a patent airway and spontaneous ventilation may be inadequate. Cardiovascular function is usually maintained.

4. Anesthesia: Consists of general anesthesia and spinal or major regional anesthesia. It does not include local anesthesia. General anesthesia is a drug-induced loss of consciousness during which patients are not arousable, even by painful stimulation. The ability to independently maintain ventilatory function is often impaired. Patients often require assistance in maintaining a patent airway, and positive pressure ventilation may be required because of depressed spontaneous ventilation or drug-induced depression of neuromuscular function. Cardiovascular function may be impaired.

annually   One year from the date of the last event, plus or minus 30 days. Synonymous with every 12 months, once a year, or every year.

annual visits   A summation of outpatient visits made by patients within a 12-month period. For example, in a physician's office, outpatient visits are counted as one visit for each patient day and per provider. If a patient visits a physician and has x-rays and a procedure performed, this is counted as one visit. If a patient visits two different providers within the same practice, this is counted as two visits.

appeal process   The process afforded to an organization that receives a Preliminary Denial of Accreditation decision, which includes the organization's right to make a presentation to the Review Hearing Panel before accreditation is denied.

applicant organization   An organization that is seeking either accreditation for the first time or re-accreditation.

application for accreditation   *See* E-App.

assessment   An objective evaluation or appraisal of an individual's health status, including acute and chronic conditions. The assessment gathers information through collection of data, observation, and physical examination.

autologous tissue   Tissue intended for transplantation into the individual from whom the tissue was recovered. The recipient and donor are the same individual.

behavioral health care and human services   A broad array of care, treatment, or services for individuals with mental health issues, child welfare needs, addictive behaviors, chemical dependency issues, or intellectual/developmental disabilities. Care, treatment, or services can be provided in a wide variety of settings, such as inpatient crisis stabilization, residential, day program, outpatient, and community-based settings.

behaviors that undermine a culture of safety   Conduct by staff working in the organization that intimidates others to the extent that quality and safety could be compromised. These behaviors, as determined by the organization, may be verbal or nonverbal, may involve the use of rude language, may be threatening, or may involve physical contact.

best practices Clinical, scientific, or professional practices that are recognized by a majority of professionals in a particular field as being exemplary. These practices are typically evidence based and consensus driven.

biologicals Medicines made from living organisms and their products, including serums, vaccines, antigens, and antitoxins.

blind specimen A sample with known value tested by personnel who do not know the expected result.

block charting A documentation method that can be used when rapid titration of medication is necessary in specific urgent/emergent situations defined in organizational policy. A single "block" charting episode does not extend beyond a four-hour time frame. If a patient's urgent/emergent situation extends beyond four hours and block charting is continued, a new charting "block" period must be started. The following minimum elements must be documented in each block charting episode:

- Time of initiation of the charting block
- Name(s) of medications administered during the block
- Starting rates and ending rates of medications administered during the charting block
- Maximum rate (dose) of medications administered during the charting block
- Time of completion of the charting block

- Physiological parameters evaluated to determine the administration of titratable medications during the charting block

blood component A fraction of separated whole blood (for example, red blood cells, plasma, platelets, granulocytes).

caregiver A family member, a significant other, a friend, a volunteer, or an individual employed by the patient or resident to provide services in the home.

care planning (or planning for care) Individualized planning and provision of care, treatment, or services that address the needs, safety, and well-being of the patient or individual served. The plan, which formulates strategies, goals, and objectives, may include narratives, policies and procedures, protocols, practice guidelines, clinical paths, care maps, or a combination of these.

certification For purposes of Joint Commission certification, determination by The Joint Commission that an eligible program or service complies with applicable Joint Commission certification requirements.

certified electronic health record A computerized medical record system that enables the documentation, sharing, and secure storage of patient data in a structured format which allows the information to be easily retrieved and transferred between settings of care and those participating in patient care. The system must meet criteria and comply with standards established by the Centers for Medicare & Medicaid Services and the Office of the National Coordinator for Health Information Technology.

child   A person between 0 and 12 years of age, or as determined by applicable law and regulation.

chronic care   The provision of care to individuals with long-standing, persistent diseases or conditions. It includes oversight and education activities specific to a disease or condition, and measures to encourage patient self-care, promote health, and prevent loss of function.

clinical decision support   Software designed to assist in clinical decision making. A clinical decision support system matches two or more characteristics of an individual patient to a computerized clinical knowledge base and provides patient-specific assessments or recommendations to the clinician. The clinician makes decisions based on clinical expertise, knowledge of the patient, and the information provided through the clinical decision support system. A clinical decision support system can be used at different points in the care process such as diagnosis, treatment, and posttreatment care, including the prediction of future events.

Clinical Laboratory Improvement Amendments of 1988 (CLIA '88)   Federal legislation that created uniform federal standards for regulating laboratory testing. CLIA '88 unified the disparate federal and state standards regulating clinical laborato-ries and extended government oversight to all testing facilities, including physician offices.

clinical leader   An individual with essential clinical knowledge who sets expectations, develops plans, and implements procedures to assess and improve the quality of the organization's clinical and support functions and processes.

clinical practice guidelines   Tools that describe a specific procedure or processes found, through clinical trials or consensus opinion of experts, to be the most effective in evaluating and/or treating a mother and/or newborn, patient, resident, or individual served who has a specific symptom, condition, or diagnosis. Synonyms include practice parameter, protocol, clinical practice recommendation, preferred practice pattern, and guideline.

clinical privileges   Authorization granted by the appropriate authority (for example, the governing body) to a practitioner to provide specific care, treatment, or services in the organization within well-defined limits, based on the following factors: license, education, training, experience, competence, health status, and judgment.

clinical staff   Individuals such as employees, licensed independent practitioners, contractors, volunteers, or temporary agency personnel who provide or have provided clinical services to the organization's patients, residents, or individuals served. *See also* staff.

close call   A patient safety event that did not reach the patient but posed a risk of harm; also called *near miss* or *good catch*.

community-based exercise   The goal of this exercise is that health care organizations collaborate with state and local entities within their community to promote an integrated emergency response. Conducting integrated planning with state and local entities could identify potential gaps in their capabilities that can then be addressed in advance of an emergency.

compartmentalization   The concept of using various building components (for example, fire walls and doors, smoke barriers, fire-rated floor slabs) to prevent the spread of fire and combustion and to provide a safe means of egress to an approved exit. The presence of these features varies depending on the building occupancy classification.

complex organization   An organization accredited by The Joint Commission under more than one accreditation manual.

comprehensive systematic analysis   A process for identifying basic or causal factors underlying variation in performance, including the occurrence or possible occurrence of a sentinel event. A root cause analysis is one type of comprehensive systematic analysis.

computed tomography dose index (CTDI or CTDIvol)   A measure of the radiation output of a computed tomography (CT) scanner. It represents CT radiation exposure to a test object and therefore does not represent the patient radiation dose.

computerized order entry system   An electronic method of documentation that enables the entry of clinical information such as orders for care, treatment, or services into a computer. It may also be referred to as a computerized provider order entry (CPOE) system.

confidentiality   Protection of data or information from being made available or disclosed to any unauthorized person(s) or process(es).

consultation   1. Provision of professional advice or services. 2. A review of an individual's problem by a second practitioner and the rendering of an opinion and advice to the referring practitioner. In most instances, the review involves the independent examination of the individual by the consultant. 3. For purposes of Joint Commission accreditation, advice that is given to staff members of surveyed organizations relating to compliance with standards and requirements that are the subject of the survey.

consultation report   1. A written opinion by a consultant that reflects, when appropriate, an examination of the individual and the individual's medical record(s). 2. Information given verbally by a consulting practitioner to a care provider that reflects, when appropriate, an examination of the individual. The individual's care provider usually documents those opinions in the medical record.

continuing care   Care provided over time in various settings, programs, or services and spanning the illness-to-wellness continuum.

continuity   The degree to which the care of individuals is coordinated among health care professionals, among organizations, and over time.

contract   A formal agreement for care, treatment, or services with an organization, agency, or individual that specifies the services, personnel, products, or space provided by, to, or on behalf of the organization and specifies the consideration to be expended in exchange.

contracted services   Services provided through a written agreement with another organization, agency, or person. The agreement specifies the services or personnel to be provided on behalf of the applicant organization and the fees to provide these services or personnel.

contractual agreement   An agreement with any organization, group, agency, or individual for services or personnel to be provided by, to, or on behalf of the organization. Such agreements are defined in written form, such as in a contract, letter of agreement, or memorandum of understanding.

Cooperative Accreditation Initiative   An initiative under which The Joint Commission relies on the process, findings, and decisions of other oversight accrediting organizations in circumstances where The Joint Commission would otherwise conduct potentially duplicative surveys of organizations seeking accreditation. Cooperative agreements are comparable to those of The Joint Commission. Entities that focus more on technical or clinical aspects of departments or services (for example, laboratory, rehabilitation units) are eligible for cooperative agreements because their accreditation requirements complement The Joint Commission's by covering additional or more detailed aspects of care delivery.

coordination of care   The process of coordinating care, treatment, or services provided by a health care organization, including referral to appropriate community resources and liaison with others (such as the individual's physician, other health care organizations, or community services involved in care or services) to meet the ongoing identified needs of individuals, to ensure implementation of the plan of care, and to avoid unnecessary duplication of services.

corrective maintenance   *See* maintenance.

credentialing   The process of obtaining, verifying, and assessing the qualifications of a practitioner to provide care or services in or for a health care organization.

credentials   Documented evidence of licensure, education, training, experience, or other qualifications.

credentials verification organization (CVO) Any organization that provides information on an individual's professional credentials. An organization that bases a decision in part on information obtained from a CVO should have confidence in the completeness, accuracy, and timeliness of information. To achieve this level of confidence, the organization should evaluate the agency providing the information initially and then periodically as appropriate. The 10 principles that guide such an evaluation include the following:

1. The agency makes known to the user the data and information it can provide.

2. The agency provides documentation to the user describing how its data collection, information development, and verification process(es) is performed.

3. The user is given sufficient, clear information on database functions, including any limitations of information available from the agency (such as practitioners not included in the database), the time frame for agency responses to requests for information, and a summary overview of quality control processes related to data integrity, security, transmission accuracy, and technical specifications.

4. The user and agency agree on the format for transmitting credentials information about an individual from the CVO.

5. The user can easily discern what information transmitted by the CVO is from a primary source and what is not.

6. For information transmitted by the agency that can go out of date (for example, licensure, board certification), the CVO provides the date the information was last updated from the primary source.

7. The CVO certifies that the information transmitted to the user accurately represents the information obtained by it.

8. The user can discern whether the information transmitted by the CVO from a primary source is all the primary source information in the CVO's possession pertinent to a given item or, if not, where additional information can be obtained.

9. The user can engage the CVO's quality control processes when necessary to resolve concerns about transmission errors, inconsistencies, or other data issues that may be identified from time to time.

10. The user has a formal arrangement with the CVO for communicating changes in credentialing information.

critical result Test result that is abnormal to a degree that may indicate a life-threatening situation (also known as critical value).

critical test A test or examination that always requires rapid communication of results, whether those results are normal or abnormal.

data integrity The accuracy, consistency, and completeness of data that are protected in some way from corruption, misuse, or accidental exposure to unauthorized users.

data source A primary source used for data collection (for example, physical health and behavioral health information, personnel records, written agreements, safety incident log).

deemed status Status conferred by the Centers for Medicare & Medicaid Services (CMS) on an organization whose standards and survey process are determined by CMS to be equivalent to those of the Medicare program or other federal laws, such as the Clinical Laboratory Improvement Amendments of 1988 (CLIA '88). Accreditation is voluntary and seeking deemed status through accreditation is an option, not a requirement.

dental services Services provided by a dentist, or a qualified individual under the supervision of a dentist, to improve or maintain the health of an individual's teeth, oral cavity, and associated structures.

dentist An individual who has received either a doctor of dental surgery degree or a doctor of dental medicine degree and who is licensed to practice dentistry.

designated equivalent source Selected agencies that have been determined to maintain a specific item(s) of credential(s) information that is identical to the information at the primary source. Some of the agencies may provide credential(s) information and services beyond what is identified below. Listing the names of these agencies does not constitute an endorsement.
Designated equivalent sources include, but are not limited to, the following:

- The American Medical Association (AMA) Physician Masterfile for verification of a physician's United States and Puerto Rican medical school graduation and postgraduate education completion
- The American Board of Medical Specialties (ABMS) for verification of a physician's board certification
- The Educational Commission for Foreign Medical Graduates (ECFMG) for verification of a physician's graduation from a foreign medical school
- The American Osteopathic Association (AOA) Physician Database for pre-doctoral education accredited by the AOA Bureau of Professional Education; post-doctoral education approved by the AOA Council on Postdoctoral Training; postdoctoral education approved by the Accreditation Council for Graduate Medical Education (ACGME); and Osteopathic Specialty Board Certification
- The Federation of State Medical Boards (FSMB) for all actions against a physician's medical license
- The American Academy of Physician Assistants (AAPA) Profile for physician assistant education, provided through the AMA Physician Profile Service (https://profiles.ama-assn.org/amaprofiles/)
- National Commission on Certification of Physician Assistants (NCCPA) certification

disaster A type of emergency that, due to its complexity, scope, or duration, threatens the organization's capabilities and requires outside assistance to sustain care, safety, or security functions.

discharge The point at which an individual's active involvement with an organization or program ends, and the organization or program no longer maintains active responsibility for the care of the individual. In ambulatory or office-based settings where episodes of care occur even though the organization continues to maintain active responsibility for the care of the individual, discharge is the point at which any encounter or episode of care (that is, an office or clinic visit for the purpose of diagnostic evaluation or testing, procedures, treatment, therapy, or management) ends.

discharge planning A formalized process in a health care organization through which a program of continuing and follow-up care is planned and carried out for each patient.

dispensing *See* medication management.

disruptive and inappropriate behavior *See* behaviors that undermine a culture of safety.

do-not-use abbreviations *See* prohibited abbreviations.

dose length product (DLP) A measure of the radiation output of a computed tomography (CT) scanner. It factors in the length of the CT scan as well as the computed tomography dose index (CTDI).

It provides an estimate of the radiation dose to a volume of tissue for a given patient in a clinical setting.

drug *See* medication.

drug allergy *See* medication allergy.

E-App An electronic form used for collecting information pertaining to the applicant organization. Information collected on this form will be used to determine the accreditation requirements applicable to the organization, the types of surveyors needed, the length of survey, and the survey fee.

Early Survey Policy A policy that permits an organization to achieve accreditation in a two-survey process. The first survey is limited in scope, and successful completion results in Preliminary Accreditation. Organizations receiving Preliminary Accreditation under this policy are not recognized by the Centers for Medicare & Medicaid Services (CMS) to meet the requirements for Medicare certification. The second survey addresses all accreditation requirements, and successful completion results in full accreditation and recognition by CMS if requesting deemed status. The CMS Regional Office makes the final determination regarding an organization's Medicare participation and the effective date of participation.

electronic prescribing The use of an automated data entry system by an authorized prescriber to transmit a prescription directly to a participating pharmacy. It is also referred to as e-prescribing.

element of performance (EP) Specific action(s), process(es), or structure(s) that must be implemented to achieve the goal of a standard. The scoring of EP compliance determines an organization's overall compliance with a standard.

emergency An unexpected or sudden event that significantly disrupts the organization's ability to provide care, treatment, or services or the environment of care itself or that results in a sudden, significantly changed or increased demand for the organization's services. Emergencies can be either human-made or natural (such as an electrical system failure or a tornado), or a combination of both, and they exist on a continuum of severity.

emergency, life-threatening A situation (for example, cardiac arrest, respiratory arrest) in which an individual may require resuscitation or other support to sustain life.

Emergency Management Plan (EMP) The organization's written document that describes the process it would implement for managing the consequences of emergencies, including natural and human-made disasters, that could disrupt the organization's ability to provide care, treatment, or services.

entry The process by which an individual comes into a setting, including screening and/or assessment by the organization or the practitioner to determine the capacity of the organization or practitioner to provide the care, treatment, or services required to meet the individual's needs.

epidemic A disease, such as influenza, that spreads rapidly, attacks many people in a geographic area, causes a high rate of morbidity or mortality, and then subsides. Epidemic applies especially to infectious diseases, as in an epidemic of cholera, but is also applied to any disease, injury, or other health-related event, such as an epidemic of teenage suicide.

every 36 months Three years from the date of the last event, plus or minus 45 days.

every 6 months Six months from the date of the last event, plus or minus 20 days.

evidence-based guidelines Guidelines that have been scientifically developed based on recent literature review and are consensus driven.

Evidence of Standards Compliance (ESC) report A report submitted by a surveyed organization, which details the action(s) that it took to bring itself into compliance with an accreditation requirement or clarifies why the organization believes that it was in compliance with the accreditation requirement for which it received a Requirement for Improvement. An ESC report must address compliance at the element of performance level.

exploitation Taking unjust advantage of another for one's own advantage or benefit.

family A person or persons who play a significant role in an individual's life. A family is a group of two or more persons united by blood or adoptive, marital, domestic partnership, or other legal ties. The family may also be a person or persons not legally related to the individual (such as a significant other, friend, support person, or caregiver) whom the individual personally considers to be family. A family member may be the surrogate decision-maker if authorized to make care decisions for the individual should the individual lose decision-making capacity or choose to delegate decision making to another.

ferromagnetic object An item that is highly attracted to magnets. Such items pose a significant risk if allowed to enter the magnetic resonance imaging (MRI) scanner room or the area immediately preceding it. Ferromagnetic objects can become projectiles when they are rapidly drawn with considerable force toward the MRI unit. Examples of ferromagnetic items are those containing iron and nickel.

fire-rated Material that has undergone a test and is fire protection rated or fire resistance rated.

Two examples of the concept of fire-rated include the following:

■ **fire resistance rating** The time, in minutes or hours, that materials or assemblies have withstood a fire exposure, as determined by tests, or methods based on tests, prescribed by the National Fire Protection Association (NFPA).

■ **fire protection rating** A designation indicating the duration of fire test exposure to which a fire door assembly or fire window assembly was exposed and for which it met all the acceptance

criteria, as determined in accordance with NFPA 252, Standard Methods of Fire Tests of Door Assemblies, or NFPA 257, Standard on Fire Test for Window and Glass Block Assemblies.

fire watch The assignment of a person or persons to an area for the express purpose of protecting occupants from fire or similar emergencies. Examples of this protection include:

■ Notifying the fire department, the building occupants, or both of an emergency

■ Preventing a fire from occurring

■ Extinguishing small fires

Focused Standards Assessment (FSA) A requirement of the accreditation process whereby an organization reviews its compliance with a selected subset of applicable Joint Commission accreditation requirements (including the applicable National Patient Safety Goals, a selection of standards that address accreditation program-specific high-risk areas, and the organization's Requirements for Improvement [RFIs] from its last triennial survey); completes and submits to The Joint Commission a Plan of Action (POA) for any accreditation requirement with which it is not in full compliance; and chooses whether to engage in a telephone discussion with a member of the Standards Interpretation Group staff to determine the acceptability of the POA or discuss any other area of concern. Alternatives for a Full FSA submission include FSA Option 1 (attestation that an FSA was completed, but not submitted to The Joint Commission), Option 2 (on-site survey with documented findings), and Option 3 (on-site survey without documented findings). The FSA encourages organizations to be in continuous compliance with Joint Commission accreditation requirements and helps them to identify and manage risk. The organization retains the option to complete self-assessment with all applicable accreditation standards in the FSA tool, available on the organization's *Joint Commission Connect*° extranet site. *See also* Intracycle Monitoring (ICM). The FSA tool can also be used as a self-assessment tool by an organization preparing for its initial accreditation survey.

full-scale exercise An operations-based exercise that tests many facets of preparedness. The exercise involves planning and response partners (for example, state and local agencies) and takes place at the health care organization's location using, as much as possible, the individuals and equipment that would be called upon in a real event. The emergency operations plan and integration of operational elements are tested in scripted emergency scenarios intended to mimic realistic situations. Through this exercise, participants utilize rapid problem solving in high-stress situations.

full survey A survey that assesses an organization's compliance with all applicable Joint Commission accreditation requirements. *See also* accreditation survey.

functional exercise An exercise that validates the coordination of the emergency response activities within the organization, including collaboration with planning and response partners. It is an operations-based exercise that is action-oriented and designed to validate plans, policies, agreements, and procedures; clarify roles and responsibilities; and identify resource gaps in an operational environment.

governance The individual(s), group, or agency that has ultimate authority and responsibility for establishing policy; maintaining quality of care, treatment, or services; and providing for organization management and planning. Governance may be a separate entity or it may fall within the medical advisory or executive committee. Other names for this group include the board, board of trustees, board of governors, board of commissioners, and partnership.

hazardous materials and waste Materials whose handling, use, and storage are guided or defined by local, state, or federal regulation, such as the Occupational Safety and Health Administration's Regulations for Bloodborne Pathogens regarding the disposal of blood and blood-soaked items and the Nuclear Regulatory Commission's regulations for the handling and disposal of radioactive waste. This also includes hazardous vapors (for example, glutaraldehyde, ethylene oxide, nitrous oxide) and hazardous energy sources (for example, ionizing or nonionizing radiation, lasers, microwave, ultrasound). Although

The Joint Commission considers infectious waste as falling into this category of materials, federal regulations do not define infectious or medical waste as hazardous waste.

hazard vulnerability analysis (HVA) A process for identifying potential emergencies and the direct and indirect effects these emergencies may have on the organization's operations and the demand for its services.

health care–associated infection (HAI) An infection acquired concomitantly by an individual who is receiving or who has received care, treatment, or services from a health care organization. The infection may or may not have resulted from the care, treatment, or services.

health information Any information, oral or recorded, in any form or medium, that is created by a health care provider, health plan, public health authority, employer, life insurer, school or university, or health care clearinghouse that relates to past, present, or future physical or mental health or condition; the provision of health care; or payment for the provision of health care to an individual.

health literacy The degree to which individuals have the capacity to obtain, process, and understand basic health information and services needed to make appropriate health decisions.

health risk behaviors Activities undertaken by an individual that have a negative impact on their health and increase the risk of disease or injury. Examples of health risk behaviors include substance abuse, tobacco use, inadequate exercise, poor dietary practices, and unsafe sexual activity.

high-risk procedures or processes A procedure or process that, if not planned and/or implemented correctly, has a significant potential for affecting the safety of a patient or an individual served.

history and physical Information gathered about an individual using a holistic approach for the purpose of establishing a diagnosis and developing a plan for care, treatment, or services to address physical health issues. The history may include information about previous illnesses; previous medical or surgical interventions and response to treatment; family health history; and social, cultural, economic, and lifestyle issues that may affect the individual's health and well-being. The physical involves the physical examination of the individual's body by the following means: inspection, palpation, percussion, and auscultation. When used in concert with behavioral health care and human services, the history and physical may be used to rule out physical causes for behavioral health conditions or to assess the impact of a medical diagnosis or treatment on a behavioral health condition or current situation.

home care The term that is generally used to refer to services provided in the home or in the community to recovering, disabled, or chronically ill persons and their families. These services may include some combination of professional health care services and personal care and supportive services. Professional health care services (also known as "skilled care") may include physical and/or psychological assessment, nursing and medical care, medication teaching and administration, wound care, pain management, disease education and management, physical therapy, speech therapy, or occupational therapy. Home supportive care services (also known as "non-skilled care") may include such things as light housekeeping, meal preparation, medication reminders, dressing, laundry, shopping, transportation, and companionship. In addition, home care can provide palliative care, respite care, hospice care, and other related services to those in need, including provision of medical equipment, medications, and supplies.

human subject research The use of humans in the systematic study, observation, or evaluation of factors for preventing, assessing, treating, and understanding an illness. The term applies to all behavioral and medical experimental research that involves human beings as experimental subjects.

imaging protocol The collection of settings and parameters used in the acquisition of medical images. Examples of settings and parameters include the clinical indication for the imaging exam, the use of contrast, patient positioning, and expected radiation dose ranges.

Immediate Threat to Health or Safety A threat that represents immediate risk and has or may potentially have serious adverse effects on the health or safety of the patient, resident, or individual served. These threats are identified by the surveyor.

infection The transmission of a pathogenic microorganism to a host, with subsequent invasion and multiplication, with or without resulting symptoms of disease.

infection, epidemic *See* epidemic.

informed consent Agreement or permission accompanied by full notice about the care, treatment, or service that is the subject of the consent. A patient must be apprised of the nature, risks, and alternatives of a medical procedure or treatment before the physician or other health care professional begins any such course. After receiving this information, the patient then either consents to or refuses such a procedure or treatment.

initial survey An accreditation survey of an organization that has not been accredited by The Joint Commission for at least four months or an accreditation survey of an organization undergoing its first Joint Commission survey.

in-service Organized educational activity designed to enhance the skills of clinical staff relevant to their disciplines and job responsibilities.

instrument, waived testing A waived testing device used for recording, measuring, or controlling. The levels of operation vary from manual steps to full automation, and specialized knowledge and skill are required.

instrument-based waived testing   Tests with analysis steps that rely on the use of an instrument to produce a test result of a patient, resident, or individual served.

integrity   The property that data or information have not been altered or destroyed in an unauthorized manner.

interdisciplinary   An approach to care that involves two or more disciplines or professions (for example, social services, specialist consultation, nursing, medicine, therapies, spiritual support) collaborating to plan, treat, or provide care or services to a mother and/or newborn, patient, resident, or individual served and/or that person's family.

interdisciplinary team   An interdependent group of individuals representing two or more disciplines or professions working collaboratively to achieve the common goal of providing patient-centered, comprehensive care in the primary care medical home. The composition of the team will vary based on patient need. The interdisciplinary team within a Primary Care Medical Home must include a doctor of medicine or doctor of osteopathy, whose involvement in a patient's care is determined by the needs of the patient. Other members of the team may include registered nurses, front office staff, care coordinators, and specialists.

interpreting services   A trans-language rendition of a spoken message in which the interpreter comprehends the source language and can speak comprehensively in the target language to convey the meaning intended in the source language. The interpreter knows health and health-related terminology and provides accurate interpretations by choosing equivalent expressions that convey the best matching and meaning to the source language and captures, to the greatest possible extent, all nuances intended in the source message.

interval-based maintenance   *See* maintenance.

Intracycle Monitoring (ICM)   A process to help accredited organizations at various touch points in the triennial accreditation cycle with their continuous compliance efforts. The process involves access to an ICM Profile available on the organization's *Joint Commission Connect*® extranet site. The ICM Profile identifies high-risk areas and related standards areas and displays them within a Focused Standards Assessment (FSA) tool, which allows organizations to conduct a self-assessment of standards to identify and manage risk in the organization. *See also* Focused Standards Assessment (FSA).

intravenous (IV) admixture   A pharmaceutical product whose preparation requires the measured addition of a medication to a 50 mL or greater bag or bottle of IV fluid. It does not include the drawing up of medications into a syringe, the addition of medication to a buretrol, or the assembly and activation of an IV system that does not involve the measurement of the additive.

invasive procedure   The puncture or incision of the skin, insertion of an instrument, or insertion of foreign material into the body for diagnostic or treatment-related purposes. Examples of invasive procedures include central line and chest tube insertions, and cardiac catheterization. Venipuncture is not categorized as an invasive procedure.

investigational medication A medication used as part of a research protocol or clinical trial.

knowledge-based information A collection of stored facts, models, and information that can be used for ongoing staff development, for designing and redesigning processes, and for solving problems. Knowledge-based information is found in the clinical, scientific, and management literature.

laboratory A facility that is equipped to examine material derived from the human body to provide information for use in the diagnosis, prevention, or treatment of disease; also called clinical laboratory or medical laboratory.

leader An individual who sets expectations, develops plans, and implements procedures to assess and improve the quality of the organization's governance, management, and clinical and support functions and processes. At a minimum, leaders include members of the governing body and medical staff, the chief executive officer and other senior managers, the nurse executive, clinical leaders, and staff members in leadership positions within the organization.

licensed independent practitioner An individual permitted by law and by the organization to provide care, treatment, and services without direction or supervision. A licensed independent practitioner operates within the scope of their license, consistent with individually granted clinical privileges. When standards reference the term licensed independent practitioner, this language is not to be construed to limit the authority of a licensed independent practitioner to delegate tasks to other qualified health care personnel (for example, physician assistants and advanced practice registered nurses) to the extent authorized by state law or a state's regulatory mechanism or federal guidelines and organizational policy.

licensure A legal right that is granted by a government agency in compliance with a statute governing an occupation (such as medicine, nursing, psychiatry, or clinical social work) or the operation of an activity in a health care occupancy (for example, skilled nursing facility, residential treatment center, hospital).

Life Safety Code[*] A set of standards for the construction and operation of buildings intended to provide a reasonable degree of safety during fires. These standards are prepared, published, and periodically revised by the National Fire Protection Association and adopted by The Joint Commission to evaluate health care organizations under its life safety management program. *See also* occupancy.

life-support equipment Any device used for the purpose of sustaining life and whose failure to perform its primary function, when used according to the manufacturer's instructions and clinical protocol, will lead to patient death in the absence of immediate intervention (for example, ventilators, anesthesia machines, heart-lung bypass machines, defibrillators).

long term care *See* nursing care center.

look-alike/sound-alike medications Similar medication names, either written or spoken, which may lead to potentially harmful medication errors when confused with each other.

magnetic resonance (MR) conditional An item that has been demonstrated to pose no known hazards in a specific magnetic resonance (MR) environment under specific conditions of use. Conditions that define the MR environment include static magnetic field strength, radiofrequency fields, specific absorption rate, and other factors. The item label must include the results of testing that characterize the behavior of the item in the MR environment. Any parameter that affects the safety of the item should be listed, and any condition that is known to produce an unsafe condition must be described.

magnetic resonance (MR) safe An item that poses no known hazards in all magnetic resonance (MR) environments. MR safe items are nonconducting, nonmetallic, and nonmagnetic items, such as a plastic Petri dish.

maintenance There are five types of maintenance — predictive, metered, corrective, interval-based, and reliability-centered:

1. Predictive maintenance - A type of maintenance strategy that provides the means to achieve reliability levels that exceed the performance of a piece of equipment or system. This strategy is designed to measure and track data significant to the piece of equipment or system. It confirms possible faults with the equipment, and specific repairs are completed before the equipment fails. Predictive analysis can be performed using advanced monitoring instruments and predictive software that collects data and performs an analysis. The data collected are analyzed, and corrective maintenance is performed when the equipment is performing outside the desired operating parameters.

2. Metered maintenance - Maintenance strategy based on the hours of run time or the number of times the equipment is used (for example, number of images processed).

3. Corrective maintenance - Maintenance strategy that restores a piece of equipment to operational status after equipment failure.

4. Interval-based maintenance - Maintenance done according to specific intervals (for example, calendar time, running hours). A number of periodic inspections or restoration tasks are completed, based on information/data obtained from the last equipment check.

5. Reliability-centered maintenance - A type of maintenance that begins with a failure mode and effects analysis to identify the critical equipment failure modes in a systematic and structured manner. The process then requires the examination of each critical failure mode to determine the optimum maintenance policy to reduce the severity of each failure.

The chosen type of maintenance strategy must take into account cost, safety, and environmental and operational consequences. Some functions are not critical and may be allowed to "run to failure," while other functions must be preserved at all cost. Reliability-centered maintenance emphasizes the use of predictive maintenance techniques in addition to traditional preventive measures (metered, corrective, and interval based).

means of egress   A continuous and unobstructed way of travel from any point in a building or other structure to a public way consisting of three separate and distinct parts: the exit access, the exit, and the exit discharge.

medical device   An instrument, apparatus, implement, machine, contrivance, implant, in vitro reagent, or another similar or related article, including a component part or accessory that is

(1) recognized in the official National Formulary or the United States Pharmacopeia or any supplement to them;
(2) intended for use in the diagnosis of disease or other conditions or in the cure, mitigation, treatment, or prevention of disease in humans or other animals; or (3) intended to affect the structure or any function of the body of humans or other animals and that does not achieve any of its primary intended purposes through chemical action within or on the body of humans or other animals and that is not dependent on being metabolized for the achievement of any of its primary intended purposes.

medical equipment   Fixed and portable equipment used for the diagnosis, treatment, monitoring, and direct care of individuals.

medical history   A component of the medical record consisting of an account of an individual's physical health history, obtained whenever possible from the individual, and including at least the following information: chief complaint, details of the present illness or care needs, relevant past history, and relevant inventory by body systems.

medical record   *See* record.

Medical Reserve Corps (MRC)   Units comprised of locally-based medical and public health volunteers who can assist their communities during emergencies, such as an influenza epidemic, a chemical spill, or an act of terrorism.

medical staff   The group of all licensed independent practitioners and other practitioners privileged through the organized medical staff process that is subject to the medical staff bylaws. This group may include others, such as retired practitioners who no longer practice in the organization but who wish to continue their membership in the group, courtesy staff, scientific staff, and so forth. *See also* medical staff, organized.

medical supplies Medical items, usually of a disposable nature, such as bandages, sterile drapes, and suture materials. These supplies differ from permanent or durable items, such as medical equipment and devices.

medication Any prescription medications, sample medications, herbal remedies, vitamins, nutraceuticals, vaccines, or over-the-counter drugs; diagnostic and contrast agents used on or administered to persons to diagnose, treat, or prevent disease or other abnormal conditions; radioactive medications, respiratory therapy treatments, parenteral nutrition, blood derivatives, and intravenous solutions (plain, with electrolytes and/or drugs); and any product designated by the Food and Drug Administration (FDA) as a drug. This definition of medication does not include enteral nutrition solutions (which are considered food products), oxygen, and other medical gases.

medication allergy A state of hypersensitivity induced by exposure to a particular drug antigen resulting in harmful immunologic reactions on subsequent drug exposures, such as a penicillin drug allergy. *See also* medication.

medication error A preventable event that may cause or lead to inappropriate medication use or patient or resident harm while the medication is in the control of the health care professional, patient, resident, or consumer. Such events may be related to professional practice, health care products, procedures, and systems, including prescribing; order communication; product labeling, packaging, and nomenclature; compounding; dispensing; distribution; administration; education; monitoring; and use. *See also* significant medication error.

medication expiration date The last date that a medication or product is to be used or administered.

medication management The process an organization uses to provide medication therapy to individuals served by the organization. The components of the medication management process include the following:

- **procurement** The task of obtaining selected medications from a source outside the organization. It does not include obtaining a medication from the organization's own pharmacy, which is considered part of the ordering and dispensing processes.
- **storage** The task of appropriately maintaining a supply of medications on the organization's premises.
- **secure** In locked containers, in a locked room, or under constant surveillance.
- **prescribing or ordering** The process of a licensed independent practitioner or prescriber transmitting a legal order

GL – 21

or prescription to an organization, directing the preparing, dispensing, and administration of a specific medication to a specific individual. It does not include requisitions for medication supplies.

■ **transcribing** The process by which an order from a licensed independent practitioner is documented either in writing or electronically.

■ **preparing** Compounding, manipulating, or in some way getting a medication ready for administration, exactly as ordered by the licensed independent practitioner.

■ **dispensing** Providing, furnishing, or otherwise making available a supply of medications to the individual for whom it was ordered (their representative) by a licensed pharmacy according to a specific prescription or medication order, or by a licensed independent practitioner authorized by law to dispense. Dispensing does not involve providing an individual a dose of medication previously dispensed by the pharmacy.

■ **administration** The provision of a prescribed and prepared dose of an identified medication to the individual for whom it was ordered to achieve its pharmacological effect. This includes directly introducing the medication into or onto the individual's body.

medication reconciliation The process of identifying the medications currently being taken by an individual. These medi-

cations are compared to newly ordered medications, and discrepancies are identified and resolved.

medications, high-alert Medications that bear a heightened risk of causing significant harm to individuals when they are used in error.

mental abuse Intentional mistreatment of an individual that may cause psychological injury. Examples include humiliation, harassment, exploitation, and threats of punishment or deprivation.

metered maintenance *See* maintenance.

mitigation, emergency Those activities an organization undertakes in attempting to reduce the severity and impact of a potential emergency. *See also* emergency.

mobile delivery of health care services The provision of health care services, staff, or equipment in the presence of the patient through a transportable or relocatable platform. This definition does not include telehealth, telemedicine, health care staffing, or mobile health technology services.

multidisciplinary team A group of staff members composed of representatives from a range of professions, disciplines, or service areas.

near miss *See* close call.

neglect The absence of the minimal services or resources required to meet basic needs. Neglect includes withholding or inadequately providing medical care and, consistent with usual care, treatment, or services, food and hydration (without approval from the individual, physician, or surrogate), clothing, or good hygiene. It may also include placing an individual in unsafe or unsupervised conditions. *See also* abuse.

nursing The health profession dealing with nursing care and services as (1) defined by the Code of Ethics for Nurses with Interpretive Statements, Nursing's Social Policy Statement, Nurses' Bill of Rights, Scope and Standards of Nursing Practice of the American Nurses Association and specialty nursing organizations and (2) defined by relevant state, commonwealth, or territory nurse practice acts and other applicable laws and regulations.

nursing care center Individuals receiving care in this setting require rehabilitative, supportive, or palliative care. This care may include time-limited medically complex or rehabilitative care, dementia-specific memory care, long term nursing care, and other specialty care services. These services may be provided within a hospital, in an organization affiliated with a hospital, or in a freestanding organization. Synonyms used by the health care field for this setting include nursing home, long term care facility, and skilled nursing facility (SNF).

nutrition, parenteral Nutrients (such as protein, sugar, fat, and added vitamins and minerals as needed) that are provided intravenously, bypassing the digestive tract. Related terms are total parenteral nutrition (TPN), partial parenteral nutrition (PPN), and hyperalimentation (HA).

occupancy The purpose for which a building or portion thereof is used or intended to be used. Depending on the organization, occupancies may include ambulatory health care occupancy, business occupancy, health care occupancy, and residential occupancy.

- **ambulatory health care occupancy** An occupancy used to provide services or treatment to four or more patients (or one or more patients in an ambulatory surgical center that elects to use The Joint Commission deemed status option) at the same time that either (1) renders them incapable of providing their own means of self-preservation in an emergency or (2) provides outpatient surgical treatment requiring general anesthesia.

- **business occupancy** An occupancy used to provide outpatient care, treatment, day treatment, or other services that does not meet the criteria in the ambulatory health care occupancy definition (for example, three or fewer individuals at the same time who are either rendered incapable of self-preservation in an emergency or are undergoing general anesthesia). For ambulatory surgical centers that elect to use The Joint Commission deemed status option, treatment of one or more incapacitated patients renders the area an ambulatory health care occupancy.

- **health care occupancy** An occupancy used for purposes such as medical or other treatment or care of persons suffering from physical or mental illness, disease, or infirmity; and for the care of infants, convalescents, or infirm aged persons. Health care occupancies provide sleeping facilities for four or more occupants and are occupied by persons who are mostly incapable of self-preservation because of age, physical or mental disability, or security measures not under the occupant's control. Health care occupancies include hospitals, critical access hospitals, skilled nursing homes, and limited care facilities.

office-based surgery practice   A surgeon-owned or -operated organization (for example, a professional services corporation, private physician office, small group practice) that provides invasive procedures and administers local anesthesia, minimal sedation, conscious sedation, or general anesthesia that renders three or fewer patients incapable of self-preservation at any time, and is classified as a business occupancy.

operative or other high-risk procedures   Operative or other invasive or noninvasive procedures that place the patient at risk; these procedures are performed to remedy an injury, ailment, defect, or dysfunction. The focus is on procedures and is not meant to include medications that place the patient at risk.

organizational and functional integration   The degree to which a component of an organization is overseen and managed by the applicant organization. Organizational integration exists when the applicant organization's governing body,

either directly or ultimately, controls budgetary and resource allocation decisions for the component or, where separate corporate entities are involved, there is greater than 50% common governing board membership on the board of the applicant organization and the board of the component. Functional integration exists when the entity meets at least three of the following eight criteria:

1. The applicant organization and the component use the same process for determining membership of licensed independent practitioners in practitioner panels or medical or professional staff and/or use the same process for credentialing and assigning of privileges or clinical responsibilities to licensed independent practitioners, and/or share a common organized medical or professional staff between the applicant organization and the component.

2. The applicant organization's human resources function hires and assigns staff at the component and has the authority to terminate staff at the component, to transfer or rotate staff between the applicant organization and the component, and to conduct performance appraisals of the staff who work in the component.

3. The applicant organization's policies and procedures are applicable to the component with few or no exceptions.

4. The applicant organization manages all operations of the component (that is, the component has little or no management authority or autonomy independent of the applicant organization).

5. The component's clinical records are integrated into the applicant organization's clinical record system.

6. The applicant organization applies its performance improvement program to the component and has authority to implement actions intended to improve performance at the component.

7. The applicant organization bills for services provided by the component under the name of the applicant organization.

8. The applicant organization and/or the component portrays to the public that the component is part of the organization through the use of common names or logos; references on letterheads, brochures, telephone book listings, or websites; or representations in other published materials.

orientation   A process used to provide initial training and information while assessing the competence of clinical staff relative to job responsibilities and the organization's mission and goals.

orthotics   Corrective appliances designed to provide external control, correction, or support of the body typically for the prevention or control of deformities that may hinder a person's ease of movement.

outbreak   The occurrence of more than the expected number of cases of disease, injury, or other health conditions among a specific group during a specified time frame.

outcome measure   A tool used to assess data which indicates the results of performance or nonperformance of a function or procedure.

ownership   The entity that has ultimate control of resources and operation of the organization applying for accreditation.

panel (primary care medical home)   For organizations that elect The Joint Commission Primary Care Medical Home option: A designated group of patients assigned to a specific primary care clinician.

patient   An individual who receives care, treatment, or services. Synonyms used by various health care fields include resident, patient and family unit, individual served, consumer, health care consumer, customer, or beneficiary.

patient identifiers   Information directly associated with an individual that reliably identifies the individual as the person for whom the service or treatment is intended. Acceptable identifiers may be the individual's name, an assigned identification number, telephone number, or other person-specific identifier.

patient safety event   An event, incident, or condition that could have resulted or did result in harm to a patient. *See also* adverse event, close call, sentinel event.

peer recommendation   Information submitted by a practitioner(s) in the same professional discipline as an applicant, reflecting their perception of the applicant's clinical practice, ability to work as part of a team, and ethical behavior; or the documented peer evaluation of practitioner-specific data collected from various sources for the purpose of evaluating current competence.

performance improvement The systematic process of detecting and analyzing performance problems, designing and developing interventions to address the problems, implementing the interventions, evaluating the results, and sustaining improvement.

phantom An object used in medical imaging that simulates features of the human body. It is scanned or imaged and used to evaluate and analyze imaging equipment performance.

pharmacist An individual who has a degree in pharmacy and is licensed and registered to prepare, preserve, compound, and dispense drugs and other chemicals.

pharmacy services Pharmaceutical care and services involving the preparation and dispensing of medications and medication-related devices and supplies by a licensed pharmacy, with or without the provision of clinical or consultant pharmacist services.

physical abuse Intentional mistreatment of an individual that may cause physical injury. Examples include hitting, slapping, pinching, or kicking, and may also include attempts to control behavior through corporal punishment.

physician As defined by the Centers for Medicare & Medicaid Services in Sec. 1861.[42 U.S.C.1395x] of the Social Security Act:

The term "physician," when used in connection with the performance of any function or action, means

(1) A doctor of medicine or osteopathy legally authorized to practice medicine and surgery by the State in which he performs such function or action (including a physician within the meaning of section 1101(a)(7)),

(2) A doctor of dental surgery or of dental medicine who is legally authorized to practice dentistry by the State in which he performs such function and who is acting within the scope of his license when he performs such functions,

(3) A doctor of podiatric medicine for the purposes of subsections (k), (m), (p)(1), and (s) of this section and sections 1814(a), 1832(a)(2)(F)(ii), and 1835 but only with respect to functions which he is legally authorized to perform as such by the State in which he performs them,

(4) A doctor of optometry, but only for purposes of subsection (p)(1) with respect to the provision of items or services described in subsection (s) which he is legally authorized to perform as a doctor of optometry by the State in which he performs them, or

(5) A chiropractor who is licensed as such by the State (or in a State which does not license chiropractors as such, is legally authorized to perform the services of a chiropractor in the jurisdiction in which he performs such ser-

vices), and who meets uniform minimum standards promulgated by the Secretary, but only for the purpose of sections 1861(s)(1) and 1861(s)(2)(A) and only with respect to treatment by means of manual manipulation of the spine (to correct a subluxation) which he is legally authorized to perform by the State or jurisdiction in which such treatment is provided. For the purposes of section 1862(a)(4) and subject to the limitations and conditions provided in the previous sentence, such term includes a doctor of one of the arts, specified in such previous sentence, legally authorized to practice such art in the country in which the inpatient hospital services (referred to in such section 1862(a)(4)) are furnished.

physician assistant   An individual who practices medicine with supervision by licensed physicians, providing services ranging from primary medicine to specialized surgical care. The scope of practice is determined by state law, the supervising physician's delegation of responsibilities, the individual's education and experience, and the specialty and setting in which the individual works. When standards reference the term "licensed independent practitioner," this language is not to be construed to limit the authority of a licensed independent practitioner to delegate tasks to other qualified health care personnel (for example, physician assistants and advanced practice registered nurses) to the

extent authorized by state law or a state's regulatory mechanism or federal guidelines and organizational policy.

Plan for Improvement (PFI)   For purposes of Joint Commission accreditation, an organization's written statement that details the procedures to be taken and time frames to correct existing *Life Safety Code®* deficiencies. *See also Life Safety Code*, Statement of Conditions™ (SOC).

Plan of Action (POA)   A plan detailing the action(s) that an organization will take in order to come into compliance with a Joint Commission accreditation requirement. A POA must be completed for each element of performance associated with a noncompliant accreditation requirement.

podiatrist   An individual who has received the degree of doctor of podiatry medicine and who is licensed to practice podiatry.

point-of-care testing   Analytical testing performed at sites outside the traditional laboratory environment, usually at or near where care is delivered to individuals. Testing may be categorized as waived, moderate, or high complexity under the Clinical Laboratory Improvement Amendments of 1988 (CLIA '88). Testing may range from simple waived procedures, such as fecal occult blood, to more sophisticated chemical analyzers. Guided by CLIA requirements this testing may be under the control of the main laboratory, another specialized laboratory (for example, for arterial blood gas), or the nursing service (for example, for glucose meters). Point-of-care testing may also be known as alternative site testing, decentralized laboratory testing, or distributed site testing.

population-based care   The assessment, monitoring, and management of the health care needs and outcomes of identified groups of patients and communities, rather than individual patients. The goal of population-based care is to improve the health of the population, increase awareness of behavior-related health risks, promote healthy lifestyle activities and patient self-management, and decrease health care inequities.

practice guidelines   *See* clinical practice guidelines.

practitioner   Any individual who is licensed and qualified to practice a health care profession (for example, physician, nurse, social worker, clinical psychologist, psychiatrist, respiratory therapist) and is engaged in the provision of care, treatment, or services. *See also* licensed independent practitioner.

predictive maintenance   *See* maintenance.

preparedness, emergency   Activities an organization undertakes to build capacity and identify resources that may be used if an emergency occurs. *See also* emergency.

prescribing or ordering   *See* medication management.

preventive care   The provision of health care that focuses on disease prevention and health maintenance. It includes early diagnosis of disease as well as discovery and identification of individuals at risk for the development of specific health problems or in need of counseling or other necessary interventions to avert a health problem. Screening tests, health education, and immunization programs are common examples of preventive care.

primary care clinician   A clinician operating within the primary care medical home who works collaboratively with an interdisciplinary team and in partnership with the patient to address the patient's primary health care needs. Primary care clinicians have the educational background, broad-based knowledge, and experience necessary to handle most medical and other health care needs of the patients who have selected them, including resolving conflicting recommendations for care. The primary care clinician is selected by the patient and serves as the primary point of contact for the patient and family. A primary care clinician operating within the primary care medical home is a doctor of medicine or doctor of osteopathy, or an advanced practice nurse or physician assistant practicing in collaboration with a doctor of medicine or doctor of osteopathy. The term "collaboration" in this context means that health care providers work together to meet the needs of the patient. It is not the intent of this requirement to impose additional restrictions on the scope of practice of an advanced practice nurse, nor is it meant to preempt applicable state law.

primary care medical home (PCMH) A model of primary health care that is based on five operational characteristics: patient-centered care; comprehensive care; coordinated care; superb access to care; and a system-based approach to quality and safety. They address the roles and functions of the patient, organization, primary care clinician, and interdisciplinary team. PCMH Certification is an optional certification that requires compliance with accreditation requirements plus an additional set of PCMH-specific requirements.

primary source The original source or an approved agent of that source of a specific credential that can verify the accuracy of a qualification reported by an individual practitioner. Examples include medical schools, nursing schools, graduate education, state medical boards, federal and state licensing boards, universities, colleges, and community colleges.

primary source verification Verification of an individual practitioner's reported qualifications by the original source or an approved agent of that source. Methods for conducting primary source verification of credentials include direct correspondence, documented telephone verification, secure electronic verification from the original qualification source, or reports from credentials verification organizations (CVOs) that meet Joint Commission requirements. *See also* credentials verification organization (CVO).

privacy (of information) The right of an individual to limit the disclosure of personal information.

privileging The process whereby the specific scope and content of patient care services (that is, clinical privileges) are authorized for a health care practitioner by a health care organization based on evaluation of the individual's credentials and performance. *See also* licensed independent practitioner.

prohibited abbreviations A list of abbreviations, acronyms, symbols, and dose designations that are not to be used throughout the organization. For accreditation purposes, the prohibited list applies, at a minimum, to all orders and all medication-related documentation that is handwritten (including free-text computer entry) or on preprinted forms.

prosthetics An artificial extension that replaces a missing part of the body. Examples include, but are not limited to, customized prostheses and breast prostheses.

protected health information Health information that contains information such that an individual person can be identified as the subject of that information.

psychosocial Pertaining to the influence of social factors on an individual's mind or behavior and to the interrelation of behavioral and social factors.

Public Information Policy A Joint Commission policy which specifies the information that The Joint Commission may release about accredited organizations. By submitting a signed accreditation contract, the organization is acknowledging that The Joint Commission may make available to the public the accreditation-related information in accordance with this policy.

qualifications   Knowledge, education, training, experience, competency, licensure, registration, or certification related to specific responsibilities.

quality control   A set of activities or techniques whose purpose is to ensure that all quality requirements are being met. The organization monitors processes and solves performance problems to achieve this purpose.

quality of care, treatment, or services The degree to which care, treatment, or services for individuals and populations increases the likelihood of desired health or behavioral health outcomes. Considerations include the appropriateness, efficacy, efficiency, timeliness, accessibility, and continuity of care; the safety of the care environment; and the individual's personal values, practices, and beliefs.

Quality Report   A publicly available report that includes relevant and useful information about the provision of safe quality care provided in individual Joint Commission–accredited and –certified organizations. Quality Reports are created at the organization level and contain information regarding an organization's accreditation or certification status. These reports provide detailed information about an organization's performance and how it compares to

that of similar organizations; the organization's accreditation and/or certification decision and the effective dates of the accreditation/certification award; the last full survey/review date and last survey/review date; programs accredited and/or services certified by The Joint Commission, and programs or services accredited by other accrediting bodies; compliance with The Joint Commission's National Patient Safety Goals; special quality awards, and for hospitals, performance on National Quality Improvement Goals. If an organization has achieved both Joint Commission certification and accreditation, its Quality Report will contain both certification and accreditation information; the organizations will also have a separate Certification Quality Report.

quantitative result   A test result that is measured as a discrete number.

quarterly   Every three months, plus or minus 10 days.

range orders   Orders in which the dose or dosing interval varies over a prescribed range, depending on the situation or the individual's status.

rationale for a standard   A short paragraph that explains the justification for a standard; that is, why the standard is important or how it contributes to quality and/ or safety. A rationale is not scored, and not every standard has a rationale.

read-back   A method used to ensure understanding of information being communicated, often used between members of a care, treatment, or service team. The process involves the receiver of a verbal or telephone order writing down the complete order or test result or entering it into a computer and then reading it back and receiving confirmation from the person who gave the order or test result.

reassessment Ongoing data collection, which begins on initial assessment, comparing the most recent data with the data collected at earlier assessments.

record 1. An account compiled by physicians and other health care professionals of a variety of health information, such as assessment findings, treatment details, and progress notes. 2. Data obtained from the records or documentation maintained on a patient or resident in any health care setting (for example, hospital, home care, nursing care center, practitioner office). The record includes automated and paper medical record systems.

recovery, emergency The final phase of emergency management, related to strategies, actions, and individual responsibilities necessary to restore the organization's services after an emergency. *See also* emergency.

registered nurse (RN) A person who is licensed to practice professional nursing.

reliability-centered maintenance *See* maintenance.

reportable range The range of test values over which the relationship between the instrument, kit, or system's measurement response is shown to be valid.

Requirement for Improvement (RFI) A recommendation that is required to be addressed in an organization's Evidence of Standards Compliance in order for the organization to retain its accreditation. Failure to adequately address an RFI after two opportunities may result in a recommendation to place the organization in Accreditation with Follow-up Survey.

response, emergency Actions taken and procedures implemented by the organization when an emergency occurs. *See also* emergency.

Review Hearing Panel A panel of three individuals, including one member of The Joint Commission's Board of Commissioners, which evaluates the facts of an organization appealing a Preliminary Denial of Accreditation.

risk assessment, proactive An assessment that examines a process in detail including sequencing of events, actual and potential risks, and failure or points of vulnerability and that prioritizes, through a logical process, areas for improvement based on the actual or potential impact (that is, criticality) of care, treatment, or services provided.

root cause analysis (RCA) *See* comprehensive systematic analysis.

SAFER Matrix The Survey Analysis for Evaluating Risk (SAFER™) Matrix gives a visual representation of the risk level of each Requirement for Improvement (RFI). Each observation reported by a surveyor is plotted on the SAFER Matrix according to the risk level of the finding. The risk level is determined according to two factors: (1) the likelihood of the finding to cause harm to patients, staff, and/or visitors, and (2) the scope at which the finding was observed.

safety The degree to which the risk of an intervention (for example, use of a drug, or a procedure) and risk in the care environment are reduced for a patient and other persons, including health care practitioners. Safety risks may arise from the performance of tasks, from the structure of the physical environment, or from situations beyond the organization's control (such as weather).

safety management Activities selected and implemented by the organization to assess and control the impact of environmental risk, and to improve general environmental safety.

sampling Selecting a subset from a larger group of units or observations that provides information that may be used to decide about the larger quantity.

scope of services The activities performed by governance, managerial, clinical, or support staff.

secure In a locked container, in a locked room, or under constant surveillance.

security Protection of people and property against harm or loss (for example, workplace violence, theft, access to medications). Security incidents may be caused by persons from outside or inside the organization.

security, information Administrative, physical, and technical safeguards to prevent unauthorized access, use, disclosure, modification, or destruction of information or interference with system operations in an information system.

self-administration Independent use of a medication by a patient, resident, or individual served, including medications that may be held by the organization for independent use.

self-management Activities performed by patients with one or more chronic conditions that enable them to take an active role in the management of their health care and improve their clinical outcomes.

semi-quantitative result Results of tests that are more precise than qualitative tests (negative/positive results) but less precise than quantitative tests (numerical value), usually scored on a graded scale (for example, 1+, 2+, 3+).

sentinel event A patient safety event (not primarily related to the natural course of the patient's illness or underlying condition) that reaches a patient and results in death, permanent harm, or severe temporary harm. Sentinel events are a subcategory of adverse events.

sexual abuse Intentional mistreatment of a sexual nature of an individual that may cause physical and/or psychological injury. Examples include sexual harassment, sexual coercion, and sexual assault.

significant adverse drug reaction (ADR) An adverse medication reaction experienced by an individual that required intervention to preclude or mitigate harm or that requires monitoring to confirm that it resulted in no harm to the individual.

significant adverse medication reaction *See* significant adverse drug reaction (ADR).

significant medication error A medication error that reached an individual that required intervention to preclude or mitigate harm and/or that required monitoring to confirm that it resulted in no harm to the individual.

size-specific dose estimate (SSDE) A measure of the radiation output of a computed tomography scanner. Along with the computed tomography dose index (CTDI), it factors in the patient's size to provide a better estimate of the radiation dose to a volume of tissue for a given patient in a clinical setting.

social worker An individual who provides a range of counseling, case management, and advocacy services to individuals served in various settings. Social workers may work in or with community-based programs, schools, residential and foster care programs, or independently as private practice psychotherapists. A social worker has at least a bachelor's degree in social work plus documentation of any additional training, education, or experience commensurate with their responsibilities.

staff As appropriate to their roles and responsibilities, all people who provide care, treatment, or services in the organization, including those receiving pay (for example, permanent, temporary, part-time personnel, as well as contract employees), volunteers and health profession students. The definition of staff does not include licensed independent practitioners who are not paid staff or who are not contract employees.

standard A principle of patient safety and quality of care that a well-run organization meets. A standard defines the performance expectations, structures, or processes that must be substantially in place in an organization to enhance the quality of care, treatment, or services.

Statement of Conditions™ (SOC) A proactive document that helps an organization do a critical self-assessment of its current level of compliance and describe how to resolve any *Life Safety Code* deficiencies. The SOC was created to be a "living, ongoing" management tool that should be used in a management process that continually identifies, assesses, and resolves *Life Safety Code* deficiencies.

sterilization The use of a physical or chemical procedure to destroy all microbial life, including highly resistant bacterial endospores.

stored emergency power supply systems (SEPSS) Systems that automatically supply illumination or power to critical areas and equipment essential for safety to human life. Included are systems that supply emergency power for such functions as illumination for safe exiting, ventilation where it is essential to maintain life, fire detection and alarm systems, public safety communications systems, and processes where the current interruption would produce serious life safety or health hazards to patients, residents, individuals served, the public, or staff. Note: Other non-SEPSS battery back-up emergency power systems that an organization has determined to be critical for operations during a power failure (for example, laboratory equipment, electronic medical records) should be properly tested and maintained in accordance with manufacturer recommendations.

support services   Services provided in an individual's place of residence on a per-visit or per-hour basis to meet the identified needs of an individual who requires assistance in the maintenance and management of household routines, such as cleaning or shopping. These services may include, but are not limited to, those provided by homemakers, chore service workers, or companions. These services may be provided directly or through contract with another organization or individual.

surveillance   Systematic method of collecting, consolidating, and analyzing data concerning the frequency or pattern of, and causes or factors associated with, a given disease, injury, or other health condition. Data analysis is followed by the dissemination of that information to those who can improve outcomes. Examples of surveillance data can include ventilator associated pneumonia, antibiotic prophylaxis, hemodialysis catheter infections, implant infections, surgical site infections, hand hygiene, drug resistant organisms (MRSA, VRE), equipment sterile processing, vaccinations, urinary tract infections, and health care worker immunization.

survey   A key component in the accreditation process whereby a surveyor(s) conducts an evaluation of an organization's compliance with Joint Commission accreditation requirements.

surveyor   For purposes of Joint Commission accreditation, a health care professional who meets The Joint Commission's surveyor selection criteria, evaluates compliance with accreditation requirements, and provides education regarding compliance with accreditation requirements to surveyed organizations or systems. The type of surveyor(s) assigned is determined by the accreditation program and its services. A surveyor may be, but is not limited to, a licensed physician, surgeon, podiatrist, dentist, nurse, physician assistant, pharmacist, medical technologist, respiratory therapist, administrator, social worker, psychologist, or behavioral health care professional.

tabletop exercise   An exercise that involves key personnel discussing simulated scenarios and is used to assess plans, policies, and procedures. It is a discussion-based exercise that familiarizes participants with current plans, policies, agreements, and procedures, or may also be used to develop new plans, policies, agreements, and procedures.

telehealth The use of electronic information and telecommunications technologies to support long-distance clinical health care, patient and professional health-related education, public health, and health administration.

telemedicine The use of medical information exchanged from one site to another via electronic communication to improve patients' health status. Telemedicine is a subcategory of telehealth.

The Joint Commission An independent, not-for-profit organization dedicated to improving the safety and quality of health care through standards development, public policy initiatives, accreditation, and certification. The Joint Commission accredits and certifies more than 20,000 health care organizations and programs in the United States.

time-out, invasive procedure An immediate pause by the entire surgical team to confirm the correct patient, procedure, and site.

tissue Any group of cells that perform specific functions.

tracer methodology A process surveyors use during the survey to analyze an organization's systems or processes for delivering safe, high-quality care by following an individual patient or resident through the organization's care process in the sequence experienced by each individual.

Depending on the setting, this process may require surveyors to visit multiple care programs and services within an organization or within a single program or service to "trace" the care rendered.

transfer agreement A written understanding that provides for the reciprocal transfer of individuals between health care organizations.

translation services A trans-language rendition of a written document in which the translator comprehends the source language and can write comprehensively in the target language to convey the meaning intended in the source language. The translator knows health and health-related terminology and provides accurate translations by choosing equivalent expressions that convey the best matching and meaning to the source language and captures, to the greatest possible extent, all nuances intended in the source document.

transmission-based precautions Infection prevention and control measures to protect against exposure to a suspected or identified pathogen. These precautions are specific and based on the way the pathogen is transmitted. Categories include contact, droplet, airborne, and a combination of these.

uniform data set An agreed-on and accepted set of terms and definitions constituting a core of data; a collection of related data items.

unit dose Medication to be given to a particular patient at a specific time packaged in the exact dosage required for that time.

urgent care The delivery of ambulatory medical care to patients who have an injury or illness that requires immediate care but is not serious enough to warrant a visit to an emergency room. Urgent care centers often have extended hours and typically *see* patients on a walk-in basis without a scheduled appointment. Care may include diagnostic and therapeutic services, on-site x-ray, laboratory testing, pharmacy, and laceration and fracture care.

utility systems Building systems that provide support to the environment of care, including electrical distribution and emergency power; vertical and horizontal transport; heating, ventilating, and air conditioning (HVAC); plumbing, boiler, and steam; piped gases; vacuum systems; and communication systems, including data exchange systems.

variance A measure of the difference in a set of observations; statistically, the square of the standard deviation.

waived testing Tests that meet the Clinical Laboratory Improvement Amendments of 1988 (CLIA '88) requirements for waived tests and are cleared by the Food and Drug Administration for home use. These tests employ methodologies that are so simple and accurate that the likelihood of erroneous results is negligible, or they pose no risk of harm to the patient, resident, or individual served if the test is performed incorrectly. *See also* Clinical Laboratory Improvement Amendments of 1988 (CLIA '88).

Index (IX)

A

Abbreviations, acronyms, symbols, and dose designations, do-not-use list (IM.02.02.01), IM-8–IM-9
ABHR (alcohol-based hand rub) requirements (LS.03.01.30), LS-14–LS-17
ABMS (American Board of Medical Specialties), HR-16
Abuse or neglect
  assessment for (PC.01.02.09), PC-8
  protection from (RI.01.06.03), RI-12–RI-13
Accreditation award, marketing and communication guidelines for publicizing, APR-6
Accreditation Council for Graduate Medical Education (ACGME), HR-16
Accreditation decision categories
  Accreditation with Follow-up Survey, APR-3
  Denial of Accreditation, APR-1
  Preliminary Denial of Accreditation (PDA), APR-1
Accreditation Participation Requirements (APRs)
  accreditation status, representation of (APR.08.01.01), APR-6
  applicability grids, SAP-3
  chapter focus, overview, and outline, APR-1–APR-2
  compliance with
    assessment of, APR-1
    requirement for improvement for noncompliance, APR-1
  consultants, Joint Commission employees as (APR.06.01.01), APR-5
  external evaluations, sharing results of (APR.05.01.01), APR-5
  Immediate Threat to Health or Safety, care treatment, and services pose no risk of (APR.09.04.01), APR-7–APR-8
  observers of on-site surveys (APR.07.01.01), APR-5–APR-6
  Quality Report, adherence to guidelines for describing information in (APR.09.03.01), APR-7
  safety and quality concerns
    reporting of, how to contact Joint Commission or organization management (APR.09.01.01), APR-1, APR-6
    reporting of by staff (APR.09.02.01), APR-1, APR-7

scope of services and facilities, representation of (APR.08.01.01), APR-6
  submission of information
    accuracy of information (APR.01.02.01), APR-1, APR-3–APR-4
    changes in information (APR.01.03.01), APR-4–APR-5
    timely submission (APR.01.01.01), APR-3
  survey performance at Joint Commission's discretion (APR.02.01.01), APR-1, APR-5
Accreditation program–specific risk areas and risk icon, INTRO-2
Accreditation status
  marketing and publicizing accreditation award, APR-6
  representation of (APR.08.01.01), APR-6
  requirement for improvement, failure to resolve, APR-1
  submission of information, timely (APR.01.01.01), and, APR-3
Accreditation with Follow-up Survey
  submission of information, timely (APR.01.01.01), APR-3
Accrediting bodies, sharing results of evaluations by (APR.05.01.01), APR-5
Accuracy of information
  APR on (APR.01.02.01), APR-1, APR-3–APR-4
  E-App, APR-3
    length of survey and, APR-3
  falsification of information, APR-1, APR-3–APR-4
  marketing and publicizing accreditation award, APR-6
  Quality Report, adherence to guidelines for describing information in (APR.09.03.01), APR-7
ACGME (Accreditation Council for Graduate Medical Education), HR-16
Acquired immunodeficiency syndrome (AIDS), IC-1
Acronyms, do-not-use list (IM.02.02.01), IM-8–IM-9
ADA (Americans with Disabilities Act), HR-14, RI-6
Administration of medications (MM.06.01.01), MM-16–MM-17
Administrative responsibilities (LD.04.01.05), LD-22–LD-23
Admission to care (PC.01.01.01), PC-4
Advance directives
  inclusion of in clinical record (RC.02.01.01), RC-5–RC-7
  policies and procedures on (RI.01.05.01), RI-12

2022

SAC

Index (IX)

SAC

Standards Applicability Process (SAP)

2022

SAC

Waived Testing (WT)